# New Frontiers in HIV/AIDS Research

# New Frontiers in HIV/AIDS Research

Edited by Seth Phelps

AMERICAN
MEDICAL PUBLISHERS
www.americanmedicalpublishers.com

American Medical Publishers,
41 Flatbush Avenue,
1st Floor, New York,
NY 11217, USA

Visit us on the World Wide Web at:
www.americanmedicalpublishers.com



ISBN: 978-1-63927-206-8



**Cataloging-in-Publication Data**

New frontiers in HIV/AIDS research / edited by Seth Phelps.
p. cm.
Includes bibliographical references and index.
ISBN 978-1-63927-206-8
1. HIV infections. 2. AIDS (Disease). 3. HIV-positive persons. 4. AIDS (Disease)--Patients. I. Phelps, Seth.
RC606.6 .N49 2022
616.979 2--dc23

# Table of Contents

# Preface

HIV transmission occurs through sexual contact, vertical transmission from mother to baby, and through exposure to infected body fluids and tissues. The viral load of an HIV-infected person is an important factor in mother to child and sexual transmission. A person in the later stages of infection is more likely to transmit infection compared to another in the initial stages. In many parts of the world, HIV/AIDS is a chronic condition rather than a terminal disease. Without treatment, an individual can survive for an average of 9 to 11 years, depending on the type of HIV, and between 6 to 19 months after the diagnosis of AIDS. Research in HIV/AIDS explores the clinical management of the disease as well as investigates the nature of HIV as an infectious agent. Research is also being undertaken to develop HIV vaccines, antiretroviral drugs and microbicides for sexually transmitted diseases. Other strategies such as circumcision, and pre-exposure and post-exposure prophylaxis are being studied for their role in lowering HIV risk. This book includes some of the vital pieces of work being conducted across the world, on various topics related to HIV/AIDS research. It provides significant information of this condition to help develop a good understanding of AIDS, its modes of transmission and its management and control. It aims to equip students and experts with the advanced topics and upcoming concepts in this domain.

The researches compiled throughout the book are authentic and of high quality, combining several disciplines and from very diverse regions from around the world. Drawing on the contributions of many researchers from diverse countries, the book's objective is to provide the readers with the latest achievements in the area of research. This book will surely be a source of knowledge to all interested and researching the field.

In the end, I would like to express my deep sense of gratitude to all the authors for meeting the set deadlines in completing and submitting their research chapters. I would also like to thank the publisher for the support offered to us throughout the course of the book. Finally, I extend my sincere thanks to my family for being a constant source of inspiration and encouragement.

**Editor**

1

# Sexual Behavior of Perinatally Infected Youth in Northwest Ethiopia: Implication for HIV Prevention Strategy

**Nurilign Abebe Moges and Habtamu Mellie Bizuayehu**

*Public Health Department, Medicine and Health Sciences College, Debre Markos University, Debre Markos, Ethiopia*

Correspondence should be addressed to Nurilign Abebe Moges; nurel13@gmail.com

Academic Editor: Seble Kassaye

*Background.* The major mode of HIV transmission in many resource-limited settings is via heterosexual intercourse, but the primary risk factor for youth is primarily through perinatal infection. With the maturing of the HIV epidemic, youth who acquired the virus perinatally are now reaching adolescence and becoming young adults. There is a paucity of data on the sexual practices of perinatally infected youth in Ethiopia. *Methods.* This a cross-sectional study among 343 HIV positive youths receiving HIV care and treatment in the two hospitals in northwest Ethiopia. A self-administered questionnaire was administered among those who were able to read and write, and the questionnaire was administered by a trained study team member for those who were illiterate. Data were entered using Epi data version 3.5 and analyzed using SPSS. Sexual behaviors of the two groups were compared using bivariate logistic regression and the significant ones were further analyzed using multivariate logistic regression. Statistical significance was declared at 95% confidence interval and P-value less than 0.05. *Result.* About (63.3%) were females, and 177 (51.6%) were between 20 and 24 years of age. The modes of HIV acquisition were 133 (35%) through perinatal HIV infection, 120 (35%) through sexual contact, 27 (7.9%) through exposure to HIV infected sharp materials, and 63 (18.4%) unsure how they acquired HIV. More than half 155 (59.3%) had multiple sexual partners, and 50 (63.3%) of their sexual partners were HIV negative. Among those who were sexually active, only 77 (56.2%) use a condom consistently. *Conclusions.* More children who acquired HIV from their mothers are joining the youth population. Their sexual behavior is similar to those youth with behaviorally acquired HIV. There is significant risky sexual behavior among both groups. There is great urgency to effectively address the HIV the prevention strategy to break the cycle of "transgenerational" infection.

## 1. Background

Globally, there were a total of 36.7 million (30.8 million-42.9 million) people living with Human Immunodeficiency Virus (HIV) with an estimate of 5000 new infections daily. Among these, 64% are from sub-Saharan Africa, and 37% of new infections are among young people aged 15–24 years [1]. In Ethiopia, new HIV infections are increasing; in 2016 there were 30,000 (19,000–41,000) compared to 2010 when there was an estimate of 23,000 (16,000–31,000) infections, thus reverting to the peak of the epidemic in 2005 when an estimate of 30,000 (23,000–39,000) new infections was reported [1]. In eastern and southern Africa, young women aged 15–24 years accounted for 26% of new HIV infections in 2016 despite making up just 10% of the population [1]. These surveillance data indicate that youths remain at risk of HIV in this region. It has been more than 33 years since HIV was noted for the first time in 1984 in Ethiopia [2]. Most HIV infections in Ethiopia are the result of heterosexual intercourse and currently the percentage of young females age 15–24 who have had their sexual debut before age of 15 has decreased from 16% in 2005 and 11% in 2011 to 9% in 2016 [3]. Currently, there are 710, 000 (570,000–880,000) living with HIV in Ethiopia, and 61% of adults and 35% of children are on treatment [1].

Young people living with HIV are often in discordant sexual relationships, with potential for HIV transmission to their HIV-negative partner. A study in central Uganda revealed that 40% preferred negative partners for marriage and only 31% boy or girl relationships had disclosed their

HIV status to their partners. A reported 57% of participants in this study did not consistently use condoms, and 30% had more than one sexual partner in the past six months [4].

There are some studies on the sexual risks behaviors of adolescents in Ethiopia [5–9] but there are limited data among HIV positive youth entering adulthood, ages 15–24, where the highest risk of new HIV infections is observed. Further, there are no data on the sexual behaviors regarding the sexual behaviors among those who acquired HIV through perinatal exposure. In the Gondar region of Ethiopia, 25% of the youth had previous sexual intercourse and reported at least one high risk sexual behavior [5]. Knowledge about HIV prevention among young people (15–24) was low 28.4%, and condom use at last higher-risk sex (with a nonmarital, noncohabiting partner) was 65.8% and 28% among males and females respectively [1]. A high number of children are orphaned due to HIV/AIDS in Ethiopia [10] and there were 3% HIV positive children among 15–24 age youth in Ethiopia [11]. We are now seeing perinatally HIV infected children now surviving long enough to join the population of youth and reaching their sexual debut. In this study, we aim to fill the information gap on the sexual behaviors of youth with perinatal and behaviorally acquired HIV infection in northwest Ethiopia.

## 2. Methods

*2.1. Study Design and Setting.* A cross-sectional study among HIV seropositive youths (15–24 years) was conducted in Felege Hiwot referral hospital, Bahrdar, and Debre Markos referral hospital, Debre Markos, Northwest Ethiopia. These hospitals were selected purposively for high client flow and these two big hospitals in west and East Gojjam zones. Felege Hiwot referral hospital is found in the regional city (Bahrdar) which is 555 kilometer from the capital city Addis Ababa and Debre Markos referral hospitals 299 kilometers away from Addis Ababa and 265 kilometers from Bahrdar. The study was undertaken from December 1, 2016, to February 28, 2017.

*2.2. Study Population.* All HIV seropositive youth ages 15–24 years who were receiving medical care and support in the two hospitals were eligible for inclusion in the study. Those youths who were lost to follow up due to drop out transfer out and defaulter status did not enroll in the study.

*2.3. Sample Size Determination.* The sample size was calculated based on the assumption of 95% confidence interval, 5% margin of error, and 50% proportion with high risky sexual practices. The required sample size was calculated using EPI INFO version 3.5, and 384 participants were required to have sufficient power based on the underlying assumptions stated above. However, there were only 350 youths during the study period, and all are included in the study. Study participants were taken during their regular medical follow-up period. Since the data collection period was for three months, almost all youths receiving care at the study sites were enrolled into the study.

*2.4. Data Collection.* Data collection tool was developed from reviewing existing tools in the literature. The questionnaire was translated into Amharic (local language) and back-translated into English to maintain consistency. Ten percent of the tools were pretested in none-selected ART centers and errors identified during the pretest were corrected accordingly. Data were collected by trained interviewers and self-administered questionnaire for illiterate and literate participants respectively. Five case managers (those HIV positive people who had specialized training on HIV case management and working in the hospitals) served as data collectors were recruited and trained by the study team. The training was focused on the objective of the study, confidentiality of information, and the contents of the questionnaire in detail. The primary outcome variable was means of HIV acquisition and youth sexual behavior. For the explanatory variable, sociodemographic characteristics, sexual and other practices that may affect HIV risk, perceived peer-pressure, attending religious ceremony status, the frequency of Religious attending, type of music to which the participant usually listens, knowing another HIV positive person, and HIV/AIDS-related knowledge and attitude were assessed for all youths.

*2.5. Operational Definitions.* Mode of HIV transmission was determined based on respondents answer as (from sexual intercourse, mother to child transmission, using sharp materials (nonoccupational), or I do not know the cause).

Risky sexual practice: inconsistent condom use and or having two or more sexual partners in the last six months were considered as risky sexual behavior [12].

*2.6. Data Processing and Analysis.* Each questionnaire was coded and entered into Epi data version 3.5 statistical package, and it was exported to SPSS version 20.0 statistical package for analysis of statistical inferences. Data cleaning and editing were made before analysis. The result of the study is presented using descriptive statistics (percent, mean, and median values) and analytic statistics (odds ratios).

Before running the multiple logistic regressions assumption of multicolinearity was checked using Pearson correlation and tolerance/variance inflation factor. Binominal logistic regressions were used to calculate the univariate and multivariate-adjusted odds ratio and to determine independent predictors of the dependent variable. Only those variables which were associated with dependent variable with p-value $< 0.05$ in univariate analysis that were not collinear were used in the multivariate logistic regression model.

*2.7. Data Quality Management.* To maintain data quality training was given for data collectors. Adequately designed data collection material was developed by reviewing different kinds of literature. Supervision is carried out on a daily base to check completeness, consistency both by the supervisor and by investigators. Completed questionnaires were reviewed by the principal investigators. At the completion of data entry, data cleaning was done using frequencies, cross-tabulations, sorting, and listing to check missed values and outliers.

Table 1: sociodemographic characteristics of HIV positive youths by HIV acquisition status in North West Ethiopia, 2017.

| Characteristics | HIV acquisition through (%) | | Total (%) | P-value |
|---|---|---|---|---|
| | Mother to child | Behavioral | | |
| **Sex** | | | | |
| Male | 67 (53.2) | 59 (46.8) | 126 (36.7) | 0.001 |
| Female | 156 (71.9) | 61 (28.1) | 217 (63.3) | |
| **Age** | | | | |
| 15–19 | 54 (32.5) | 112 (67.5) | 166 (48.4) | 0.001 |
| 20–24 | 169 (95.5) | 8 (4.5) | 177 (51.6) | |
| **Current residence** | | | | |
| Rural | 51 (32.5) | 8 (13.6) | 59 (17.2) | 0.001 |
| Urban | 172 (60.6) | 112 (39.4) | 284 (82.8) | |
| **Marital status** | | | | |
| Married/cohabited | 97 (90.7) | 10 (9.3) | 107 (31.2) | 0.001 |
| Single | 78 (42.4) | 106 (57.6) | 184 (53.6) | 0.001 |
| Divorced | 38 (95) | 2 (5) | 40 (11.7) | 0.001 |
| Widowed | 10 (83.3) | 2 (16.7) | 12 (3.5) | 0.093 |
| **Have monthly income** | | | | |
| Yes | 131 (84.5) | 24 (15.5) | 155 (44.9) | 0.001 |
| No | 92 (48.9) | 96 (51.1) | 188 (55.1) | |
| **Amounts of monthly income** | | | | |
| 50–700 birr | 64 (78) | 18 (22) | 82 (53.2) | 0.016 |
| >700 birr | 66 (91.7) | 6 (8.3) | 72 (46.8) | |
| **Currently living with** | | | | |
| Nuclear family | 52 (40.3) | 77 (59.7) | 129 (37.6) | 0.001 |
| Relatives | 23 (42.6) | 31 (57.4) | 54 (15.7) | 0.001 |
| Alone | 84 (9.3) | 9 (9.7) | 93 (27.1) | 0.001 |
| Husband/wife | 64 (95.5) | 3 (4.5) | 67 (19.5) | 0.001 |
| **Parents residence** | | | | |
| Urban | 109 (51.4) | 103 (48.6) | 212 (61.8) | 0.001 |
| Rural | 114 (87) | 17 (3) | 131 (38.2) | |
| **Education status** | | | | |
| Cannot read and Write | 45 (97.8) | 1 (2.2) | 46 (13.4) | 0.001 |
| Can read and write only | 36 (94.7) | 2 (5.3) | 38 (11.1) | 0.001 |
| Complete primary education | 80 (51.3) | 76 (48.7) | 156 (45.5) | 0.001 |
| Complete secondary education | 62 (60.2) | 41 (39.8) | 103 (30) | 0.001 |

Errors that were identified in the data base were corrected by referring to the original paper-based questionnaire. This information in the questionnaires with disagreement with entered data was corrected. But questionnaires with incomplete information were discarded.

*2.8. Ethical Considerations.* The proposal was submitted to Debre Markos University ethics committee for ethical approval and clearance. Permission was also obtained from the hospitals' administrators. For the sake of confidentiality, no personal identifier was recorded in the questionnaire, and data collectors were health professionals working in ART clinic. For children less than 18 years the parents or care givers gave consent. All consents were written informed consent. The participants were informed of the potential risk and benefits of participating in the study and participants were reassured that no personal identifiers would be collected. Those study participants who had symptoms concerning for a sexually transmitted disease (STD) at the time of data collection were referred for clinical care and treatment.

## 3. Result

*3.1. Socio-Demographic Characteristics.* A total of 343 youth were included in this study. More than half 217 (63.3%) were females and mean age of 19.83 (SD of +/- 3.5 years), and 177 (51.6%) were in the age group of 20–24. About 284 (82.8%) were living in urban areas. About 154 (44.9%) receive monthly pocket money. Most of the females, 156 (71.9%), acquired HIV prenatally. (Table 1).

*3.2. Clinical Characteristics of Youths.* The majority of participants 324 (94.5%) were on antiretroviral therapy (ART). About 240 (70%) of them have been told of their HIV status

Table 2: Sociodemographic characteristics among HIV positive youths in North West Ethiopia, 2017.

| Characteristics | Response (frequency and percentage) |
|---|---|
| **ART status** | |
| On ART | 324 (94.5) |
| Pre ART | 19 (5.5) |
| **Who tolled their HIV status** | |
| Parents | 81 (23.6) |
| Health professionals | 240 (70) |
| Their friends | 22 (6.4) |
| **HIV acquired through** | |
| Sexual intercourse | 133 (38.8) |
| Mother to child | 120 (35) |
| Sharp materials | 27 (7.9) |
| did not know | 63 (18.4) |

by health professionals in the healthcare facility. Means of HIV acquisition from mother to child was the second most common next to HIV acquired through sexual intercourse (Table 2).

The magnitude of early sexual initiation by age of 15 years is 90 (46.6%) (CI=95% CI (39.2–53.6). Among those with early sexual debut, 94 (90.4%) acquired HIV through perinatal transmission. The majority of youth with perinatal HIV infection reported being sexually active 194 (56.6%) and the average age in years was 17 (SD+/- 3). A larger proportion of the youth reported multiple lifetime sexual partners, 115 (59.3%), with an average of 2 sexual partners. The overall reported HIV status of partners was HIV negative for 50 (63.3%) individuals who had one partner and 67 (58.3%) among those with two or more sexual partners (Table 3).

*3.3. Factors Associated with Risky Sexual Behavior.* Bivariate logistic regressions was run using risky sexual behavior as dependent variable. Independent variables form sociodemographic, clinical, and sexual characteristics. In the bivariate analysis, four variables namely, sex, resident, age and mode of HIV acquisitions were significant. Then in the multivariate logistic regressions revealed that females were 3.09 times more likely to engage in risky sexual practice compared to males AOR, 3.09 (95% CI, 1.41–7.19). Similarly, those acquired HIV through behaviorally were 4.73 times more likely to practice risky sexual behavior AOR, 4.73 (95% CI, 1.32–16.57) Table 4.

## 4. Discussion

This study determines the proportion of youth perinatally acquired HIV in the two large clinical practices and describes the sexual behaviors of these youth. The proportion of youth with perinatally acquired HIV among the 15–24-year olds we studied was high, 35%, minimally lower than the proportion of youth with sexually acquired HIV infection, 38.8%. The high proportion of perinatally acquired infection in this age group is higher than data reported from elsewhere in the world where the majority of HIV acquisition in this age group is related to sexual activity [13–15]. It was estimated that 90% of HIV transmission among children 15 years and younger was from mother to child among HIV infected children [16]. These children are now surviving into their late teens, and as they engage in sexual relations, have the potential to transmit HIV to their HIV-negative sexual partners and, among female youths, perinatal HIV transmission remains possible. This makes effective HIV prevention strategies critically important to address both of these possible modes of transmission, and to break the cycle of ongoing HIV transmission that has contributed to the resurgence of new HIV cases that continue to be reported in our national surveillance data. Our approach to HIV prevention should include a nuanced approach to prevent "transgenerational" HIV infection as this may contribute to increased incidence of new HIV infections that is being reported in many developing countries including Ethiopia. This was indicated where HIV incidence was not decreased as per expected. In 2016, the incidence was similar to what was in 2005 though it was decreased up to 2010 in Ethiopia [1]. Therefore, policymakers better to devise HIV transmission strategy for both sexual and "transgenerational" HIV transmission.

Sexual behavior of HIV-positive youth has not been studied in Ethiopia unlike the general youth in general [6–9]. Further, the differences in sexual behaviors and social characteristics of those who acquired HIV from their mothers has not been previously described. In this study, we describe the contributions of various modes of transmission among HIV-positive youth receiving care.

Majority of females acquired HIV from their mother compared to males. That may explain the higher HIV burden among women among whom HIV prevalence is higher compared with men in Ethiopia [5, 17]. It was also demonstrated that females were more likely to be engaged in risky sexual behavior than males. Majority of youth with perinatally acquired HIV were from rural areas although the majority of HIV-positive youth in the programs are urban residents. This explains the difference in the observed HIV disease burden that is generally higher in urban areas than rural areas. Ninety-one percent of youths in the age group of 20–24 were not perinatally acquired compared to those aged 15–19. With increasing age, there is a higher likelihood of engaging in risky sexual behavior.

Though there is the difference in sex, current residence, monthly pocket money, number of sexual partners, age, and living arrangement, there was no difference by early initiation of sexual intercourse, consistent condom use and ever use a condom comparing youth with perinatally acquired HIV infection and youth with sexual and other modes of HIV acquisition. This study did not find a causal relationship between mode of HIV acquisition and other youth characteristics.

## 5. Conclusion

More children who acquired the virus from their mother are joining the youth population than ever. Most of their sexual behavior is similar to those who acquired HIV through sexual and sharp material and those who did know the source.

TABLE 3: Self-reported sexual behavior by HIV acquisition status among HIV positive youths in North West Ethiopia, 2017.

| Characteristics | HIV acquisition status | | Total (%) |
|---|---|---|---|
| | Mother to child | Others means | |
| **Had sex in the last six months** | | | |
| Yes | 30 (83.33%) | 6 (16.67%) | 36 (10.50) |
| No | 193 (62.87%) | 114 (37.13%) | 307 (89.5) |
| **Ever had sex** | | | |
| Yes | 172 (88.7% | 22 (11.3%) | 194 (56.6) |
| No | 51 (34.2%) | 98 (65.8%) | 149 (43.4) |
| **First sexual initiation started** | | | |
| Less than 18 years | 94 (90.4%) | 10 (9.6%) | 90 (46.4) |
| Greater than or equal to 18 years | 78 (86.7% | 12 (13.3%) | 104 (53.6) |
| **Numbers of lifetime sexual partner** | | | |
| single | 63 (79.7%) | 16 (11.3%) | 79 (40.7) |
| multiple | 110 (95.7) | 15 (4.3%) | 115 (59.3) |
| **HIV status of sexual partner (have only 1)** | | | |
| HIV positive | 14 (82.4%) | 3 (17.6%) | 17 (21.5) |
| HIV negative | 40 (80%) | 10 (20%) | 50 (63.3) |
| Unknown | 12 (100%) | 0 | 12 (15.2) |
| **HIV status of sexual partner (more than 1)** | | | |
| HIV positive | 19 (90.5%) | 2 (9.5) | 21 (18.3) |
| HIV negative | 63 (94%) | 4 (6%) | 67 (58.3) |
| Unknown | 23 (88.9% | 3 (11.1%) | 27 (23.5) |
| **Ever use condom** | | | |
| Yes | 119 (86.9%) | 18 (13.1%) | 137 (70.6) |
| No | 54 (94.4%) | 3 (5.3%) | 57 (29.4) |
| **Consistent condom use** | | | |
| Yes | 65 (84.4%) | 12 (15.6%) | 77 (56.2) |
| No | 54 (90%) | 6 (10%) | 60 (43.8) |

TABLE 4: Univariate and multivariate logistic regression of risky sexual behaviors of HIV positive youths in northwest Ethiopia, 2017.

| Characteristics | Risky sexual behavior | | Crud odds ratio at 95% CI | Adjusted odds ratio at 95% CI |
|---|---|---|---|---|
| | Yes | No | | |
| **Sex** | | | | |
| Male | 35 | 14 | 1 | 1 |
| Female | 79 | 66 | 2.09 (1.04–4.21) | **3.18 (1.41–7.19)** |
| **Residence** | | | | |
| Rural | 33 | 11 | 1 | 1 |
| Urban | 81 | 69 | 2.56 (1.20–4.43) | 2.14 (0.97–4.69) |
| **Age** | | | | |
| 15–19 | 12 | 23 | 1 | 1 |
| 20–24 | 102 | 57 | 0.29 (0.14–0.63) | 0.49 (0.20–1.18) |
| **Mode of HIV acquisitions** | | | | |
| MTCT | 109 | 64 | 1 | 1 |
| behavioral | 5 | 16 | 5.45 (1.91–15.58) | **4.73 (1.35–16.57)** |

Youths above 20 years and those with multiple sexual partners who acquired HIV were less likely to have acquired HIV through perinatal HIV transmission. Youths in urban setting and living with relatives were less likely to receive the virus from their mother.

## Conflicts of Interest

Both authors declare that there are no financial and authorship conflicts of interest.

## Authors' Contributions

Both authors contributed to the conception, design, and execution of this study. Nurilign Abebe Moges initiate the idea and participated in proposal development, data collection, analysis, manuscript preparation, and revision. Habtamu Mellie Bizuayehu was also involved in the study activities starting from the conception of the idea to the revision of the manuscript throughout the whole process of the study.

## Acknowledgments

The authors would like to acknowledge Debre Markos University for funding the research for data collection. We would also like to extend our appreciation to data collectors and study participants.

## References

[1] U. AIDSinfo, *Joint United Nations Programme on HIV/AIDS (UNAIDS Accessed*, vol. 16, 2017, http://aidsinfo.unaids.org.

[2] G. Okubagzhi and S. Singh, "Establishing an HIV/AIDS programme in developing countries: The Ethiopian experience," *AIDS*, vol. 16, no. 12, pp. 1575–1586, 2002.

[3] ICF. CSACEa, "Ethiopia Demographic and Health Survey," *CSA and ICF*, 2016.

[4] R. Ankunda, L. M. Atuyambe, and N. Kiwanuka, "Sexual risk related behaviour among youth living with HIV in central Uganda: Implications for HIV prevention," *Pan African Medical Journal*, vol. 24, article no. 49, 2016.

[5] Y. Shiferaw, A. Alemu, A. Girma et al., "Assessment of knowledge, attitude and risk behaviors towards HIV/AIDS and other sexual transmitted infection among preparatory students of Gondar town, north west Ethiopia," *BMC Research Notes*, vol. 4, article 505, 2011.

[6] D. Kebede, A. Alem, G. Mitike et al., "Khat and alcohol use and risky sex behaviour among in-school and out-of-school youth in Ethiopia," *BMC Public Health*, vol. 5, article no. 109, 2005.

[7] H. Alemu, D. H. Mariam, K. A. Belay, and G. Davey, "Factors predisposing out-of-school youths to HIV/AIDS-related risky sexual behaviour in northwest Ethiopia," *Journal of Health, Population and Nutrition*, vol. 25, no. 3, pp. 344–350, 2007.

[8] M. T. Malaju and G. A. Asale, "Association of Khat and alcohol use with HIV infection and age at first sexual initiation among youths visiting HIV testing and counseling centers in Gamo-Gofa Zone, South West Ethiopia," *BMC International Health and Human Rights*, vol. 13, no. 1, 2013.

[9] A. Seme, D. H. Mariam, and A. Worku, "The association between substance abuse and HIV infection among people visiting HIV counselling and testing centres in Addis Ababa, Ethiopia," *Ethiopian Journal of Health Development*, vol. 19, no. 2, 2005.

[10] T. Menna, A. Ali, and A. Worku, "Prevalence of "HIV/AIDS related" parental death and its association with sexual behavior of secondary school youth in Addis Ababa, Ethiopia: A cross sectional study," *BMC Public Health*, vol. 14, no. 1, 2014.

[11] N. Taffa, J. Sundby, C. Holm-Hansen, and G. Bjune, "HIV prevalence and socio-cultural contexts of sexuality among youth in Addis Ababa, Ethiopia," *Ethiopian Journal of Health Development*, vol. 16, no. 2, 2002.

[12] I. CSA, "Ethiopia demographic and health survey," in *Proceedings of the Central Statistical Agency and ICF International*, pp. 2012-430, Addis Ababa, Ethiopia and Calverton, Maryland, USA, 2011.

[13] R. Dominicana, HIV MODES OF TRANSMISSION MODEL;Analysis of the distribution of new HIV infections in the Dominican Republic and recommendations for prevention,.

[14] PHAo. Canada, "HIV TRANSMISSION RISK: A SUMMARY OF THE EVIDENCE. , Canada," in *HIV TRANSMISSION RISK: A SUMMARY OF THE EVIDENCE. , Canada*, IDPA. CONTROL, Ed., 14 Canada PHAo. HIV TRANSMISSION RISK, A SUMMARY OF THE EVIDENCE. in. CONTROL IDPA, 2012.

[15] KNAC. Council, "IV PREVENTION RESPONSE AND MODES OF TRANSMISSION ANALYSIS".

[16] oUNPo. HIV/AIDS, A review of HIV transmision through breat feeding,.

[17] A. Y. Mohammed, "Knowledge, Attitude and Practice On HIV/AIDS Prevention Among Batu Terara Preparatory School Students in Goba Town, Bale Zone, Southeast Ethiopia," *Primary Health Care Open Access*, vol. 05, no. 01, 2015.

# 2

# Reproduction and Fertility Beliefs, Perceptions, and Attitudes in People Living with HIV

**Vaidehi Mujumdar,[1] Doris Berman ,[1] and Katherine R. Schafer [2]**

[1] *Wake Forest School of Medicine, 1 Medical Center Blvd, Winston-Salem, NC 27157, USA*
[2] *Section on Infectious Diseases, Wake Forest University Health Sciences, Winston-Salem, NC, USA*

Correspondence should be addressed to Doris Berman; dberman@wakehealth.edu

Academic Editor: Mwiya I. Liamunga

People living with HIV (PLWH) have distinct needs when it comes to reproductive health, specifically regarding fertility, family planning, and pregnancy, and these needs are often complicated by HIV status. While there is ample research that focuses on reproductive health in PLWH through a quantitative lens, there is a lack of research using qualitative methods, namely, the narrative interview model. We searched PubMed and relevant abstracts to identify 72 articles published from 1997 to 2016 that described a qualitative framework for exploring the behaviors and perceptions regarding family planning, abortion, pregnancy, parenthood, fertility, and forced sterility in PLWH. The inclusion criteria initially showed 147 articles, which were further screened to exclude those that did not address fertility and family planning specifically. Our final sample of articles included articles related to qualitative research on reproductive attitudes, beliefs, and behaviors of PLWH. Several of these articles were mixed-methods analyses, but our focus was on the qualitative portion only. Further qualitative works in this area will not only contribute to gaps quantitative research in the field cannot capture by design, but also inform clinical practice, policy, and interventions through systematic, in-depth evaluation.

## 1. Introduction

Qualitative research on reproductive behaviors and perceptions of people living with HIV (PLWH) is lacking compared to quantitative studies. Often in HIV research, qualitative studies are embedded within larger quantitative studies to further elucidate the data of the larger study [1–6].

Theories of reproductive health in HIV populations increasingly appear in the literature on individual and community health, especially in relation to racial and ethnic minority populations and groups that experience significant health disparities. The vast majority of these studies are conducted using traditional, standard quantitative research methodology such as data coding and content analysis [7, 8].

However, there is a dearth of qualitative studies in the United States that explore the reproductive narratives of PLWH. PLWH encounter many challenges in their interactions with reproductive health services, often impacting their pregnancy decisions [9, 10]. In this review, we summarize the existing qualitative literature on reproductive health perceptions and decision-making for PLWH. This article will contribute knowledge to an area of increasing needs for patient care and best practices because PLWH can now engage in healthy, safe sexual relationships and make informed decisions surrounding safe reproduction with decreased risk of HIV transmission.

## 2. Materials and Methods

We identified articles in the English language literature using PubMed using the following MeSH terms: *HIV-positive, HIV seropositive, reproductive behavior, fertility, pregnancy, and qualitative*. We also examined the references of articles identified through the selected articles. Though comprehensive, this process was not a formal systematic review. We chose not to conduct a formal systematic review because of the limited amount of qualitative research on reproductive behavior targeted to fertility, family planning (FP), and pregnancy in the United States. Included studies were primarily qualitative or mixed-methods with a qualitative component. Studies could involve behaviorally infected or perinatally infected participants, of both sexes. We focused on findings presented for females and males, but found that there were not as many studies focused on men. We did not limit our results to a particular geographic location, ethnic group, or country.

Because the purpose of this article and in general of qualitative, semistructured interviews is to explore participants' perspectives and experiences, we did not formally grade the strength or weakness of the evidence of the articles synthesized. Below, we summarize the key themes and findings across the identified articles, each in three primary areas of interest: (1) family planning, (2) pregnancy, and (3) fertility. We familiarized ourselves with the data by a thorough review of articles that met inclusion criteria and then, based on key conclusions from each article, identified major themes that unified the body of work. The three themes that we have focused on for this review were identified and conceptualized through the principles of Grounded Theory. Important findings from the literature were identified and grouped into themes.

We identified articles that met inclusion criteria from the past twenty years: 1997 to 2016. A majority of the studies were conducted outside of the United States (US), including Argentina, Brazil, India, Iran, Ireland, Kenya, Malawi, Mexico, South Africa, Uganda, and Zimbabwe. Sample sizes ranged from 10 to over 100 participants. In-depth, semistructured interview was the primary method of data collection. Most studies used Grounded Theory as a form of data collection and analysis [11, 12]. Results of these studies were analyzed using descriptive qualitative measures, specifically data coding to generate theory on the lived experiences of the participants. Age ranges of participants varied, with all studies including only men and women of reproductive ages. All studies were primarily focused on heterosexual couples and individuals, with no specific investigations of men who have sex with men (MSM), women who have sex with women (WSW), or any other gender identities or sexual orientations. While women were the majority of participants, men as individuals with HIV or as part of a serodiscordant couple were also included in some of the interviews.

## 3. Results and Discussion

*3.1. Family Planning.* Results from studies discussing family planning (FP) among individuals, couples, and communities noted the importance of childbearing and the right to have children, regardless of the HIV status of the parents in their cultural context. However, HIV stigma, fear of HIV transmission to partner or child, lack of healthcare provider's support, lack of negotiating power for safer sex, and a lack of knowledge or education about safer conception and pregnancy interventions were barriers to having children [9, 13–20].

Among adolescents living with HIV, the desire to possibly have children is high [21]. In one US-based study, 11 youths discussed pregnancy (10 females and one male) and all expressed interest in having a child in the future. Out of the 11, none reported concern about HIV transmission to a partner; they were more concerned about possible vertical transmission [22]. A mixed-methods study on HIV-positive women in Spain interviewed 134 women and found that 49% of the participants expressed a desire to reproduce. This finding was positively associated with (1) lower age (women under 30 had higher reproductive desire than those aged 30–39), (2) having no children, (3) being an immigrant, and (4) not receiving antiretroviral treatment (ART) [23].

Integrating FP services into HIV care can improve contraceptive uptake among women living with HIV in resource-limited settings [24, 25]. However, there is a lack of research examining preconception experiences of HIV-positive men. Findings from in-depth interviews with 21 men living with HIV seeking care at HIV clinics in Kenya suggest that MLWH appear invested in FP. Inclusion of these men in FP decision-making could strengthen both female and male agency in making such decisions [26–28].

When Highly Active Antiretroviral Therapy (HAART) first became available, it was found that the availability of this treatment encouraged patients to have children as their risk of transmitting the virus was substantially decreased, as evidenced by studies in Zimbabwe and Tanzania [29, 30]. Motivation for mothers to follow more intensive and long-term drug regimens often arose from concern for their children's welfare [31]. Similarly, although the idea of assisted reproduction as a way of minimizing the risk of HIV transmission was often initially met with negative reactions, one study, conducted in Kenya, found that once patients learned more about this option, they were interested in it being available in their community [32].

Another South African study explored the attitudes and behaviors of pregnant women and their partners who participated in a behavioral risk reduction intervention. HIV prevalence in the clinics studied ranged from 15 to 40%, and 44 of the 472 study participants were HIV-positive, although less than half had shared that result with their partners. The results suggested that men value and understand the importance of being involved in women's reproductive health. The men interviewed were interested in acquiring information about safe FP with HIV to support their partners [26, 33].

Perceived gender roles around antenatal and delivery care also vary across communities and may play a significant part in the FP process. A study on antenatal and delivery care in Kenya found that male partners of HIV-positive women, while encouraging of their partners to attend antenatal or delivery care, did not generally accompany their wives. Three main barriers were identified, including (1) viewing pregnancy support as a female role, (2) negative healthcare worker attitudes towards male involvement, and (3) antenatal and delivery unit infrastructure that was not friendly for couples [18]. The first barrier was also a common theme in a multisite study in Cameroon, the Dominican Republic, Georgia, and India [34].

Family planning decisions may depend heavily on gendered power dynamics framed by the local sociocultural context. A qualitative study in western Kenya showed a different picture of men's involvement than studies in other communities. Seventy-six in-depth interviews were conducted with 38 couples, of which 22 couples were concordant HIV-positive. Results suggested that FP use signified female promiscuity and infidelity, indicating a need for gender transformative approaches to work within a male-dominated reproductive decision cultural context [35, 36]. A study that compared couples' experiences in a matrilineal and patrilineal community in rural Malawi found that in both communities the husbands' desires were the driving factor for further pregnancies, even when the women were worried about the risks of pregnancy [37].

Timing of childbirth was another significant factor in pregnancy desires and intentions. In-depth interviews with 36 Kenyan heterosexual HIV-serodiscordant couples who had recently conceived found that conception was an urgent matter, largely stemming from a desire for both partners to raise children together while the HIV-infected partner was healthy [38]. Similar findings were seen in a study of HIV-positive women in Tamil Nadu, India. The main factors distinguishing women who wanted to have a child and those who did not were their levels of anxiety about their future health and available family support. Women who decided to have a child did so based on family support, especially when family members offered to take care of the child if one or both of the parents died [39]. A Brazilian study indicated that many women made provisions with their family for the care of their children. Thinking about the possibility of their children becoming orphans made women feel impotent and guilty. Such painful feelings were minimized through defense mechanisms such as compensation, denial, rationalization, and projection [40].

The nature of providers' attitudes towards pregnancy and FP in HIV care was beyond the scope of this paper. However, available studies revealed provider ambivalence regarding childbearing among PLWH and some placed judgment on this population's reproduction in general. Providers recognized the sexual and reproductive rights of PLWH but struggled with concerns about spreading infection [41, 42]. Many providers also believed that reproductive technologies that do not maintain biological and cultural linkage are not acceptable options to their patients [43, 44]. In an Argentinian study, participants reported that healthcare professionals did not acknowledge their reproductive health wishes or provide useful information or referral [17]. Appropriate training is needed to create a more patient-centered approach and to enable providers to better understand the relationship and social realities surrounding their patients' childbearing intentions. As discussed in the pregnancy and fertility sections, the common perception of a provider as inherently powerful shows the dangers of unequal power dynamics between providers and patients. Although a significant number of HIV-positive women intend to have children in the future, few work with providers to safely plan pregnancy [45, 46].

Studies on HIV-related pregnancy counseling suggested that PLWH preferred having HIV-specific services because of better confidentiality and reduced opportunities for unwanted disclosure that could lead to stigma [47]. Interestingly, in one study in Ireland, women diagnosed with HIV during the course of their pregnancy were encouraged by their pregnancy to achieve stability. The diagnosis of HIV, while traumatic, was also a motivating factor [48]. HIV diagnosis during pregnancy and subsequent disclosure to a partner were noted as a common trigger of intimate partner violence among HIV-positive women [43, 49].

*3.2. Fertility.* Understanding how PLWH perceive the significance of maintaining their fertility or having that fertility forcibly taken away is crucial in providing supportive care for these individuals and their partners. To improve the reproductive care for women and men with HIV, it is necessary to explore and understand their fertility constructs and desires within their local context.

We found 12 studies exploring this issue, all of which used qualitative methods. A study in Botswana suggested that cultural norms, specifically the belief that reproduction signifies a full and productive adult, increase risky reproductive and sexual choices. For women, negative themes that emerged included uncertainties about their health futures and the perception of unpleasant experiences in pregnancy [50]. Similarly, a study in Ethiopian women with HIV cited factors such as age, marital length, partner's sexual preferences and views on contraception, duration of HIV diagnosis, and community pressure as factors that influenced fertility desire [51]. Misconceptions about HIV and its effects on fertility were pervasive in a sample of HIV-positive women; most couples stated that unintentional pregnancy occurred because they believed the HIV-positive partner(s) to be infertile [52].

Although partners seemed to make fertility decisions more as a unit, female preferences carried more influence when individual fertility and conception desires differed [53]. This was also true in a study in Durban, South Africa, that showed that women were the dominant decision-makers about fertility, whether they involved their partners or not [54].

Forced sterilization, as a counterpoint to fertility, came up as a theme for women who were HIV-positive [55]. The experiences of HIV-positive women in two South African provinces suggested the rampancy of coercion and pressure on women with HIV to undergo sterilization. One study interviewed twenty-two women who reported their sterilization between 1996 and 2010 without their informed consent or without their knowledge. They cited three issues leading to the subjugation of their reproductive rights: (1) lack of respect for their autonomy, (2) lack of information given about what sterilization entailed, and (3) subtle or overt pressure to sign the consent [56].

Furthermore, a mixed-methods study on HIV-positive women in Latin America found that 23% of the 285 women in the study experienced pressure to undergo sterilization after diagnosis [57]. Healthcare providers who knew their pregnant patients' HIV diagnosis were six times more likely to coerce or force sterilization than with pregnant patients without a known HIV diagnosis. The providers' coercive tactics included misinformation about pregnancy risks and denying medical services needed to prevent vertical transmission, mainly during caesarean delivery. In addition, many of the interviewed women reported losing the rights to choose number of pregnancies or type of contraception after they were diagnosed with HIV. Studies in Mexico and Tanzania cited similar experiences for the women they interviewed. Many of these women were also advised to undergo tubal ligation or abortions [57–61].

*3.3. Conception and Pregnancy.* Wanting and having a child at some point in their lives was a common theme among PLWH in studies worldwide [9, 62]. The desire to have a child versus intentional pregnancy was mediated by sociocultural and health perceptions and beliefs about conception, pregnancy, and postnatal life with children. Having children was seen as a reason to have hope in the future [63].

A study on pregnancy intentions in South Africa and Malawi among HIV-positive women and their partners, seroconcordant and serodiscordant, found that a partner's expectations for pregnancy, finances, and family composition were key factors in negotiating pregnancy desires. The majority of participants did not actively plan for a pregnancy and challenged the notion that reproductive decisions are always conscious actions [64]. Women's conscious decisions, cited in another study, were based on their judgment of the positive aspects of motherhood versus the negative pressures of social stigma [65].

A sample of ten individuals in serodiscordant relationships interviewed in Northern Ireland reported a willingness to accept the biological risk of infection through unprotected sex in order to meet their desires to conceive without medical interventions, which included but were not limited to ART. This decision-making was also influenced by negative experiences with healthcare providers who were unwilling to support their HIV-positive patients' attempts to conceive [53].

The experiences of a repeat pregnancy are also important in how PLWH view having additional children. Akelo et al. interviewed 40 HIV-positive Kenyan women about their experiences of repeat pregnancy [66]. Qualitative analysis revealed concerns about modern contraception methods as having negative side effects that "ruined the womb." Having the "right" number of children was another important theme for these women and was reinforced by religious leaders, family, and the broader community. A multisite study conducted in South Africa found that pregnancy desires are motivated by whether or not the participant has had any children with his/her current partner rather than by the number of living children. Interviews conducted were with both men (37%) and women (63%) [67].

The presence of HIV-related stigma inevitably affects the women's experience of pregnancy and care. Positive experiences of pregnancy care in Ireland were associated with empathy and understanding of unique needs, continuity of care, and normalizing pregnancy with HIV as much as possible [4, 68]. A literature review of studies focused on the pregnancy decisions of HIV-positive women showed that neonatal outcomes often received more attention than the health of the HIV-positive mother pre-, peri-, and postnatally. It also highlighted the impact of social stigma, discrimination, and, in many countries, the criminalization of HIV transmission that pregnant HIV-positive women must navigate throughout their pregnancies [69].

Having an HIV diagnosis also complicates abortion intentions and decisions. Women living with HIV in Cape Town, South Africa, reported stigma for both becoming pregnant and terminating a pregnancy. This stigma was both self-imposed and from external sources, including family members, partners, community members, and healthcare providers. Despite South Africa's liberal abortion law, abortion is potentially more stigmatizing than pregnancy for women living with HIV [70, 71]. In countries where abortion laws are more restrictive, like Nigeria and Zambia, community attitudes heavily favor continuing childbearing over abortion for women living with HIV [72].

For women living with HIV, their HIV status is an important part of the decision-making around pursuing an abortion. Other factors considered in terminating the pregnancy included stage of life when pregnancy occurred and the level of support from partners and/or families [73, 74].

## 4. Discussion

There is a small but rich pool of qualitative studies that provide some insight into how an HIV diagnosis may complicate beliefs, perceptions, and behaviors related to reproductive health. The findings described suggest a need for better understanding of the complex psychosocial milieu surrounding fertility, family planning, and reproduction for PLWH.

Because there were no qualitative studies of reproductive beliefs of PLWH who identify as LGBTQ*, the findings in this paper reflect only heterosexual PLWH. Research is needed to build an understanding of reproductive health perceptions for PLWH who identify as LGBTQ* in order to best meet these patients' needs.

This review highlights the importance of developing and leveraging trusted provider and community-based relationships and assessing patients' beliefs and values in a sociocultural context, to ensure clear, consistent, and relevant communications. Based on the available literature, PLWH may benefit from more intentional integration of reproductive health in existing HIV care provision programs. Additionally, perceptions, beliefs, and preferences around fertility, family planning, conception, pregnancy, and termination rely heavily on gender roles and the sociocultural context in which the patient lives. The necessary next step will be to identify, implement, and evaluate policies and practices addressing reproductive health in HIV populations that are culturally congruent and accessible.

Qualitative research is a valuable tool to begin understanding patients' perspectives on reproductive health and to generate hypothesis-driven quantitative research to support the reproductive health for PLWH. This review illustrates the value of qualitative narratives in building a more comprehensive understanding of reproductive health perceptions for PLWH. Integrating qualitative interviews into components of HIV research on reproductive health will move clinical care, policy, and interventions forward, as well as providing an opportunity to empower patients to talk about their experiences. It is crucial to produce further published research demonstrating that the patient is the expert in this area of healthcare.

## Disclosure

The findings and conclusions of this report are those of the authors.

## Conflicts of Interest

No competing financial interests exist.

## Acknowledgments

Both Vaidehi Mujumdar and Doris Berman received Medical Student Research Program funding from Wake Forest School of Medicine and Dr. Katherine R. Schafer received funding from NIA, Grant 1R03AG048033-01A1, to complete this literature review.

## References

[1] A. C. Gielen, K. A. McDonnell, P. J. O'Campo, and J. G. Burke, "Suicide risk and mental health indicators: Do they differ by abuse and HIV status?" *Women's Health Issues*, vol. 15, no. 2, pp. 89–95, 2005.

[2] A. C. Gielen, R. M. Ghandour, J. G. J. G. Burke, P. Mahoney, K. A. McDonnell, and P. O'Campo, "HIV/AIDS and intimate partner violence: Intersecting women's health issues in the United States," *Trauma, Violence, & Abuse*, vol. 8, no. 2, pp. 178–198, 2007.

[3] A. D. S. Rossi, E. Amaral, and M. Y. Makuch, "Access of people living with HIV to infertility services: Perspective of Brazilian healthcare professionals," *AIDS Care Psychological and Socio-medical Aspects of AIDS/HIV*, vol. 23, no. 10, pp. 1329–1335, 2011.

[4] J. Heys, G. Jhangri, T. Rubaale, and W. Kipp, "Infection with the human immunodeficiency virus and fertility desires: results from a qualitative study in rural Uganda.," *World health & population*, vol. 13, no. 3, pp. 5–17, 2012.

[5] A. C. Gielen, K. A. McDonnell, J. G. Burke, and P. O'Campo, "Women's lives after an HIV-positive diagnosis: disclosure and violence.," *Maternal and Child Health Journal*, vol. 4, no. 2, pp. 111–120, 2000.

[6] E. Schatz and J. Williams, "Measuring gender and reproductive health in Africa using demographic and health surveys: The need for mixed-methods research," *Culture, Health and Sexuality*, vol. 14, no. 7, pp. 811–826, 2012.

[7] M. W. Carter, J. M. Kraft, K. Hatfield-Timajchy et al., "The reproductive health behaviors of hiv-infected young women in the United States: A literature review," *AIDS Patient Care and STDs*, vol. 27, no. 12, pp. 669–680, 2013.

[8] L. J. Koenig, L. Espinoza, K. Hodge, and N. Ruffo, "Young, seropositive, and pregnant: epidemiologic and psychosocial perspectives on pregnant adolescents with human immunodeficiency virus infection," *American Journal of Obstetrics & Gynecology*, vol. 197, no. 3, pp. S123–S131, 2007.

[9] B. C. Gombachika, E. Chirwa, A. Malata, J. Sundby, and H. Fjeld, "Reproductive decisions of couples living with HIV in Malawi: What can we learn for future policy and research studies?" *Malawi Medical Journal*, vol. 25, no. 3, pp. 65–71, 2013.

[10] P. A. Lee King and D. J. Pate, "Perinatal HIV testing among African American, Caucasian, Hmong and Latina women: Exploring the role of health-care services, information sources and perceptions of HIV/AIDS," *Health Education Research*, vol. 29, no. 1, pp. 109–121, 2014.

[11] J. M. Corbin and A. Strauss, *Basics of Qualitative Research: Techniques and Procedures for Developing Grounded Theory*, SAGE, Thousand Oaks, Calif, USA, 1998.

[12] C. Auerbach and LB. Silverstein, *Qualitative Data: An Introduction to Coding and Analysis*, NYU Press, 2003.

[13] N. L. Beckerman, S. Letteney, and K. Lorber, "Key emotional issues for couples of mixed HIV status," *Social Work in Health Care*, vol. 31, no. 4, pp. 25–41, 2000.

[14] S. B. Kirshenbaum, A. E. Hirky, J. Correale et al., "'Throwing the dice': pregnancy decision-making among HIV-positive women in four U.S. cities," *Perspectives on Sexual and Reproductive Health*, vol. 36, no. 3, pp. 106–113, 2004.

[15] J. Beyeza-Kashesya, F. Kaharuza, F. Mirembe, S. Neema, A. M. Ekstrom, and A. Kulane, "The dilemma of safe sex and having children: Challenges facing HIV sero-discordant couples in Uganda," *African Health Sciences*, vol. 9, no. 1, pp. 2–12, 2009.

[16] M. L. Giles, M. E. Hellard, S. R. Lewin, and M. L. O'Brien, "The work of women when considering and using interventions to reduce mother-to-child transmission (MTCT) of HIV," *AIDS Care Psychological and Socio-medical Aspects of AIDS/HIV*, vol. 21, no. 10, pp. 1230–1237, 2009.

[17] M. L. Gogna, M. M. Pecheny, I. Ibarlucía, H. Manzelli, and S. B. López, "The reproductive needs and rights of people living with HIV in Argentina: health service users' and providers' perspectives," *Social Science & Medicine*, vol. 69, no. 6, pp. 813–820, 2009.

[18] P. Kawale, D. Mindry, S. Stramotas et al., "Factors associated with desire for children among HIV-infected women and men: A quantitative and qualitative analysis from Malawi and implications for the delivery of safer conception counseling," *AIDS Care Psychological and Socio-medical Aspects of AIDS/HIV*, vol. 26, no. 6, pp. 769–776, 2014.

[19] Y. A. Sofolahan and C. O. Airhihenbuwa, "Cultural expectations and reproductive desires: experiences of South African women living with HIV/AIDS (WLHA)," *Health Care for Women International*, vol. 34, no. 3-4, pp. 263–280, 2013.

[20] S. B. Garko, "Sexual and family planning practices and needs of people living with HIV/AIDS in Nigeria: A rapid ethnographic assessment," *Annals of African Medicine*, vol. 6, no. 3, pp. 124–127, 2007.

[21] E. E. Ezeanolue, A. P. Wodi, R. Patel, A. Dieudonne, and J. M. Oleske, "Sexual behaviors and procreational intentions of adolescents and young adults with perinatally acquired human immunodeficiency virus infection: experience of an urban tertiary center," *Journal of Adolescent Health*, vol. 38, no. 6, pp. 719–725, 2006.

[22] A. D. Leonard, C. M. Markham, T. Bui, R. Shegog, and M. E. Paul, "Lowering the Risk of Secondary HIV Transmission: Insights From HIV-Positive Youth and Health Care Providers," *Perspectives on Sexual and Reproductive Health*, vol. 42, no. 2, pp. 110–116, 2010.

[23] V. Hernando, B. Alejos, D. Álvarez et al., "Reproductive desire in women with HIV infection in Spain, associated factors and motivations: a mixed-method study," *BMC Pregnancy and Childbirth*, vol. 14, no. 1, article no. 194, 2014.

[24] F. Laher, C. S. Todd, M. A. Stibich et al., "A qalitative assessment of decisions affecting contraceptive utilization and fertility intentions among HIV-positive women in Soweto, South Africa," *AIDS and Behavior*, vol. 13, no. 1, pp. S47–S54, 2009.

[25] F. Laher, C. S. Todd, M. A. Stibich et al., "Role of menstruation in contraceptive choice among HIV-infected women in Soweto, South Africa," *Contraception*, vol. 81, no. 6, pp. 547–551, 2010.

[26] R. Patel, S. Baum, D. Grossman et al., "HIV-positive men's experiences with integrated family planning and HIV services in western Kenya: Integration fosters male involvement," *AIDS Patient Care and STDs*, vol. 28, no. 8, pp. 418–424, 2014.

[27] T. K. Kwambai, S. Dellicour, M. Desai et al., "Perspectives of men on antenatal and delivery care service utilisation in rural western Kenya: a qualitative study," *BMC Pregnancy and Childbirth*, vol. 13, article no. 134, 2013.

[28] A. R. Tao, M. Onono, S. Baum et al., "Providers' perspectives on male involvement in family planning in the context of a cluster-randomized controlled trial evaluating integrating family planning into HIV care in Nyanza Province, Kenya," *AIDS Care Psychological and Socio-medical Aspects of AIDS/HIV*, vol. 27, no. 1, pp. 31–37, 2015.

[29] V. Ndlovu, "Considering childbearing in the age of highly active antiretroviral therapy (HAART): Views of HIV-positive couples," *Sahara J*, vol. 6, no. 2, pp. 58–68, 2009.

[30] E. J. Mmbaga, G. H. Leyna, M. J. Ezekiel, and D. C. Kakoko, "Fertility desire and intention of people living with HIV/AIDS in Tanzania: a call for restructuring care and treatment services," *BMC Public Health*, vol. 13, article 86, 2013.

[31] M. Ngarina, E. A. M. Tarimo, H. Naburi et al., "Women's preferences regarding infant or maternal antiretroviral prophylaxis for prevention of mother-to-child transmission of HIV during breastfeeding and their views on option B+ in Dar es Salaam, Tanzania," *PLoS ONE*, vol. 9, no. 1, Article ID e85310, 2014.

[32] B. T. Breitnauer, O. Mmeje, B. Njoroge, L. A. Darbes, A. Leddy, and J. Brown, "Community perceptions of childbearing and use of Safer conception strategies among HIV-discordant couples in Kisumu, Kenya," *Journal of the International AIDS Society*, vol. 18, no. 1, Article ID 19972, 2015.

[33] M. E. Shikwane, O. M. Villar-Loubet, S. M. Weiss, K. Peltzer, and D. L. Jones, "HIV knowledge, disclosure and sexual risk among pregnant women and their partners in rural South Africa," *Sahara J*, vol. 10, no. 2, pp. 105–112, 2013.

[34] J. Orne-Gliemann, P. T. Tchendjou, M. Miric et al., "Couple-oriented prenatal HIV counseling for HIV primary prevention: an acceptability study," *BMC Public Health*, vol. 10, article 197, 2010.

[35] E. K. Harrington, S. Dworkin, M. Withers, M. Onono, Z. Kwena, and S. J. Newmann, "Gendered power dynamics and women's negotiation of family planning in a high HIV prevalence setting: a qualitative study of couples in western Kenya," *Culture, Health and Sexuality*, vol. 18, no. 4, pp. 453–469, 2016.

[36] E. K. Harrington, S. J. Newmann, M. Onono et al., "Fertility intentions and interest in integrated family planning services among women living with HIV in nyanza province, Kenya: A qualitative study," *Infectious Diseases in Obstetrics and Gynecology*, vol. 2012, Article ID 809682, 8 pages, 2012.

[37] B. C. Gombachika and H. Fjeld, "In search of a face: Childbearing decisions among couples living with HIV from rural southern Malawi," *African Journal of AIDS Research*, vol. 13, no. 1, pp. 21–29, 2014.

[38] J. Pintye, K. Ngure, K. Curran et al., "Fertility Decision-Making among Kenyan HIV-Serodiscordant Couples Who Recently Conceived: Implications for Safer Conception Planning," *AIDS Patient Care and STDs*, vol. 29, no. 9, pp. 510–516, 2015.

[39] S. Kanniappan, M. J. Jeyapaul, and S. Kalyanwala, "Desire for motherhood: exploring HIV-positive women's desires, intentions and decision-making in attaining motherhood," *AIDS Care: Psychological and Socio-medical Aspects of AIDS/HIV*, vol. 20, no. 6, pp. 625–630, 2008.

[40] E. M. Hebling and E. Hardy, "Feelings related to motherhood among women living with HIV in Brazil: A qualitative study," *AIDS Care Psychological and Socio-medical Aspects of AIDS/HIV*, vol. 19, no. 9, pp. 1095–1100, 2007.

[41] J. Moodley, D. Cooper, J. E. Mantell, and E. Stern, "Health care provider perspectives on pregnancy and parenting in HIV-positive individuals in South Africa," *BMC Health Services Research*, vol. 14, no. 1, article no. 384, 2014.

[42] J. M. Turan, S. Miller, E. A. Bukusi, J. Sande, and C. R. Cohen, "HIV/AIDS and maternity care in Kenya: How fears of stigma and discrimination affect uptake and provision of labor and delivery services," *AIDS Care Psychological and Socio-medical Aspects of AIDS/HIV*, vol. 20, no. 8, pp. 938–945, 2008.

[43] A. M. Hatcher, N. Woollett, C. C. Pallitto et al., "Bidirectional links between HIV and intimate partner violence in pregnancy: Implications for prevention of mother-to-child transmission," *Journal of the International AIDS Society*, vol. 17, Article ID 19233, 2014.

[44] P. Kawale, D. Mindry, A. Phoya, P. Jansen, and R. M. Hoffman, "Provider attitudes about childbearing and knowledge of safer conception at two HIV clinics in Malawi," *Reproductive Health*, vol. 12, no. 1, article no. 17, 2015.

[45] S. Finocchario-Kessler, N. Mabachi, J. K. Dariotis, J. Anderson, K. Goggin, and M. Sweat, "'We weren't using condoms because we were trying to conceive': the need for reproductive counseling for HIV-positive women in clinical care," *AIDS Patient Care and STDs*, vol. 26, no. 11, pp. 700–707, 2012.

[46] S. Finocchario-Kessler, M. D. Sweat, J. K. Dariotis et al., "Childbearing motivations, pregnancy desires, and perceived partner response to a pregnancy among urban female youth: does HIV-infection status make a difference?" *AIDS Care*, vol. 24, no. 1, pp. 1–11, 2012.

[47] M. Colombini, R. Mutemwa, J. Kivunaga et al., "Experiences of stigma among women living with HIV attending sexual and reproductive health services in Kenya: A qualitative study," *BMC Health Services Research*, vol. 14, no. 1, article no. 412, 2014.

[48] C. Kelly, F. Alderdice, M. Lohan, and D. Spence, "Creating continuity out of the disruption of a diagnosis of HIV during pregnancy," *Journal of Clinical Nursing*, vol. 21, no. 11-12, pp. 1554–1562, 2012.

[49] C. Mulrenan, M. Colombini, N. Howard, J. Kikuvi, and S. H. Mayhew, "Exploring risk of experiencing intimate partner violence after HIV infection: A qualitative study among women with HIV attending postnatal services in Swaziland," *BMJ Open*, vol. 5, no. 5, Article ID e006907, 2015.

[50] R. L. Upton and E. M. Dolan, "Sterility and stigma in an era of HIV/AIDS: narratives of risk assessment among men and women in Botswana.," *African Journal of Reproductive Health*, vol. 15, no. 1, pp. 95–102, 2011.

[51] D. B. Demissie, B. Tebeje, and T. Tesfaye, "Fertility desire and associated factors among people living with HIV attending antiretroviral therapy clinic in Ethiopia," *BMC Pregnancy and Childbirth*, vol. 14, no. 1, article no. 382, 2014.

[52] R. King, K. Khana, S. Nakayiwa et al., "'Pregnancy comes accidentally-like it did with me': reproductive decisions among women on ART and their partners in rural Uganda," *BMC Public Health*, vol. 11, article 530, 2011.

[53] C. Kelly, M. Lohan, F. Alderdice, and D. Spence, "Negotiation of risk in sexual relationships and reproductive decision-making amongst HIV sero-different couples," *Culture, Health and Sexuality*, vol. 13, no. 7, pp. 815–827, 2011.

[54] H. M. Marlow, S. Maman, A. K. Groves, and D. Moodley, "Fertility Intent and Contraceptive Decision-Making Among HIV Positive and Negative Antenatal Clinic Attendees in Durban, South Africa," *Health Care for Women International*, vol. 33, no. 4, pp. 342–358, 2012.

[55] K. Hopkins, R. M. Barbosa, D. R. Knauth, and J. E. Potter, "The impact of health care providers on female sterilization among HIV-positive women in Brazil," *Social Science & Medicine*, vol. 61, no. 3, pp. 541–554, 2005.

[56] A. Strode, S. Mthembu, and Z. Essack, ""She made up a choice for me": 22 HIV-positive women's experiences of involuntary sterilization in two South African provinces," *Reproductive Health Matters*, vol. 20, no. 39, pp. 61–69, 2012.

[57] T. Kendall and C. Albert, "Experiences of coercion to sterilize and forced sterilization among women living with HIV in Latin America," *Journal of the International AIDS Society*, vol. 18, no. 1, Article ID 19462, 2015.

[58] L. Campero, T. Kendall, M. Caballero, A. L. Mena, and C. Herrera, "The exercise of sexual and reproductive rights: a qualitative study of heterosexual people with HIV in Mexico," *Salud Pública de México*, vol. 52, no. 1, pp. 61–69, 2010.

[59] S. C. Keogh, M. Urassa, M. Roura et al., "The impact of antenatal HIV diagnosis on postpartum childbearing desires in northern Tanzania: a mixed methods study," *Reproductive Health Matters*, vol. 20, no. 39, pp. 39–49, 2012.

[60] T. Kendall, "Falling short of universal access to reproductive health: Unintended pregnancy and contraceptive use among Mexican women with HIV," *Culture, Health and Sexuality*, vol. 15, no. 2, pp. S166–S179, 2013.

[61] M. G. Van Dijk, K. S. Wilson, M. Silva, X. Contreras, H. D. Fukuda, and S. G. García, "Health care experiences of HIV-infected women with fertility desires in Mexico: a qualitative study," *Journal of the Association of Nurses in AIDS Care*, vol. 25, no. 3, pp. 224–232, 2014.

[62] D. Cooper, J. Harries, L. Myer, P. Orner, H. Bracken, and V. Zweigenthal, "Corrigendum to " "Life is still going on": Reproductive intentions among HIV-positive women and men in South Africa". [Soc. Sci. Med. 65 (2007) 274-283] (DOI:10.1016/j.socscimed.2007.03.019)," *Social Science & Medicine*, vol. 65, no. 10, p. 2186, 2007.

[63] Z. Behboodi-Moghadam, Z. Khalajinia, A.-R. N. Nasrabadi, M. Mohraz, and M. Gharacheh, "Pregnancy through the Lens of Iranian Women with HIV," *Journal of the International Association of Providers of AIDS Care*, vol. 15, no. 2, pp. 148–152, 2016.

[64] E. Evens, E. Tolley, J. Headley et al., "Identifying factors that influence pregnancy intentions: evidence from South Africa and Malawi," *Culture, Health and Sexuality*, vol. 17, no. 3, pp. 374–389, 2015.

[65] D. B. Barnes and S. Murphy, "Reproductive decisions for women with HIV: Motherhood's role in envisioning a future," *Qualitative Health Research*, vol. 19, no. 4, pp. 481–491, 2009.

[66] V. Akelo, E. McLellan-Lemal, L. Toledo et al., "Erratum: Determinants and experiences of repeat pregnancy among HIV-positive kenyan women-A mixed-methods analysis (PLoS ONE)," *PLoS ONE*, vol. 10, no. 7, Article ID e0134536, 2015.

[67] D. L. Mindry, T. L. Crankshaw, P. Maharaj et al., ""We have to try and have this child before it is too late": Missed opportunities in client-provider communication on reproductive intentions of people living with HIV," *AIDS Care Psychological and Socio-medical Aspects of AIDS/HIV*, vol. 27, no. 1, pp. 25–30, 2015.

[68] C. Kelly, F. Alderdice, M. Lohan, and D. Spence, "'Every pregnant woman needs a midwife'-The experiences of HIV affected women in maternity care," *Midwifery*, vol. 29, no. 2, pp. 132–138, 2013.

[69] S. MacCarthy, J. J. K. Rasanathan, L. Ferguson, and S. Gruskin, "The pregnancy decisions of HIV-positive women: the state of knowledge and way forward," *Reproductive Health Matters*, vol. 20, supplement 39, pp. 119–140, 2012.

[70] P. Orner, J. Harries, D. Cooper, and M. De Bruyn, "A qualitative exploration of HIV-positive pregnant women's decision-making regarding abortion in Cape Town, South Africa," *Sahara J*, vol. 7, no. 2, pp. 44–51, 2010.

[71] P. Orner, M. de Bruyn, and D. Cooper, "'It hurts, but I don't have a choice, I'm not working and I'm sick': Decisions and experiences regarding abortion of women living with HIV in Cape Town, South Africa," *Culture, Health and Sexuality*, vol. 13, no. 7, pp. 781–795, 2011.

[72] M. L. Kavanaugh, A. M. Moore, O. Akinyemi et al., "Community attitudes towards childbearing and abortion among HIV-positive women in Nigeria and Zambia," *Culture, Health and Sexuality*, vol. 15, no. 2, pp. 160–174, 2013.

[73] R. M. Barbosa, A. A. Pinho, N. S. Santos, and W. V. Villela, "Exploring the relationship between induced abortion and HIV infection in Brazil," *Reproductive Health Matters*, vol. 20, no. 39, pp. 80–89, 2012.

[74] W. V. Villela, R. M. Barbosa, A. P. Portella, and L. A. de Oliveira, "Motives and circumstances surrounding induced abortion among women living with HIV in Brazil," *Ciencia & Saúde Coletiva*, vol. 17, no. 7, pp. 1709–1719, 2012.

# HIV Epidemic in Tanzania: The Possible Role of the Key Populations

**Bonaventura C. T. Mpondo,[1] Daniel W. Gunda,[2] and Semvua B. Kilonzo[2]**

[1]*Department of Internal Medicine, School of Medicine, College of Health Sciences, The University of Dodoma, Dodoma, Tanzania*
[2]*Department of Internal Medicine, School of Medicine, Catholic University of Health and Allied Sciences, Mwanza, Tanzania*

Correspondence should be addressed to Bonaventura C. T. Mpondo; boniempondo@gmail.com

Academic Editor: David Katzenstein

HIV remains a public health concern in Tanzania and other Eastern and Southern African countries. Estimates show that there were about 1.4 million people living with HIV in Tanzania in the year 2013. HIV is a generalized epidemic in Tanzania with heterosexual transmission being the main route of transmission. Recently, however, there has been growing concern on the potential role of the key populations in HIV epidemic in the country. Studies done have shown significantly higher HIV prevalence in these populations compared to the general population. These studies have also reported high risky behaviors among members of these populations. This review aims at discussing the possible role of the key populations in the HIV epidemic in Tanzania.

## 1. Background

HIV remains a public health concern in many sub-Saharan African countries including Tanzania. In the year 2013, it was estimated that there were a total of 1.4 million people living with HIV in Tanzania [1]. The national prevalence among people aged 15–49 years in Tanzania was estimated to be 5.1% in 2011, which is a drop of approximately 2% compared to the year 2003 [2]. In Tanzania, HIV is a generalized epidemic affecting both urban and rural populations with approximately over 80% of HIV infections resulting from heterosexual transmission [3].

Key populations (KPs) are defined by World Health Organization (WHO) as both vulnerable populations and populations at higher risk of acquiring HIV infection [4]. They usually have both legal and social issues related to their behaviors which increase their vulnerability to HIV. Members of the KPs include people who inject drugs (PWID), men who have sex with men (MSM), transgender persons, female sex workers (FSW), and prisoners. KPs are important to the dynamics of HIV transmission in a given setting and are essential partners in an effective response to the epidemic [5, 6]. There is evidence of overlapping sexual network between KPs and general population [7]. This indicates that HIV among key populations is not isolated; if not properly addressed it could risk the national responses.

Research worldwide shows that HIV disproportionately affects members of the key populations (KPs) as compared to the general population. When compared to the general population, global data shows that on average PWID are 22 times more likely to be HIV-positive [1], transgender 49 times [8], sex workers 14 times [9], MSM 13 times [10, 11], and prisoners 6–50 times, depending on specific contexts [8]. Despite the small number of studies done in Tanzania, evidence indicates HIV prevalence of 42% among PWID [12], 31.4% among female sex workers [13], and 30.2% among MSM [14]. HIV prevalence among transgender people is not known and official data from prisons is not available.

Despite the high HIV prevalence in these populations, there are also reports of multiple sexual partners and high frequency of partner change with low condom usage in these populations [13, 15–17]. According to the sexually transmissible infections (STIs) transmission model as described by Anderson, people who have high rates of partner change have high chances of transmitting HIV and other STIs [18]. These individuals with high frequency change of sexual partners and other risky behaviors form the "core group" with their sexual partners forming the "adjacent group"; this group can serve as "bridging population" between the core group and the general population. This mini-review aims at highlighting the possible role of KPs in HIV epidemic in Tanzania.

## 2. Estimates on Key Population Size in Tanzania

In April 2014, the Ministry of Health of Tanzania together with the Tanzania Commission for AIDS (TACAIDS) met with stakeholders to estimate the HIV prevalence and population estimates of the key populations in mainland Tanzania. The stakeholders reviewed the existing evidence and identified the limitations and knowledge gaps in the studies. They then used a Delphi method [19] to come to a consensus on the estimated population size and HIV prevalence on the three groups of key populations: female sexual workers, men who have sex with men, and people who use/inject drugs [20].

For the female sex workers (FSWs), the population size was estimated to be 155,450 individuals (range: 128,610–198,050). The HIV prevalence in this group was estimated to be 26 percent (range: 14–37%). For men who have sex with men, the population in urban mainland Tanzania was estimated to be 49,700 individuals (range: 41,000–71,000); the HIV prevalence was estimated to be 25 percent (range: 18–35%). Among the people who use/inject drugs, their number was estimated to be 30,000 (range: 20,000–42,500), with a consensus point prevalence estimate of 36 percent (range: 22–43%). Estimates done in Unguja island in Zanzibar in 2011/2012 using multiple methods concluded that there were 3000 PWID, 3958 FSW, and 2157 MSM [21]; the total population of Unguja was estimated to be 896,721 from the 2012 census.

Tanzania is, however, one of the countries where all these populations are criminalized. There is therefore high possibility of the population size to be underestimated; this concept has been proved in recent studies [22].

## 3. Epidemiology of HIV among KPs

*3.1. Prevalence of HIV among MSM.* MSM remain a hidden population in Tanzania because the practice is still stigmatized and criminalized. There are few reports on the possible contribution of MSM in the HIV epidemic in the country. Few studies have been done to determine the magnitude of HIV among MSM in Tanzania. In 2012, a study done in Dar es Salaam and Tanga, two regions along the coast, found that HIV prevalence was 30.2% in Dar es Salaam and 11% in Tanga [14]. In Zanzibar, an island where the prevalence in the general population is estimated to be 0.6%, a survey done in 2007 found the prevalence among the MSM to be 12.3%, which is about 20-fold higher [23]. A recent published study found that the HIV seroprevalence of this group in Dodoma which is the capital city of the country was 17%, which is approximately five times that of men in the general population [24].

*3.2. Prevalence of HIV among Female Sex Workers.* Tanzanian law criminalizes sex work practice and it is punishable by law. Despite this fact, the practice has been documented in Tanzania, especially in Dar-es-Salaam which is the economic capital of the country [13]. Globally, it is estimated that FSW are 14 times more likely to be living with HIV compared to women in the general population [9]. In Tanzania, however, data on HIV prevalence among sexual workers is scarce. Few studies have been done to estimate the magnitude of HIV in this population. A survey conducted in Dar es Salaam in 2010 reported HIV prevalence among sexual workers to be 31.4% [13] compared to the prevalence of 10.4% in the general population [2]. Another study done in the northern part of the country among hotel and bar workers who in most cases are also sexual workers found HIV prevalence of 26.3% [25]. The findings in these studies are in line with the findings from a review that reported high prevalence of around 36.9% in SSA which was the highest compared to other geographical regions [9]. Studies done elsewhere in Africa have reported a wide range of HIV prevalence among FSW: from 34% in Cameroon to 75% in Kenya [26].

*3.3. Prevalence of HIV among Injecting Drug Users.* For the past ten years, Tanzania has documented a significant increase in the number of people who inject drugs [27]. In the year 2012, through its outreach programs, the National AIDS Control Program (NACP) reported to have engaged 2530 individuals who were injecting drugs. Several studies have been done to assess the risk for HIV and determine the prevalence in this population in Tanzania. There was significantly higher HIV prevalence in this group compared to the general population. One study that was conducted in Dar es Salaam in 2006 reported the prevalence of 42% [12]. Among women injecting drugs, the prevalence was estimated to be 55% [28]. Studies on HIV prevalence among the members of the key populations in Tanzania are summarized in Table 1.

## 4. Risk Factors for HIV in the General Population

The prevalence of HIV in general population in Tanzania is estimated to be about 5.1%; however, there are geographical variations with high burden in the Southern Highland zone of the country [2] (Figure 1). Several studies have been done to determine the drivers of HIV epidemic in Tanzania. A survey that was conducted by the National Institute for Medical Research in 2009 revealed that early age for sexual debut, having multiple sexual partners, extramarital sex, and low knowledge on condoms were factors associated with HIV risk in Tanzanian communities [29]. In this survey, 85% of the respondents reported to have had their sexual debut between the ages of 10–19 years. Early sexual debut has been reported to be a predictor of having multiple sexual partners later in life [30]. Up to 25% of the respondents reported that they did not know where to get the condoms; extramarital sex was reported in 79% of the respondents. The conclusion from this survey was that high levels of multiple and concurrent

TABLE 1: Summary of studies on HIV prevalence among the different key populations in Tanzania.

| Population | Study | Study setting | Prevalence |
|---|---|---|---|
| MSM | Ross et al., 2014 [14] | Dar es Salaam | 30.2% |
| | | Tanga | 11.0% |
| | Dahoma et al., 2011 [23] | Zanzibar | 12.3% |
| | Mmbaga et al., 2017 [24] | Dodoma | 17.0% |
| FSW | NACP, 2011 [13] | Dar es Salaam | 31.4% |
| | Kapiga et al., 2002 [25] | Moshi | 26.3% |
| PWID | Williams et al., 2009 [12] | Dar es Salaam | 42.0% |
| | Atkinson et al., 2011 [28] | Dar es Salaam | 55.0% among women |

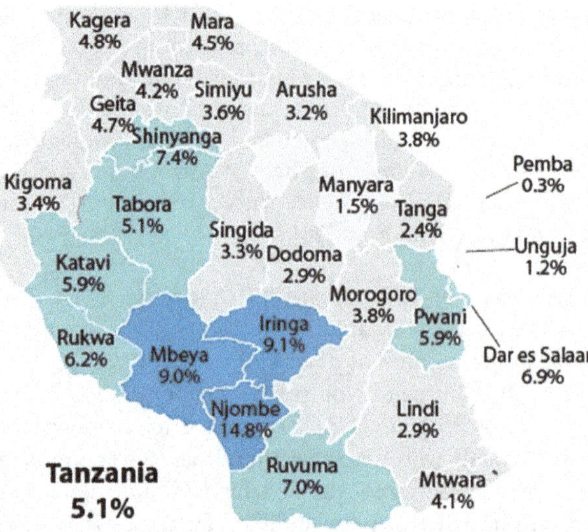


FIGURE 1: HIV prevalence among men and women aged 15–49 years in Tanzania by region [2]. *Source*: Tanzania HIV/AIDS and Malaria Indicator Survey 2011/2012.

sexual partners, intergenerational sex, and transactional sex were among the drivers of HIV epidemic in Tanzania.

Other studies have also demonstrated risk factors for HIV in Tanzania. A prospective study done in Mbeya found that younger age, low level of education, alcohol use, and number of sexual partners were associated with the risk for HIV [31]. The number of sexual partners was also found to be a risk factor in a case-control study done in the northwestern part of the country [32]. Another survey done in rural Tanzania found HIV prevalence of 5.6%; multiple sexual partners and alcohol consumption were associated with the risk for HIV [33].

Risky behaviors, however, are not the only reason for HIV transmission in the general population. Several studies have shown a discrepancy between high risky behavior and HIV prevalence, suggesting that there are other factors that explain HIV transmission. A study done in Zimbabwe and Tanzania found that the participants in Tanzania had more risky sexual behaviors and other risk factors for HIV than those in Zimbabwe; the prevalence of HIV was, however, higher in Zimbabweans [34]. The discrepancy between the HIV prevalence and risky sexual behavior has also been reported in another study done in four different African cities [35]. Concurrent sexual partnerships have also been believed to be among the major factors driving HIV epidemic in sub-Saharan Africa; however, one systematic review of the existing evidence concluded that concurrent sexual relationships do not explain the HIV epidemics in Africa [36].

## 5. Risky Behaviors among the Key Populations

*5.1. Men Who Have Sex with Men.* Evidence shows that same-sex sexual practices in Tanzania are not and have not been uncommon; they date as far back as the 19th century [40]. Studies done to assess sexual behaviors among MSM in Tanzania have identified several risks. A study done in Dar es Salaam, Tanzania, by Nyoni and Ross in 2013 found that condom usage was very low among the MSM. Only 43% of the participants reported using condom regularly with casual partners and 49% with regular partners in this study [16]. Inconsistent condom use was also found to be common in another survey done in Zanzibar in 2007; in this study, 85% of the respondents reported inconsistent condom use [23]. Majority of the MSM in the country have been reported to prefer receptive anal position (bottom position) [14–16] which is associated with higher risk of HIV transmission as compared to insertive anal position (top position) [41]. Paid sex and multiple sexual partners are also common in this population [14–16, 23, 37]. Another study in Dar es Salaam found out that up to 36% of respondents were practicing paid sex. The study also found that money-motivated MSM were more likely to identify themselves as bisexuals but also have significant number of partners of both sexes [37]. Having a female partner was a common finding in most of the studies [15, 23, 24] which increases the risk of transmission to the general population.

*5.2. Female Sex Workers.* The potential for female sexual workers transmitting HIV to the general population should not be underestimated [42]. Their clients can serve as the "bridging population" and transmit HIV to the general population [6]. A survey conducted in Dar es Salaam in 2010 estimated that the number of clients per female sexual worker in Tanzania averages at 3 [13]. The survey also found that female sexual workers were involved in risky sexual behaviors as reported elsewhere [6, 26] which include multiple sexual partners, inconsistent condom use, and the use of illicit drugs.

TABLE 2: Summary on risky behaviors and the respective studies among the key populations in Tanzania.

| Population | Risky behaviors | Study |
|---|---|---|
| MSM | Low condom use | Nyoni and Ross, 2013 [16]<br>Dahoma et al., 2011 [23] |
| | Preference of receptive anal position (bottom position) | Ross et al., 2014 [14]<br>Mmbaga et al., 2012 [15]<br>Nyoni and Ross, 2013 [16] |
| | Paid sex and multiple sexual partners | Nyoni and Ross, 2013 [16]<br>Dahoma et al., 2011 [23]<br>Ross et al., 2014 [14]<br>Bui et al., 2014 [37] |
| | Multiple sexual partners | Bui et al., 2014 [37] |
| FSW | Multiple sexual partners/high frequency of partner change<br>Inconsistent condom use<br>Alcohol and drug abuse | NACP, 2011 [13]<br>Kapiga et al., 2002 [25] |
| PWUD/PWID | Multiple sexual partners | Mlunde et al., 2016 [17]<br>Matiko et al., 2015 [38] |
| | Low and inconsistent condom use | Mlunde et al., 2016 [17]<br>Tan et al., 2015 [39]<br>Matiko et al., 2015 [38] |
| | Needle sharing | Tan et al., 2015 [39]<br>Matiko et al., 2015 [38] |

With the reported high number of sexual partners and high frequency of partner change in addition to condom use being low and inconsistent, this population has very high chance of acquiring and transmitting HIV infection to their male clients who then serve as the "bridging population" to their wives and girlfriends.

*5.3. People Who Inject Drugs (PWID).* Reports worldwide show that PWUD/PWID are at a significant risk of acquiring HIV infection when compared to the general population [43]. Their partners represent another population that can serve as a "bridging population" for HIV transmission. In 2015, UNAIDS estimated that 9% of all new infections in Eastern and Southern Africa were the clients of sex workers and other sexual partners of key populations [43]. Very few studies have been done in Tanzania to identify risky behaviors in this population. One study done in Dar es Salaam in 2014 found that this population was involved in a number of high risk behaviors that increase in their risk of acquiring HIV; however, there was low tendency for screening for HIV and other sexually transmissible infections. In this study, 37.5% of participants reported having multiple sexual partners; however, only 17% reported condom use [17]. Another study done in Mwanza, northwestern Tanzania, in 2014 also reported low condom use in this population; additionally, the study found that more than half of the participants were sharing needles and use illicit drugs during sex [39]. Needle sharing, multiple sexual partners, and low condom use were also reported in a survey done in Zanzibar [38]. Screening for HIV and other STIs was found to be low in this population in Dar es Salaam and Zanzibar [17, 38]. The role of STIs in increasing HIV transmission has been studied previously; despite some trials showing no effect in HIV transmission, most studies have shown that STIs, especially ulcerative ones, increase the risk of HIV transmission [44, 45]. Also early treatment of HIV has been shown to minimize the risk of HIV transmission [46]. The fact that this population is at increased risk for acquiring HIV with low screening rates further increases the chance of them transmitting HIV to the general population. Studies on risky behaviors among the key populations in Tanzania are summarized in Table 2.

## 6. Possible Role of Key Populations in HIV Transmission

HIV prevalence has been reported to be higher among the members of the key populations compared to the general population in Tanzania just like in other countries. As reported earlier, members of these populations have high frequency of partner change; with the high HIV prevalence, these form a "core group" in the transmission model described by Anderson [47]. According to the model, sexual partners of these individuals will serve as a "bridging population" between the members of the core groups and the general population (Figure 2). Members of the core groups and their sexual partners have been shown to be the drivers of HIV epidemic in many parts of the world [5]. Members of the key population, therefore, together with their sexual partners could be contributing to the epidemic in Tanzania.

## 7. Status of Interventions to Reduce HIV Transmission in Key Populations in Tanzania

Tanzania through scaling up HIV interventions has managed to significantly reduce the prevalence of HIV in the general

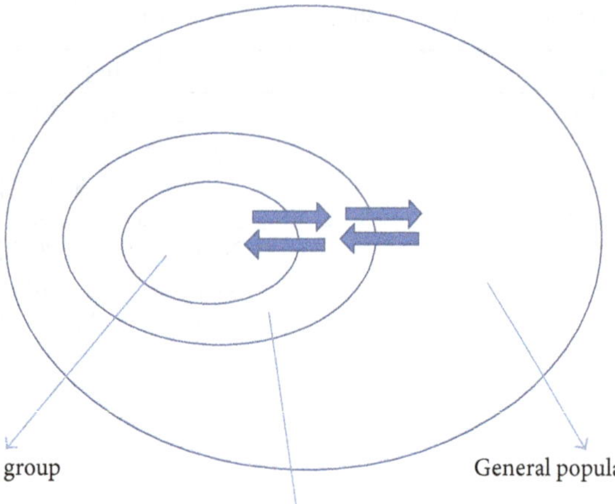


Figure 2: Sexual networks according to Anderson Transmission model [18].

population. The prevalence of HIV has been on the decline; in 2003/2004, the prevalence was estimated to be 7%. The survey done in 2007/2008 found the prevalence to be 5.7% and that in 2011/2012 found it to be 5.1%. However, the prevalence among the KPs has been found to be disproportionately high. The country therefore saw the need to have interventions among the KPs and developed a national guideline that stipulates the comprehensive package of HIV interventions for key populations [48]. The guidelines aimed at increasing access to both health-related and social services among the members of the KPs in order to minimize HIV transmission in these vulnerable and at risk groups.

The guideline among other things includes recommendations for HIV prevention, diagnosis, treatment, and care, biomedical interventions such as nonoil lubricants for MSM and medically assisted therapy (MAT) for PWID, management of comorbidities and coinfections, and finally the social and behavioral interventions for HIV prevention. The Ministry of Health committed itself to ensure implementation of this guideline by putting in place the systems and structure to support the implementation. In October 2016, the Ministry of Health decided to suspend activities for drop in centers for MSM which were responsible for differentiated service delivery for MSM; it also suspended the use of nonoil-based lubricants pending review of the existing evidence and acceptability of their use in Tanzania. The ministry aims at reviewing the package for health and HIV services for KPs and then incorporating those interventions that are internationally acceptable and in line with the country's laws, traditions, and customs.

The situation is different with PWID. Interventions for PWID have been in place before the release of the guideline. In 2010, Tanzania developed a guideline for medically assisted treatment of opioid dependence [48]; in 2011, Tanzania became the first President's Emergency Plan for AIDS Relief (PEPFAR) country in Africa to establish medically assisted therapy (MAT) as part of HIV prevention intervention for PWID by opening MAT clinic at Muhimbili National Hospital. In 2012, another pilot clinic was opened at Mwananyamala Hospital in Dar es Salaam. However, accessibility remains poor; so far such clinics are available in only one city (Dar es Salaam) in mainland Tanzania.

## 8. Conclusions and Recommendations

Members of key population have higher rates of HIV in Tanzania compared to the general population. Risky sexual behaviors have been reported to be common in these populations; interactions with the general population increase the chance of transmission of HIV to the general population. Interventions to minimize HIV prevalence and transmission risk in these populations such as promoting and providing condoms for MSM and FSW, promoting the use of water-based lubricants for MSM, screening and treating STIs, harm-reduction techniques for IDUs (e.g., needle syringe exchange programs), and HIV counseling, testing, and early treatment initiation are important measures to prevent HIV transmission in Tanzania. The country therefore needs to lay stress on the need for HIV prevention, care, and treatment among the members of the key populations.

## Conflicts of Interest

The authors declare that they have no conflicts of interest.

## Acknowledgments

The authors would like to thank Dr. Rodgers Rodriguez for his assistance in reviewing the article for any spelling and grammatical errors.

## References

[1] UNAIDS, "UNAIDS report on the global AIDS epidemic 2013," New York, USA, 2013.

[2] TACAIDS, ZAC, NBS, OCGS, and ICF, "Tanzania HIV/AIDS and Malaria Indicator Survey 2011-12," Dar es Salaam, Tanzania, 2013.

[3] National AIDS Control Programme (NACP), "National guidelines for the management of HIV and AIDS," Dar es Salaam, Tanzania, 2015.

[4] UNAIDS, "Terminology Guidelines," New York, USA, 2011.

[5] F. A. Plummer, N. J. D. Nagelkerke, S. Moses, J. O. Ndinya-Achola, J. Bwayo, and E. Ngugi, "The importance of core groups in the epidemiology and control of HIV-1 infection," *AIDS*, vol. 5, no. 1, pp. S169–S176, 1991.

[6] C. M. Lowndes, M. Alary, H. Meda et al., "Role of core and bridging groups in the transmission dynamics of HIV and STIs in Cotonou, Benin, West Africa," *Sexually Transmitted Infections*, vol. 78, no. 1, pp. i69–i77, 2002.

[7] Y. A. Amirkhanian, "Social networks, sexual networks and HIV risk in men who have sex with men," *Current HIV/AIDS Reports*, vol. 11, no. 1, pp. 81–92, 2014.

[8] S. D. Baral, T. Poteat, S. Strömdahl, A. L. Wirtz, T. E. Guadamuz, and C. Beyrer, "Worldwide burden of HIV in transgender

women: A systematic review and meta-analysis," *The Lancet Infectious Diseases*, vol. 13, no. 3, pp. 214–222, 2013.

[9] S. Baral, C. Beyrer, K. Muessig et al., "Burden of HIV among female sex workers in low-income and middle-income countries: a systematic review and meta-analysis," *The Lancet Infectious Diseases*, vol. 12, no. 7, pp. 538–549, 2012.

[10] C. Beyrer, S. D. Baral, F. Van Griensven et al., "Global epidemiology of HIV infection in men who have sex with men," *The Lancet*, vol. 380, no. 9839, pp. 367–377, 2012.

[11] S. Baral, F. Sifakis, F. Cleghorn, and C. Beyrer, "Elevated risk for HIV infection among men who have sex with men in low- and middle-income countries 2000–2006: a systematic review," *PLoS Medicine*, vol. 4, no. 12, article e339, 2007.

[12] M. L. Williams, S. A. McCurdy, A. M. Bowen et al., "HIV seroprevalence in a sample of Tanzanian intravenous drug users," *AIDS Education and Prevention*, vol. 21, no. 5, pp. 474–483, 2009.

[13] NACP, "HIV Behavioral and Biological Surveillance Survey Among Female Sex Workers in Dar es Salaam , 2010," pp. 1–64, 2011.

[14] M. W. Ross, J. Nyoni, H. O. Ahaneku, J. Mbwambo, R. S. McClelland, and S. A. McCurdy, "High HIV seroprevalence, rectal STIs and riskxy sexual behaviour in men who have sex with men in Dar es Salaam and Tanga, Tanzania," *BMJ Open*, vol. 4, no. 8, Article ID e006175, 2014.

[15] E. J. Mmbaga, M. J. Dodo, G. H. Leyna, K. Moen, and M. T. Leshabari, "Sexual practices and perceived susceptibility to HIV infection among men who have sex with men in Dar Es Salaam, mainland Tanzania," *Journal of AIDS and Clinical Research*, vol. 3, 2012.

[16] J. E. Nyoni and M. W. Ross, "Condom use and HIV-related behaviors in urban Tanzanian men who have sex with men: A study of beliefs, HIV knowledge sources, partner interactions and risk behaviors," *AIDS Care - Psychological and Socio-Medical Aspects of AIDS/HIV*, vol. 25, no. 2, pp. 223–229, 2013.

[17] L. B. Mlunde, B. F. Sunguya, J. K. Mbwambo et al., "A mismatch between high-risk behaviors and screening of infectious diseases among people who inject drugs in Dar es Salaam, Tanzania," *PLoS ONE*, vol. 11, no. 2, Article ID e0148598, 2016.

[18] R. M. Anderson, *Transmission Dynamics of Sexually Transmitted Infections*, McGraw-Hill, New York, USA, 3rd edition, 1999.

[19] T. J. Gordon, "The Delphi method," in *Futures Research Methodology*, 2009.

[20] A. Dutta, C. Barker, and N. Makyao, "Consensus Estimates on Key Population Size and HIV Prevalence in Tanzania," National AIDS Control Programme, pp. 1–34, 2014.

[21] F. J. Khalid, F. M. Hamad, A. A. Othman et al., "Estimating the number of people who inject drugs, female sex workers, and men who have sex with men, Unguja Island, Zanzibar: Results and synthesis of multiple methods," *AIDS and Behavior*, vol. 18, no. 1, pp. S25–S31, 2014.

[22] S. L. M. Davis, W. C. Goedel, J. Emerson, and B. S. Guven, "hort report Punitive laws , key population size estimates , and Global AIDS Response Progress Reports: an ecological study of 154 countries," *Journal of the International AIDS Society*, vol. 20, no. 1, pp. 1–8, 2017.

[23] M. Dahoma, L. G. Johnston, A. Holman et al., "HIV and related risk behavior among men who have sex with men in Zanzibar, Tanzania: Results of a behavioral surveillance survey," *AIDS and Behavior*, vol. 15, no. 1, pp. 186–192, 2011.

[24] E. J. Mmbaga, K. Moen, N. Makyao, R. Mpembeni, and M. T. Leshabari, "HIV and STI s among men who have sex with men in Dodoma municipality, Tanzania: a cross-sectional study," *Sexually Transmitted Infections*, vol. 93, no. 5, pp. 314–319, 2017.

[25] S. H. Kapiga, N. E. Sam, J. F. Shao et al., "HIV-1 epidemic among female bar and hotel workers in Northern Tanzania: Risk factors and opportunities for prevention," *Journal of Acquired Immune Deficiency Syndromes*, vol. 29, no. 4, pp. 409–417, 2002.

[26] L. Morison, H. A. Weiss, A. Buvé et al., "Commercial sex and the spread of HIV in four cities in sub-Saharan Africa," *AIDS*, vol. 15, no. 4, pp. S61–S69, 2001.

[27] E. A. Ratliff, S. A. McCurdy, J. K. Mbwambo et al., "An Overview of HIV Prevention Interventions for People Who Inject Drugs in Tanzania," *Advances in Preventive Medicine*, vol. 2013, pp. 1–6, 2013.

[28] J. Atkinson, S. McCurdy, M. Williams, J. Mbwambo, and G. Kilonzo, "HIV risk behaviours, perceived severity of drug use problems, and prior treatment experience in a sample of young heroin injector s in Dar es Salaam, Tanzania," *African Journal of Drug and Alcohol Studies*, vol. 10, no. 1, pp. 1–9, 2011.

[29] E. S. Maswanya, P. P. Mutalemwa, E. H. Shayo et al., "Drivers of HIV/AIDS epidemics in Tanzania mainland," Dar es Salaam, Tanzania, 2010.

[30] B. Zaba, R. Isingo, A. Wringe, M. Marston, E. Slaymaker, and M. Urassa, "Influence of timing of sexual debut and first marriage on sexual behaviour in later life: Findings from four survey rounds in the Kisesa cohort in northern Tanzania," *Sexually Transmitted Infections*, vol. 85, no. 1, pp. i20–i26, 2009.

[31] S. Geis, L. Maboko, E. Saathoff et al., "Risk factors for HIV-1 infection in a longitudinal, prospective cohort of adults from the mbeya region, Tanzania," *Journal of Acquired Immune Deficiency Syndromes*, vol. 56, no. 5, pp. 453–459, 2011.

[32] M. Quigley, K. Munguti, H. Grosskurth et al., "Sexual behaviour patterns and other risk factors for HIV infection in rural Tanzania: A case-control study," *AIDS*, vol. 11, no. 2, pp. 237–248, 1997.

[33] E. J. Mmbaga, A. Hussain, G. H. Leyna, K. S. Mnyika, N. E. Sam, and K.-I. Klepp, "Prevalence and risk factors for HIV-1 infection in rural Kilimanjaro region of Tanzania: Implications for prevention and treatment," *BMC Public Health*, vol. 7, article no. 58, 2007.

[34] M. P. Mapingure, S. Msuya, N. E. Kurewa et al., "Sexual behaviour does not reflect HIV-1 prevalence differences: A comparison study of Zimbabwe and Tanzania," *Journal of the International AIDS Society*, vol. 13, no. 1, article no. 45, 2010.

[35] A. Buvé, M. Caraël, R. J. Hayes et al., "The multicentre study on factors determining the differential spread of HIV in four african cities: Summary and conclusions," *AIDS*, vol. 15, no. 4, pp. S127–S131, 2001.

[36] L. Sawers and E. Stillwaggon, "Concurrent sexual partnerships do not explain the HIV epidemics in Africa: A systematic review of the evidence," *Journal of the International AIDS Society*, vol. 13, no. 1, article no. 34, 2010.

[37] T. C. Bui, J. E. Nyoni, M. W. Ross, J. Mbwambo, C. M. Markham, and S. A. McCurdy, "Sexual Motivation, Sexual Transactions and Sexual Risk Behaviors in Men who have Sex with Men in Dar es Salaam, Tanzania," *AIDS and Behavior*, vol. 18, no. 12, pp. 2432–2441, 2014.

[38] E. Matiko, A. Khatib, F. Khalid et al., "HIV Prevalence and Risk Behaviors Among People Who Inject drugs in Two Serial Cross-Sectional Respondent-Driven Sampling Surveys, Zanzibar 2007 and 2012," *AIDS and Behavior*, vol. 19, no. 1, pp. 36–45, 2015.

[39] A. X. Tan, S. Kapiga, K. Khoshnood, and R. D. Bruce, "Epidemiology of drug use and HIV-related risk behaviors among people who inject drugs in Mwanza, Tanzania," *PLoS ONE*, vol. 10, no. 12, Article ID e0145578, 2015.

[40] K. Moen, P. Aggleton, M. T. Leshabari, and A.-L. Middelthon, "Same-sex practicing men in Tanzania from 1860 to 2010," *Archives of sexual behavior*, vol. 43, no. 6, pp. 1065–1082, 2014.

[41] R. F. Baggaley, R. G. White, and M.-C. Boily, "HIV transmission risk through anal intercourse: systematic review, meta-analysis and implications for HIV prevention," *International Journal of Epidemiology*, vol. 39, no. 4, pp. 1048–1063, 2010.

[42] P. D. Ghys, C. Jenkins, and E. Pisani, "HIV surveillance among female sex workers," *AIDS*, vol. 15, no. 3, pp. S33–S40, 2001.

[43] UNAIDS, "Global AIDS Update," New York, USA, 2016.

[44] S. R. Galvin and M. S. Cohen, "The role of sexually transmitted diseases in HIV transmission," *Nature Reviews Microbiology*, vol. 2, no. 1, pp. 33–42, 2004.

[45] R. H. Gray, M. J. Wawer, R. Brookmeyer et al., "Probability of HIV-1 transmission per coital act in monogamous, heterosexual, HIV-1-discordant couples in Rakai, Uganda," *The Lancet*, vol. 357, no. 9263, pp. 1149–1153, 2001.

[46] M. S. Cohen, M. McCauley, and T. R. Gamble, "HIV treatment as prevention and HPTN 052," *Current Opinion in HIV and AIDS*, vol. 7, no. 2, pp. 99–105, 2012.

[47] J. Cates W. and G. Dallabetta, "The staying power of sexually transmitted diseases," *Lancet*, vol. 354, no. 9196, p. SIV62, 1999.

[48] Ministry of Health and Social Welfare (MoHSW) [Tanzania Mainland], "National guideline for comprehensive package of HIV interventions for key populations," Dar es Salaam, Tanzania, 2014.

# 4

# Conceptualising the Factors Affecting Retention in Care of Patients on Antiretroviral Treatment in Kabwe District, Zambia, Using the Ecological Framework

**Ferdinand C. Mukumbang, Joyce Chali Mwale, and Brian van Wyk**

*School of Public Health, University of the Western Cape, Cape Town, South Africa*

Correspondence should be addressed to Ferdinand C. Mukumbang; mukumbang@gmail.com

Academic Editor: Robert R. Redfield

*Background.* HIV remains a major public health challenge in Zambia. The roll-out of antiretroviral treatment (ART) has engendered new challenges in retention in care. *Objective.* To conceptualise the factors affecting retention in care of ART patients at three primary healthcare facilities using the ecological framework. *Method.* Qualitative data were collected through in-depth interviews with 45 ART patients and three focus group discussions with 20 healthcare providers from three primary healthcare facilities in Kabwe district, Zambia, and subjected to thematic content analysis. *Results.* Individual level barriers to retention in care included side effects, gaining weight, belief in faith healing, and use of herbal remedies and alcohol. Interpersonal barriers such as stigma and nondisclosure of HIV status were reported. At the institutional level, inadequate space in the clinic, long waiting times, long travel distances, and shortage of third-line drugs presented barriers to retention in care. Food shortages and patient mobility were reported as community barriers to retention in care. *Conclusion.* The ecological framework conceptualises the complex and dynamic factors affecting retention in ART care and highlights the need for multifaceted interventions that combine health education, disease management, and opportunities for income generation in a socially responsive and accountable environment.

## 1. Introduction

HIV/AIDS remains a major public health problem in sub-Saharan Africa, causing the death of millions of adults in their prime, disrupting and impoverishing families and turning millions of children into orphans [1]. At the end of 2016, 1.2 million people were living with HIV in Zambia, of whom a million were adults aged 15–49 years and 540,000 were women [2]. The Zambian Ministry of Health responded to the HIV epidemic by developing policies and treatment guidelines for the testing and treatment of people living with HIV (PLHIV). Consequently, there has been a rapid scale-up of treatment, with 671,066 PLHIV initiated on antiretroviral treatment (ART) at the end of 2014. The rapid scale-up to initiate PLHIV on ART, nevertheless, is accompanied by challenges of suboptimal retention in care and poor medication adherence [3], especially in the context of fragile healthcare systems, which characterises most low- and middle-income countries [4].

Although the number of people receiving ART continues to rise in Africa, it is estimated that approximately three-quarters of adults living with HIV in sub-Saharan Africa have not achieved viral suppression [5]. Many studies have shown that the proportion of patients that remain in care following ART initiation is low and retention in care remains a challenge in many countries with a high burden of HIV/AIDS [6]. A review of 33 patient cohorts taking ART in 13 African countries suggested that only 60% of patients remained in ART programmes after two years, with loss to follow-up (patients with unknown outcomes) accounting for 56% of all attrition [7]. Although we could not obtain actual retention-in-care rates, the Zambia Population-Based HIV Impact Assessment (ZAMPHIA) reported viral load suppression among PLHIV aged 15 to 59 years in Zambia at 59.8%–61.3% and 57.5% among females and males, respectively, by the end of 2016 [8]. These low viral load rates are suggestive of equally low retention-in-care rates.

Nonadherence to ART is identified as the most common reason for treatment failure [9]. Thus, retaining patients on ART is of public health importance as it is directly linked to access to medication and medication adherence [10]. Nonadherence to ART poses major challenges to reducing new HIV infections, addressing health disparities, and improving health outcomes [11]. Retention in care—the ability of PLHIV to adhere to critical aspects of care, such as attending regular follow-up appointments, scheduled laboratory tests, and other monitoring activities as prescribed by the healthcare provider [12]—is, therefore, an important aspect of ART programmes. In this study, retention in care was defined as patients attending their last scheduled follow-up appointment.

Issues related to the retention in care of patients on ART have been previously investigated in many regions in low- to middle-income countries [14] including Zambia. It has been observed that factors influencing retention-in-care behaviours are similar to those that influence adherence to ART [11]. If patients are not retained in care, it becomes a challenge for these patients to receive medications regularly, and thus retention in care is a critical mediator to medication adherence. Stricker and colleagues suggest that "retention in care and adherence to ART are critical elements of HIV care interventions and are closely associated with optimal individual and public health outcomes" [15]. Barriers to retention in care and adherence to medication could lead to increased morbidity and mortality in the patients through suboptimal viral suppression, increased risk of drug resistance, and increased risk of HIV transmission [16]. The spillover effect is a loss of or reduction in individual income, potentially translating to lower economic productivity at the country level and more expenditure of the health system through longer hospital stays and regimen switch to second- and third-line ART drugs [15].

Various models have also been applied to classify the factors affecting retention in ART care and adherence to treatment. For instance, Holtzman and colleagues used Andersen's Behavioural Model to map patient-identified barriers and facilitators to retention in HIV care and antiretroviral therapy adherence [17]. Other studies have classified these factors under various headings such as individual-related factors, medication-related factors, health systems related factors, socioeconomic factors, and sociocultural factors [18]. The goal of conceptualising these factors within a framework is to make sense of the complex and dynamic factors affecting retention in care of patients on ART. Nevertheless, the authors did not find any studies framing these factors on the ecological framework, a public health focus towards understanding the dynamic interrelations among various personal and environmental factors affecting retention in ART care. Therefore, our objective was to conceptualise the factors affecting retention in care of patients receiving ART at three primary health facilities in Kabwe district in Zambia using the ecological framework. Mapping the factors influencing poor retention in ART care using the ecological framework could provide a useful model for understanding and classifying these challenges, an important step towards a comprehensive and preferential solution approach in the context of resource constraints.

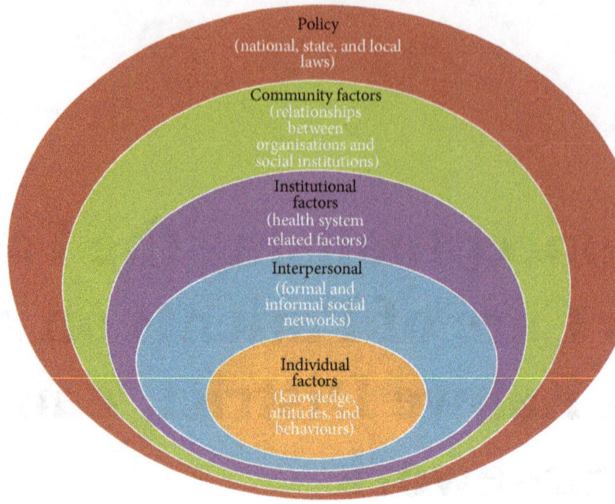


FIGURE 1: The ecological model [13].

*1.1. Conceptual Model.* The study was guided by the ecological framework, a theory-based framework for understanding the multifaceted and interactive effects of personal and environmental factors that determine behaviours. We thought that this model would be useful to understand the interaction of personal, health system, and environmental factors that affect the retention in care of PLHIV on ART in Kabwe district. Figure 1 indicates the different components (levels) that constitute the socioecological model.

The ecological perspective epidemiology emphasises the interaction between, and interdependence of, factors within and across all levels of a health problem. Two important perspectives that guide the ecological perspective are that behaviour affects and is affected by multiple levels of influence and that individual behaviour shapes and is shaped by the social environment.

As illustrated in Figure 1, these levels are (1) intrapersonal or individual factors, (2) interpersonal factors, (3) institutional or organisational factors, (4) community factors, and (5) public policy factors [13]. The ecological framework is based on evidence that no single factor can explain health seeking behaviours or a health related problem and highlights the importance of people's interactions with their physical and sociocultural environments in determining their health behaviours (or perpetuating the health problem). Therefore, the ecological framework recognises multiple levels of factors that influence a person's health behaviours. In this way, the framework considers the interaction between factors at the different levels as being of equal importance. The model assumes that appropriate changes in the social environment will produce changes in individuals and that the support of individuals in the population is essential for implementing environmental changes [13].

## 2. Research Method

*2.1. Setting.* The study was conducted in Kabwe district of the central province of Zambia. Kabwe district is one of the six districts in the central province of Zambia. Kabwe district is approximately 139 km from the capital city Lusaka and covers a surface area of 1,577 km$^2$. According to the Census of Population and Housing of 2010, Kabwe has an estimated population of 210,979 inhabitants with a population density of 128.7 persons per km$^2$. The population consists of 48.8% males and 51.2% females and the average annual rate of population growth is estimated at 1.4% [19]. According to the MoH data of 2014, the district's population has increased to 217,843. Kabwe district is a transit town with huge traffic of people moving through the Great North road to the Copperbelt and northern part of Zambia from Lusaka and vice versa. The district is comprised of multilingual ethnic groups, with Bemba being the most widely spoken local language. Economically, Kabwe district has high (64%) poverty levels due to high unemployment rates brought about by the closure of factories and mines in 1995. Economic activities are mainly informal, though a few people are formally employed.

## 3. Design

A descriptive qualitative study design was used. According to V. Lambert and C. E. Lambert [20], it allows for the "comprehensive summarisation, in everyday terms, of specific events experienced by individuals or groups of individuals." The authors suggest that this research design should be used when a straightforward description of a phenomenon is desired. A description of the different factors allowed us to classify them within the different levels of the ecological model.

*3.1. Sampling.* A sample of 65 participants participated in the study representing two groups: healthcare providers and patients. Using facility ART registers, an electronic smart care system, a pharmacy logbook, and patient locator forms, 45 patients—36 who were on ART at the time of the study and nine who had discontinued treatment (defaulted)—were purposively selected. Fifteen participants were selected from each ART site. Participants who were not able to come to the clinic were contacted and interviewed at their homes with the aid of patient locator forms and the adherence support workers. At each site (clinic), participants were recruited with the help of healthcare professionals. The characteristics of the study participants are displayed in Table 1.

The healthcare providers were also recruited purposively to provide an alternative source of information with regard to the factors influencing retention in care. Table 2 displays the number and distribution of healthcare providers included in the study.

*3.2. Data Collection.* Two data collection methods were employed: individual in-depth interviews with patients using semistructured (open-ended) questions and focus group discussions with health workers. Semistructured interviews (using interview guides) allowed us to explore why patients on ART discontinue their clinic visits. Twenty health workers participated in the focus group discussions. Three focus group discussions were held, one at each site. Nine nurses, five clinical officers, and six adherence workers participated in total.

TABLE 1: Characteristics of ART patients who participated in the study.

| Characteristics | Frequency ($N$ = 45) |
|---|---|
| Sex | |
| Female | 25 |
| Male | 20 |
| Age (in years) | |
| 18–24 | 3 |
| 25–34 | 21 |
| 35–44 | 14 |
| 45 and above | 7 |
| Marital status | |
| Single | 8 |
| Married | 23 |
| Divorced/separated | 4 |
| Widow(er) | 10 |
| Level of education | |
| None | 3 |
| Primary school | 29 |
| Secondary school | 13 |
| Tertiary | 0 |
| Source of livelihood | |
| Formal employment | 2 |
| Self-employed | 32 |
| Unemployed | 7 |
| Dependents | 4 |

TABLE 2: Healthcare workers in three FGDs.

| Category of health workers | Katondo Clinic | Ngungu Clinic | Makululu Clinic | Total |
|---|---|---|---|---|
| Nurses | 4 | 2 | 3 | 9 |
| Clinical officers | 1 | 3 | 1 | 5 |
| Adherence workers | 1 | 2 | 3 | 6 |
| Total | 6 | 7 | 7 | 20 |

The interviews and focus group discussions were conducted in Bemba, the local language, which enabled the participants to clearly understand the questions and express themselves fluently. The interviews and the focus group discussions were audio-recorded with the participants' permission. To ensure anonymity of the study participants, the participants in the focus group discussions were given numbers during the sessions by which to identify them. The recorded sessions (interviews and group discussions) were transcribed verbatim and translated from Bemba to English by the second author who is fluent in both languages. The translations were checked by a research assistant who is also fluent in both languages. Any disparities in the meanings of words or phrases were addressed through the process of reconciliation between the second author and the research assistant.

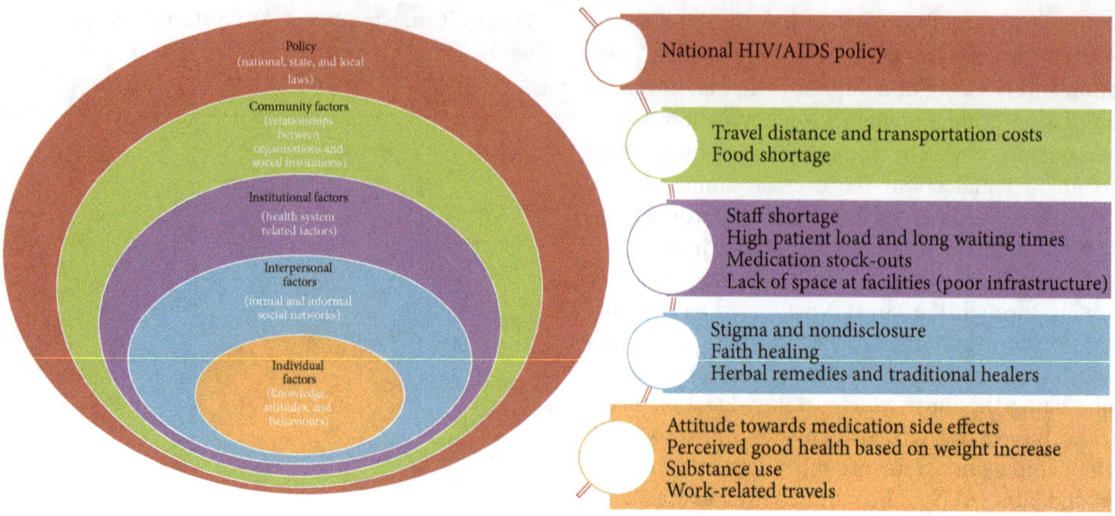


FIGURE 2: Summary of themes identified based on the components of the ecological model.

## 4. Ethical Considerations

Ethics clearance was granted by the University of the Western Cape's Senate Research Committee and the Zambian ERES Converge ethics committee. Permission to conduct the study in Kabwe was obtained from each of the participating health facilities, the Kabwe district Ministry of Health, and the District Health office.

Participation in the study was voluntary. The participants were required to sign a consent form to acknowledge their willingness to participate in the study. While conducting the focus group discussions, we asked the participants to use pseudonames that were provided at the start of each session to preserve the anonymity of the participants.

## 5. Data Analysis

The data analysis was conducted in two steps: first, we coded the data according to a predetermined coding structure based on the ecological model (individual, interpersonal, institutional, and community factors). This step of the analysis was deductive because we were guided by the framework.

Secondly, we grouped related codes to form themes for each of the levels of the ecological model. A thematic data analysis approach was employed [21]. We (1) read the transcription notes several times to become familiar with the data, (2) identified key issues and recurrent themes emanating from the data, (3) coded and organised the data into categories, and (4) interpreted the data by fitting the identified factors within the ecological framework. The data were analysed with the aid of qualitative data analysis software, Atlas.ti version 8.0.

## 6. Rigour and Trustworthiness

Rigour and trustworthiness in qualitative research relate to credibility, dependability, transferability, and conformability of data and findings. The following actions were carried out to enforce rigour and trustworthiness in the study. (1) Triangulation of data collection methods (interviews and focus groups) and information sources (patients who are retained in care, patients who have defaulted, and healthcare workers) with regard to the sources and the findings with other studies improved the trustworthiness of the study. (2) Research team members checked the key points at the end of each interview to verify their understanding with participants. (3) An audit trail of all the documents and decision-making processes during the study was kept to ensure rigour. We followed the consolidated criteria for reporting qualitative research (COREQ) outlined by Long and colleagues [22] to conduct and report this study.

## 7. Results

The study results are presented following the constructs of the ecological model (Figure 2).

*7.1. Individual Factors.* Factors identified at the intrapersonal or individual level relate to personal history and biological factors that influence the retention-in-care behaviours of the patient. Weight increase as a sign of improved health, medication side effects, and alcohol use were patient factors identified to influence retention-in-care behaviours. In addition, trust in faith healing and the use of other herbal remedies were identified as negative influences on retention in care.

*7.1.1. Weight Increase as a Sign of Good Health.* Patients stop taking their medication after they notice an increase in body weight and start to look healthy because of taking their ART. Both the healthcare workers and the patients agreed that some patients stop taking their medication because they were feeling better and physically fit. Healthcare providers and patients reported on issues around improved health and retention in care.

> *Some patients stop taking ARV medications when they notice an increase in weight and look healthy [because of taking medication]. They feel they can do away with the drugs especially when their CD4 count is high. This affects adherence and later impacts on long term retention.* (Healthcare worker)

> *Some patients feel they are healed when they gain weight and start feeling better. There is this patient in my neighbourhood. He stopped taking his ARV medication after feeling well. He said there was no need for him to continue taking the ARV drugs.* (A 37-year-old woman)

*7.1.2. Side Effects.* Both healthcare providers and patients identified medication side effects as contributing to poor retention in care. Side effects reported were nausea, vomiting, dizziness, and breast enlargement in male patients (gynaecomastia). These may affect patients' health service seeking behaviour and may lead to attrition from ART care because, for male patients, developing breasts interfered with their self-esteem.

> *Observations made were that a few patients especially men may stop their ARV medications because of side effects like developing breasts (gynaecomastia). Other patients stop their medications because of nausea, vomiting and dizziness. Such are the patients who discourage the rest of the community to stop ARV drugs.* (Healthcare worker)

> *Yes, they [medication] affected me. I have rashes on my body, and then I stopped the medication. I later felt sick, so I decided to go back to the hospital... I explained it to them [health care workers] and they changed the drugs.* (A 42-year-old woman)

*7.1.3. Alcohol Use.* Excessive beer drinking was reported to affect patient retention in care and subsequently medication adherence. Some patients reported displaying heavy drinking behaviours after registering great improvement in their health. This is what a participant said:

> *It has been now close to one year since I stopped my ARV treatment. I just stopped taking my ARV drugs because of beer drinking. When I got drunk, I used to forget to take my drugs and eventually I stopped my drugs.* (A 32-year-old woman)

*7.2. Work-Related Travels.* According to the participating health workers, patients who travel for work purposes from their hometown tend to miss clinic appointments and default ART and this contributes to nonadherence and poor retention. Two participants mentioned truck drivers who had defaulted treatment for months and then reappeared again for treatment. This is what they had to say:

> *The other reason is I have seen many truck drivers. They tend to travel when given a contract. Then you find for months they will disappear. When they appear and you ask them why they disappeared, they say they went for work.* (Healthcare worker)

> *Some patients miss treatment appointments when they travel to go and work in another town. I can attest to this. My neighbour is always traveling and when he comes back, he mentions not having taken his ARV drugs for a long time.* (Healthcare worker)

*7.3. Interpersonal Factors.* Factors classified under the interpersonal level relate to barriers that emanate as a result of patients sharing and interpersonal relationships with various persons or groups such as family, friends, intimate partners, and peers. Based on the data, the following themes could be identified under stigma and nondisclosure of HIV status.

*7.3.1. Stigma and Nondisclosure of HIV Status.* HIV related stigma was reported as one of the reasons why some patients discontinued ARV treatment or missed treatment dosage. Healthcare providers reported that patients do not want to disclose their HIV status to either their marital partners or other members of their social network for fear of domestic violence, partner abandonment, or rejection by the community. As a result, patients opt to stop attending the clinic for ART services, which affects adherence. A patient also suggested that other patients hide their HIV status to start up and sustain relationships.

> *Couples do not want to disclose their status to each other. You find that the wife is on ARVs without the husband knowing or the husband is on treatment without the wife knowing. Sometimes you find that the husband is taking drugs from the office without the partner being aware.* (Healthcare worker)

> *Some patients hide from their relatives. Some patients who look healthy and want to get married hide and give up on treatment so that their partners do not get suspicious of their HIV status since they may lead to the end of the relationship. I have a sister from my mother's sister. She is now dead. She got married and hides her HIV status from her husband and stopped taking her ARV drugs.* (A 34-year-old woman)

Additionally, healthcare workers confirmed that stigma was still highly prevalent at individual and community levels.

> *Stigma is still very high among the rich and those in business. Some of them send other people to pick their drugs for them. If the health care worker*

> *insists on seeing the patient, they would rather stop taking the ARV drugs for fear of being known. This is why they default and we admit them here when they come very sick and weak.* (Healthcare worker)

*7.3.2. Faith Healing.* Religious beliefs and practices also may lead to patient attrition from ART care. Both patients and healthcare workers agree that some church pastors in their communities who conduct healing prayers sessions persuade patients to discontinue ART because they are healed.

> *Some people go to some pastors who pray for them and tell them to stop taking their ARV drugs that they are healed. I have seen some people who discontinue treatment. One even died after stopping taking these drugs. He was my neighbour.* (A 42-year-old widow)

> *Pastors who preach the gospel of faith healing convince many patients to discontinue ART. They feel healed when they are prayed for. They have faith in these pastors and they would definitely stop taking ARVs. Sometimes when they feel sick, that is when they reveal that I had stopped because I was told to stop because I was healed.* (Healthcare worker)

*7.3.3. Herbal Remedies.* Use of herbal remedies to treat HIV related illnesses was reported by both patients and healthcare providers as a cause for discontinuation from the ART programme. Some patients were being told that herbal remedies could cure HIV and AIDS. This influences the health seeking behaviours of patients, leading to discontinuation of ART. The use of herbal medicines was also reported to have been easily accessed by some patients especially those from rural settings and that people have confidence in traditional healers.

> *My neighbour used to drink these herbal remedies called Moringa from traditional healers because he was told it heals all diseases including HIV and AIDS. Unfortunately, he died.* (A 32-year-old woman)

> *Some patients especially those from rural settings find these traditional medicines easily accessible and they have more confidence in tradition healers. Whatever they say is right. That component is also affecting patients' adherence to treatment and retention in care.* (Healthcare worker)

*7.4. Institutional Related Factors.* Institutional related factors speak to the health system factors and these factors relate to the way health services are organised and delivered and relates to access to the facility and to medication, the overall environment of the facility, the patient–provider relationship, and support services that are incorporated into care [8]. The following health system factors were identified: staff shortage, medication stock-out, congested facilities, long waiting times, and travel distance and cost of transportation.

*7.4.1. Staff Shortage.* Healthcare providers and patients identified staff shortage as a factor influencing retention in care of patients on ART. This is because staff shortages lead to long queues at the clinic waiting area and, consequently, long waiting times. Because of this, patients get frustrated and tired of waiting to be seen.

> *There are few health workers to attend to patients at ART centres. In most instances only one clinical officer or one nurse on full ART day working with two adherence support workers against a crowd of patients. Some patients get tired of waiting and go back home without being seen.* (A 36-year-old woman)

> *There is only one person remaining at ART clinic to see patients. This clinical officer is overwhelmed with work and two days a week is too much for this person. Therefore, there are many compromises. If you saw today the queue that was there. He had to review the in-patients first and then outpatients. It's too much.* (Healthcare worker)

It was also reported that several patients discontinue treatment because of long waiting times at the ART clinics. Participants complained about long waiting times, which made them more likely to stop coming to the clinic to collect their drugs. Patients reported long waiting time of four to six hours at the clinics before receiving care services.

> *The health workers are few. Sometimes there can be only one. The rest could be these volunteers. That is the reason why we even spend more time here.* (A 35-year-old widow)

> *We take a long time here. Sometimes I spend about 4 hours and sometimes 5 hours depending on the time, they start the clinic. This is frustrating. You can even stop coming to this clinic to collect ARV drugs.* (A 37-year-old widow)

The healthcare providers corroborated that high patient load at ART centres leads to long waiting times and in some instances contributes to high defaulter rates.

> *Actually, we have many patients at these clinics in relation to the health care workers. When we look at the trained adherence support counsellors they are not even enough to carter for all the patients.* (Healthcare worker)

*7.4.2. Stock-Out of Antiretroviral Medication.* Healthcare workers and patients reported that ART clinics sometimes ran low on the ARV stocks, which affects the supply of medication received by the patients. Some participants reported receiving a one-month supply of ARV drugs when a three-month supply had been prescribed, while other participants reported frequent visits to the ART centres to be tiring especially when one does not have transport money. One participant reported a stock-out of third-line drugs, which are mostly found at referral hospitals, and patients had to travel to access treatment.

> *If they say there is a shortage of ARV drugs, they write medication for three months but they will give you for one month then tell you to come and collect for remaining months. When you come, you just go straight to the pharmacy. However, this sometimes makes you tired especially where you have transport money.* (A 28-year-old man)

> *We had a stock out sometime last year but all of this year we never had a stock out. We had many challenges for third line ARV drugs. We have some patients who are on third line treatment. Those on the third line are not accessing their drugs here despite being under this clinic. Them they go to Lusaka to access treatment. Because of this, they may not have transport to go to Lusaka for drugs. For example, we had to contribute to transport for one to go to Lusaka.* (Healthcare worker)

*7.4.3. Inadequate Space for ART Clinic.* Healthcare providers reported limited space within the ART clinic as being a challenge towards the implementation of ART. This can have an impact on patient adherence and long-term retention. Participants reported using any free room or an empty office, which do not provide a waiting area for patients. In this case, confidentiality (privacy) during ART clinic is compromised because of overcrowding of patients.

> *We do not have enough space at this clinic for ART patients. Instead, we use any room not in operation during the ART day, the office either for the sister in charge or the Male circumcision room. You can just see how this passage is congested. Because of this, even space for individual counselling has become a challenge as it leads to loss of patients in ART programme because confidentiality is compromised.* (Healthcare worker)

> *Some patients tend to shun ART services where there is no confidentiality. We have many patients who are lost to follow up because of the same confidentiality due to lack of space for ART clinic.* (Healthcare worker)

*7.5. Community Related Factors.* The community, as relates to the ecological model, has three aspects: (1) mediating structures or face-to face primary groups, (2) relationships among organisations and groups within a defined area, and (3) a population with political entities [13]. Factors operative at these different levels of the community were considered. These factors include travel distance and cost of transportation, food shortage, and work-related mobility

*7.5.1. Travel Distance and Cost of Transportation.* Although ART sites do not charge for HIV related services, travel distance and additional costs incurred traveling to ART centres may contribute to nonretention in the care of patients on ART programme more so for patients who cannot afford it. While some participants reported travel distance to ART centres as a barrier to accessing treatment, others also mentioned lack of money to pay for transport:

> *Distance from home to the clinic is very long. I take one hour walking to this clinic when I am fast. I can even take an hour and 30 minutes if am not fast. Sometimes, if am not feeling well, I cannot walk this distance and if I do not have someone to come and collect the drugs for me, I miss the appointment date and come later when I feel better.* (A 42-year-old widow)

> *Some patients who stay from distant places struggle to come to the clinic because of transport costs. Sometimes they would even resist to starting treatment or when they start they will pretend they will come back to the clinic because of distance.* (Healthcare worker)

> *The other reason is about distance. Some places become impassable during the rainy season and it is not easy for them to access ARVs. You find in some areas bridges are swept away and this will cause some patients to default treatment. So, they can't find their way to the clinic.* (Healthcare worker)

*7.5.2. Food Shortage.* Food insecurity at the household level may cause patients on ART to stop their medication. Both healthcare providers and patients reported a shortage of food in the household as a reason to default treatment, which may influence adherence and long-term retention.

> *People who come from the poor settings where they have a shortage of food believe that they need to eat before they take ARV drugs. They will even tell you that I stopped because there was no one to buy food for me.* (Healthcare worker)

> *Some patients stop treatment because they do not have food in their households. My neighbour stopped taking her ARV drugs because of a shortage of food. She was afraid to take the ARV drugs on an empty stomach.* (A 25-year-old woman)

## 8. Policy Factors

Based on the ecological model, aspects of policy are very important when examining the factors affecting the implementation of the public health intervention or programme. Nevertheless, we did not explore factors at this level with the study participants because we did not consider them knowledgeable enough to respond to the questions relating to the HIV/AIDS policy environment in the Kabwe region and the national HIV programme.

## 9. Discussion

Retention in care and adherence to medication behaviours have been previously described as complex and dynamic [3, 11]. The ecological model provides an explanatory framework to understand these factors that influence retention in care and adherence, without dispelling the complex nature of these behaviours.

Individual-related factors included side effects to ARV drugs, weight increase, and feeling better as a sign of good health. The findings of this study are consistent with the findings of other studies conducted in sub-Saharan Africa and elsewhere [23, 24]. Discontinuation of ART due to gynaecomastia and perception of good health could be indicative that patients are not properly educated on the importance of adherence to their medication even if they experience certain side effects or feel better. Roura et al. [23] argue that individuals' behaviour with regard to remaining in care is influenced by factors in the immediate environment such as support (or lack thereof) from significant others, work schedule, and disclosure. Patients may fail to adhere to medication in spite of their knowledge of the importance of adhering because their personal experience may be more persuasive than medical information.

Interpersonal factors influence the health of people and communities. They affect patient lifestyle by causing stress, social isolation, and fear of rejection [25]. When a patient's emotions, opinions, or behaviours are affected by others, adherence to medication and long-term retention are affected [26]. The social factors may include experiences, interpersonal relationships with marital partners, and family members that in turn affect individual health seeking behaviour and actions [25–27]. Social factors identified include stigma, use of traditional healers with herbal remedies, faith healing, and alcohol use and nondisclosure of HIV status. The results of this study are similar to those identified in qualitative studies in developing countries. For instance, a study conducted in Zambia by Musheke et al. [28] reported "feeling better," use of herbal remedies, and faith healing as factors contributing to poor retention. A similar study conducted in Uganda by Mugisha et al. [24] also reported stigma and traditional healers as a considerable impediment to ART access, adherence, and long-term retention in care, which is at the individual, household, and community levels. The literature reveals that people living with HIV/AIDS fear to lose their social and emotional support by disclosing their HIV status to their spouses, social network, or other family members and fear of marriage breakdown in case of married people. Consequently, when social support is threatened by involuntary disclosure of HIV status, individuals abandon treatment [24].

Issues of long waiting times at health facilities due to high patient loads, staff shortages, and shortages of third-line ARV drugs were identified as health systems related factors affecting retention in care. Similar findings from the previous studies reported long waiting hours at health facilities due to high patient loads which affected patient access to treatment. Long waiting hours is among the key drivers of attrition for patients on ART [22, 29, 30]. It is recommended that adopting extended clinic hours to provide care after working hours or weekend could address the issue of clinic congestion especially for those patients that are employed [30]. Weekend clinics have been found to reduce clinic congestion and help retain patients in care.

Travel distance to ART health facilities and transport cost were reported to contribute to nonretention of patients on ART. This is mostly because ART centres are sparsely distributed within Kabwe district. In some instances, healthcare workers reported having donated transport fare to enable patients to access third-line treatment in Lusaka, approximately 139 km away from Kabwe. This study showed that distance to ART clinic is a barrier to both ARV adherence and access to care, which may affect long-term retention in care for patients in the ART programme. Similar studies from Uganda and Malawi also found the distance to ART centres as a barrier to patient retention [14, 24, 31].

The economic factors such as employment status, shortage of ARV drugs, and lack of food may influence patient retention in care. The living conditions and monitoring survey of 2006–2010 confirmed that 64% of Zambia's population falls below the national poverty line of US$1.08 per day and 90% of the labour force is in informal sector employment [19]. Even where people living with HIV are encouraged to continue accessing treatment, their health seeking behaviours are undermined by their fragile livelihoods. Concerns about the widespread poverty and food insecurity at the household level and their effect on long-term retention on ART have been previously identified [32, 33].

Stock-out of drugs was also reported by healthcare workers. Weak procurement and supply management systems in low-income countries which result in frequent shortages of ARV drugs and other essential commodities have been reported previously [1]. Similarly, many health systems are finding it difficult to ensure that there is an adequate and consistent supply of drugs and other supplies especially with the increasing number of patients initiating treatment [34].

Although healthcare workers during the focus group discussion reported intensive counselling of patients before and after ART initiation, the patients' knowledge and beliefs related to HIV and ART clearly showed that the information provided does not successfully dispel and correct the myths and misconceptions that some of the patients have. Lack of education and poor knowledge about ART and the HIV/AIDS can also lead to an inadequate understanding of the effectiveness of medications resulting in reduced adherence to treatment and poor retention of patients in care [35].

The study found factors that influence patient retention in care, which is diverse in nature and could be classified within the various spheres (levels) of the ecological model, namely, intrapersonal or individual factors, interpersonal factors, institutional or organisational factors, and community factors. This complex nature of the factors influencing retention in ART care makes it difficult to identify which of these factors is more important; even if it was possible to classify them in order of importance, the classification would have to be context-specific, thus increasing the complex nature of retention in care and adherence to medication behaviours. The study also demonstrates how individuals adjust their behaviour to their immediate social environment, which also affects their health seeking behaviour. According to Roura et al. [23], the processes through which other people's behaviours, advice, and beliefs determine health behaviour emerge as a main pathway for individual decision-making and reflect localised norms and levels of support within the individual's social networks. Roura et al. [23] also argued that the strength of social influence could severely undermine the capacity to follow through an intention to remain on treatment leading to dropping out from the treatment programme.

Following that, the ecological framework recognises multiple levels of factors that influence a person's health behaviours and the concept of reciprocal causation; addressing the challenges at one level of the framework could have a ripple effect on another area. For instance, if a patient receives effective intensive counselling and medication initiation education, he/she might refrain from using herbal treatment and other faith-based treatment options and focus on maintaining good adherence to ART. The motivation received from the counselling and educational sessions may encourage them to disclose their HIV status to their loved ones, which in turn enhances adherence based on received social support [18]. At the same time, the perceived social support also dispels perceived stigma, which enforces medication adherence. This explanation indicates a move between the intrapersonal and the interpersonal spheres of the ecological model.

In practice, addressing the community level requires taking into consideration institutional and public policy factors, as well as social networks and norms [36]. For instance, if the government of Zambia decides to open more ART service centres or implement community-based ART models to address the challenges related to long distances to the ART centres, they would have to consider the implications in terms of resources availability. In recent times, the use of community health workers to drive such initiatives as one strategy to address the growing shortage of health workers has been highlighted by various authors [37]. The application of this strategy would require the application of the policies that guide the use of community health workers. In the same way, the implementation of interventions like the community-based models would require buy-in and full participation from the community members for the intervention to work [38].

An ecological perspective shows the advantages of multilevel interventions that combine behavioural and environmental components. This resonates with the recent wave of community-based differentiated care models that are recommended for the improved management of PLHIV. Differentiated care models usually adopt a multifaceted approach towards enhancing patients' retention-in-care behaviours by embedding various strategies, including providing minimal clinical screening, quick ARV refills, health education, and adherence support within a single model [39]. Most of these models are recommended to take place in an environment that is easily accessible to the patients such as a local church, town hall, or NGO for easy medication pick-up (institutional or organisational factors). In addition to this, patients have the chance to receive continued counselling and education on the importance of remaining in care and adhering to medication (intrapersonal or personal). Group-based differentiated care models—having patients receive their care together to increase peer support among them and create an enabling treatment and care environment (intrapersonal)—could also improve their retention in care and medication behaviours. In addition, by separating the drug delivery and clinical care and reducing the intensity of the services, the care process is simplified for the providers and made much user-friendly (institutional or organisational factors). The implementation of such interventions is governed by policies at the provincial and national levels.

## 10. Limitations of the Study

While our study was focused on the factors affecting retention in ART care, we could only reach a few defaulters to participate in the study. Most of the patient participants were those currently retained in care. Limitations to the study were related to the possibility of the participants giving false responses due to the sensitive nature of the study. To reduce the chances of this occurring, the participants were reassured of confidentiality. The interviews were conducted in the Bemba local dialect and then translated to English. Translation from one language to another always introduces a chance for some meanings to be lost in the translation process. Losing meaning in translation was minimised through the process of data cleaning conducted by the first author who is fluent in both languages.

While adopting the ecological model to frame the findings of this study, we were aware of some of its limitations. For instance, it is criticised for falsely separating the social, economic, political, and cultural levels of interactions that might influence the other levels.

## 11. Recommendations

The findings of this study highlight the importance of strong community follow-up and patient support systems for all patients in the ART programme in Kabwe district [40]. There is a need to engage a wider range of partners such as community-based and faith-based organisations, local communities, and in particular people living with HIV to improve patient tracking and follow-up and, hence, retain them in care. To resolve the challenges related to the distance to the health facility and high transport cost, patients should be continually encouraged to access treatment at their nearest treatment centre.

## 12. Conclusions

The average retention rate in Kabwe district is about 65%; thus, 35% were considered to be lost to follow-up mainly due to social, economic, and structural factors. The findings of this study suggest that low retention rates are a result of complex and multidimensional factors. For easy identification and description, we have identified them following the ecological framework. These factors identified to influence retention of patients in ART programmes in Kabwe district are complex and highlight the need for multifaceted interventions that combine health education, disease management (by patient and health services), and opportunities for income generation in a socially responsive and accountable environment.

## Conflicts of Interest

The authors declare that there are no conflicts of interest regarding the publication of this manuscript.

## References


[1] World Health Organization. Retention in hiv programmes, Defining the challenges and identifying solutions, World Health Organization, 2011.

[2] Avert, Hiv and AIDS in Zambia, 2017, https://www.avert.org/professionals/hiv-around-world/sub-saharan-africa/zambiain.

[3] F. C. Mukumbang, S. Van Belle, B. Marchal, and B. Van Wyk, "Realist evaluation of the antiretroviral treatment adherence club programme in selected primary healthcare facilities in the metropolitan area of Western Cape Province, South Africa: A study protocol," *BMJ Open*, vol. 6, no. 4, Article ID 009977, 2016.

[4] A. Mills, "Health Care Systems in Low- and Middle-Income Countries," *The New England Journal of Medicine*, vol. 370, no. 6, pp. 552–557, 2014.

[5] Unaids, Treatment 2015. Unaids, 2014, http://files.unaids.org/en/media/unaids/contentassets/documents/unaidspublication/2013/JC2484_treatment-2015_en.pdf.

[6] R. Bucciardini, V. Fragola, T. Abegaz et al., "Retention in care of adult HIV patients initiating antiretroviral therapy in Tigray, Ethiopia: A prospective observational cohort study," *PLoS ONE*, vol. 10, no. 9, Article ID e0136117, 2015.

[7] M. P. Fox and S. Rosen, "Patient retention in antiretroviral therapy programs up to three years on treatment in sub-Saharan Africa, 2007-2009: Systematic review," *Tropical Medicine & International Health*, vol. 15, no. 1, pp. 1–15, 2010.

[8] Zamphia, Zambia Population-Based HIV Impact Assessment, 2016, http://phia.icap.columbia.edu/wp-content/uploads/2016/09/ZAMBIA-Factsheet.FIN_.pdf.

[9] T. Heestermans, J. L. Browne, S. C. Aitken, S. C. Vervoort, and K. Klipstein-Grobusch, "Determinants of adherence to antiretroviral therapy among HIV-positive adults in sub-Saharan Africa: a systematic review," *BMJ Global Health*, vol. 1, no. 4, p. e000125, 2016.

[10] E. Mûnene and B. Ekman, "Association between patient engagement in HIV care and antiretroviral therapy medication adherence: Cross-sectional evidence from a regional HIV care center in Kenya," *AIDS Care Psychological and Socio-medical Aspects of AIDS/HIV*, vol. 27, no. 3, pp. 378–386, 2015.

[11] I. N. Azia, F. C. Mukumbang, and B. Van Wyk, "Barriers to adherence to antiretroviral treatment in a regional hospital in Vredenburg, Western Cape, South Africa," *Southern African Journal of HIV Medicine*, vol. 17, no. 1, 2016.

[12] A. Patel, L. Hirschhorn, A. Fullem, B. Ojikutu, and R. Oser, "Adult adherence to treatment and retention in care," Arlington, VA: USAID — AIDSTAR-ONE PROJECT, Task Order 1, 2010, http://pdf.usaid.gov/pdf_docs/PNADX307.pdf.

[13] K. R. McLeroy, D. Bibeau, A. Steckler, and K. Glanz, "An ecological perspective on health promotion programs," *Health Education Journal*, vol. 15, no. 4, pp. 351–377, 1988.

[14] E. H. Geng, D. Nash, A. Kambugu et al., "Retention in care among HIV-infected patients in resource-limited settings: emerging insights and new directions," *Current HIV/AIDS Reports*, vol. 7, no. 4, pp. 234–244, 2010.

[15] S. M. Stricker, K. A. Fox, R. Baggaley et al., "Retention in Care and Adherence to ART are Critical Elements of HIV Care Interventions," *AIDS and Behavior*, vol. 18, pp. 465–475, 2014.

[16] K. L. Schaecher, "The importance of treatment adherence in HIV," *The American Journal of Managed Care*, vol. 19, pp. s231–s237, 2013, http://www.ncbi.nlm.nih.gov/pubmed/24495293.

[17] C. W. Holtzman, J. A. Shea, K. Glanz et al., "Mapping patient-identified barriers and facilitators to retention in HIV care and antiretroviral therapy adherence to Andersen's Behavioral Model," *AIDS Care Psychological and Socio-medical Aspects of AIDS/HIV*, vol. 27, no. 7, pp. 817–828, 2015.

[18] F. C. Mukumbang, S. Van Belle, B. Marchal, and B. van Wyk, "Exploring 'generative mechanisms' of the antiretroviral adherence club intervention using the realist approach: a scoping review of research-based antiretroviral treatment adherence theories," *BMC Public Health*, vol. 17, no. 1, 2017.

[19] LCMS, Living Conditions Monitoring Survey Report 2006 & 2010. Cent. Stat. Off. - Repub. Zambia, 2010, http://catalog.ihsn.org/index.php/catalog/2597.

[20] V. Lambert and C. E. Lambert, "Qualitative descriptive research: an acceptable design," *Pacific Rim International Journal of Nursing Research*, vol. 16, pp. 255-256, 2013, http://antispam.kmutt.ac.th/index.php/PRIJNR/article/download/5805/5064.

[21] M. Miles and M. Huberman, Qualitative data analysis. Second Edi. California: Sage Publications, Inc., 1994.

[22] L. Long, A. Brennan, MP. Fox, B. Ndibongo, I. Jaffray, and I. Sanne, "Review Provision of antiretroviral therapy in South Africa?: the nuts and bolts," *Journal of the International AIDS Society*, pp. 10-10, 2012.

[23] M. Roura, J. Busza, A. Wringe, D. Mbata, M. Urassa, and B. Zaba, "Barriers to sustaining antiretroviral treatment in Kisesa, Tanzania: a follow-up study to understand attrition from the antiretroviral program," *AIDS Patient Care and STDs*, vol. 23, no. 3, pp. 203–210, 2009.

[24] K. Mugisha, A. Ocero, E. Semafumu et al., Retention of HIV Positive Persons in Antiretroviral Therapy Programs in Post-Conflict Northern Uganda-Baseline Survey of 17 Health Units, pp. 1–163, 2009, http://numat.jsi.com/Resources/Docs/NUMATStudyonRetentionofHIVPositivePersonsinARTcare.pdf.

[25] S. Dewing, C. Mathews, M. Lurie, A. Kagee, T. Padayachee, and C. Lombard, "Predictors of poor adherence among people on antiretroviral treatment in Cape Town, South Africa: A case-control study," *AIDS Care Psychological and Socio-medical Aspects of AIDS/HIV*, vol. 27, no. 3, pp. 342–349, 2015.

[26] M. R. DiMatteo, "Social support and patient adherence to medical treatment: a meta-analysis," *Health Psychology*, vol. 23, no. 2, pp. 207–218, 2004.

[27] A. Adefolalu and Z. Nkosi, "The complex nature of adherence in the management of HIV/AIDS as a chronic medical condition," *Diseases*, vol. 1, no. 1, pp. 18–35, 2013.

[28] M. Musheke, V. Bond, and S. Merten, "Erratum: Individual and contextual factors influencing patient attrition from antiretroviral therapy care in an urban community of Lusaka, Zambia (Journal of the International AIDS Society, SUPPL. 1,

DOI: 10.7448/IAS.15.3.17366)," *Journal of the International AIDS Society*, vol. 16, Article ID 18590, 2013.

[29] S. T. Alamo, G. J. Wagner, J. Ouma et al., "Strategies for optimizing clinic efficiency in a community-based antiretroviral treatment programme in Uganda," *AIDS and Behavior*, vol. 17, no. 1, pp. 274–283, 2013.

[30] C. M. Miller, M. Ketlhapile, H. Rybasack-Smith, and S. Rosen, "Why are antiretroviral treatment patients lost to follow-up? A qualitative study from South Africa," *Tropical Medicine & International Health*, vol. 15, no. 1, pp. 48–54, 2010.

[31] D. M. Tuller, D. R. Bangsberg, J. Senkungu, N. C. Ware, N. Emenyonu, and S. D. Weiser, "Transportation costs impede sustained adherence and access to HAART in a clinic population in Southwestern Uganda: a qualitative study," *AIDS and Behavior*, vol. 14, no. 4, pp. 778–784, 2010.

[32] S. Young, A. C. Wheeler, S. I. McCoy, and S. D. Weiser, "A Review of the Role of Food Insecurity in Adherence to Care and Treatment Among Adult and Pediatric Populations Living with HIV and AIDS," *AIDS and Behavior*, vol. 18, pp. 505–515, 2014.

[33] A. W. Singer, S. D. Weiser, and S. I. McCoy, "Does Food Insecurity Undermine Adherence to Antiretroviral Therapy? A Systematic Review," *AIDS and Behavior*, vol. 19, no. 8, pp. 1510–1526, 2015.

[34] World Health Organization, UNAIDS U. Towards universal access:Scaling up priority HIV/AIDS interventions in the health sector, 2010, http://www.who.int/hiv/mediacentre/universal_access_progress_report_en.pdf.

[35] E. Wekesa, ART adherence in resource poor settings in sub-Saharan Africa: a multi-disciplinary review. 2008, http://uaps2007.princeton.edu/papers/70123.

[36] U.S. Department, of Health and, human services. Theory at a Glance A Guide For Health Promotion Practice (Second Edition), http://www.aub.edu.lb/fhs/heru/Documents/heru/resources/pdf/TheoryataGlance.pdf.

[37] U. Lehmann and D. Sanders, *Community Health Workers: What do we know about them?*, 2007, http://www.who.int/hrh/documents/community_health_workers.pdf.

[38] L. Baatiema, M. Skovdal, S. Rifkin, and C. Campbell, "Assessing participation in a community-based health planning and services programme in Ghana," *BMC Health Services Research*, vol. 13, no. 1, article 233, 2013.

[39] F. C. Mukumbang, S. Van Belle, B. Marchal, and B. van Wyk, "An exploration of group-based HIV/AIDS treatment and care models in Sub-Saharan Africa using a realist evaluation (Intervention-Context-Actor-Mechanism-Outcome) heuristic tool: a systematic review," *Implementation Science*, vol. 12, no. 107, 2017.

[40] J. C. Mwale, *Factors affecting retention in care of patients on antiretroviral treatment in the kabwe district, Zambia. Master's minithesis [Master's, thesis]*, 2016, http://etd.uwc.ac.za/xmlui/handle/11394/5251.

# 5

# Nasal Nitric Oxide Levels in HIV Infection: A Cross-Sectional Study

**Cecilia T. Costiniuk**[1], **Vikram Mehraj**,[1] **Jean-Pierre Routy**[1], **Christina de Castro**,[1] **Natale Wasef**,[2] **Mohammad-Ali Jenabian**,[3] **Syim Salahuddin**,[1] **Bertrand Lebouché**,[1] **Joseph Cox**,[1] **Jason Szabo**,[1] **Marina Klein**,[1] **Larry Lands**,[4] **and Adam J. Shapiro**[4]

[1]*Chronic Viral Illnesses Service and Research Institute, McGill University Health Centre (MUHC), Montreal, QC, Canada*
[2]*Department of Medicine, National University of Ireland, Galway, Ireland*
[3]*Department of Biological Sciences and BioMed Research Centre, Université du Québec à Montréal (UQAM), Montreal, QC, Canada*
[4]*Division of Pediatric Respiratory Medicine, McGill University Health Center Research Institute, Montreal, QC, Canada*

Correspondence should be addressed to Cecilia T. Costiniuk; cecilia.costiniuk@mcgill.ca

Academic Editor: Patrice K. Nicholas

*Introduction.* Low levels of nasal NO have been associated with increased propensity to rhinosinusitis and respiratory tract infections. Our objective was to describe nasal NO levels in HIV-infected individuals versus healthy controls and determine possible risk factors for reduced nasal NO levels. *Materials and Methods.* HIV-infected individuals and healthy controls were recruited. Participants underwent nasal NO testing by standardized methods using a CLD88 chemiluminescence analyzer and completed the Sinonasal Outcome Test-20 (SNOT-20) on symptoms of rhinosinusitis. *Results.* Participants included 41 HIV-infected individuals with suppressed VL on antiretroviral therapy (ART group), 5 HIV-infected individuals with detectable VL off ART (viremic group), and 12 healthy controls (HC group). Mean nasal NO level was 253 (±77) nL/min in the ART group, 213 (±48) nL/min in the viremic group, and 289 (±68) nL/min in the HC group ($p = 0.133$; ANOVA). There was no correlation between nasal NO level and VL in viremic individuals ($r = -0.200$; $p = 0.747$). Differences were observed in mean total points on the SNOT-20 which were 19 (±16)/100, 18 (±26)/100, and 4 (±4)/100 in the ART, viremic, and HC groups, respectively ($p = 0.013$; ANOVA). *Conclusion.* Healthy individuals, HIV patients on ART, and viremic individuals off ART display similar nasal NO levels. However, rhinosinusitis symptoms remain prominent despite ART-treatment.

## 1. Background

Although antiretroviral therapy (ART) reduces one's risk for various infections, rhinosinusitis remains one of the most common complications of HIV infection and is experienced by up to 68% of patients during their infection [1]. Induced by infectious stimuli, nasal nitric oxide (NO) is an important innate defense against various respiratory pathogens, and low NO levels have been associated with increased propensity to rhinosinusitis and other respiratory tract infections [2]. In a single study to explore nasal NO levels in HIV-infected individuals, performed by Palm and colleagues during the early ART era, individuals with HIV had significantly reduced levels of nasal NO [3]. Since the study by Palm and colleagues during the early ART era, no subsequent studies have examined nasal NO levels in individuals receiving long-term ART. Our objective was to describe nasal NO levels in HIV-infected individuals on modern, effective ART relative to levels observed in HIV-infected individuals not on ART and healthy controls. A secondary objective was to determine possible patient characteristics for reduced nasal NO levels in HIV-infected individuals.

## 2. Materials and Methods

Following the ethical approval by the McGill University Health Centre (MUHC) Research Ethics Board, 3 groups of participants were recruited. The ART group consisted of HIV-infected adults with a suppressed viral load for ≥1 year on ART, the viremic group consisted of HIV-infected individuals not taking ART with detectable VL, and the healthy control (HC) group was comprised of age- and sex-matched HIV-uninfected controls. HIV-infected individuals were recruited from the Chronic Viral Illness Service of the McGill University Health Centre. The exclusion criteria included acute respiratory or viral illness within two weeks of NO testing, chronic pulmonary disease, or current use of nasal/inhaled steroids or nasal decongestants. The participants were in the clinic 2 hours prior to NO testing, during which time there was no exercise, nor any food or drink consumption.

Individuals completed the Sinonasal Outcome Test-20 (SNOT-20) questionnaire, a widely used and validated quality-of-life instrument that assesses the clinical impact of chronic rhinosinusitis [4]. The clinical and laboratory parameters on HIV infection within three months of enrollment were collected from medical records. Nasal NO testing was performed by standardized methods using a CLD88 chemiluminescence analyzer (EcoPhysics, AG, Duernten, Switzerland) [5–7]. While seated with a plastic catheter and soft nasal sponge placed securely into one nostril, patients blew into a cardboard resistor in order to close their velum and prevent dilution of nasal gas (containing much higher NO levels) with gas from lower airways. Expiratory maneuvers lasted at least 10 seconds, producing an initial washout phase followed by a NO concentration plateau phase, signifying steady state NO sampling from the nasal cavity. The same procedure was done for the contralateral nostril. For each nostril, the mean of 2 separate plateau measurements were calculated, followed by the mean for both nostrils together to provide the final result [5, 6]. Nasal NO values are expressed in nanolitres/minute (nL/min), which reflects the product of the nasal NO concentration in parts per billion and the flow rate in the sampling catheter of 0.33 L/min. All NO measurements were performed with ambient NO levels <50 ppb. Descriptive and inferential analyses were performed using SPSS 23.0 and graphs were created using GraphPad Prism 7.0. Comparisons were tested at 5% level of significance using independent sample $t$-test, $\chi^2$ test, Fisher's exact test, and one-way analysis of variance (ANOVA) with LSD post hoc test where appropriate. Correlations were measured using Spearman's rank correlation coefficient. Multivariate linear regression analysis was conducted to adjust for the effect of age, gender, body mass index (BMI), eosinophil count, and time of NO measurement on nasal NO levels.

## 3. Results

A total of fifty-eight (58) individuals participated, including 41 (71%) individuals with undetectable VL and 5 (9%) viremic individuals off ART. In addition, 12 (21%) healthy, HIV-uninfected volunteers also participated in the study. The majority (76%) of participants were tested between 11 am and 5 pm, when nasal NO values are in steady state and unaffected by normal circadian changes in nasal NO [8].

The mean age of participants was 47 ± 10 years old and 62% were males. The distribution of age and sex was statistically similar across the three groups ($p > 0.05$). None of the participants had previously undergone nasal operations or sinus procedures, and none had any known history of nasal polyps. Participant characteristics are outlined in Table 1. A significantly larger proportion of individuals (42%) with HIV infection on ART were smokers compared to HIV-infected individuals off ART (20%), while none of the healthy controls were smokers ($p = 0.012$, Fisher's exact test). Furthermore, none of the healthy controls nor viremic HIV-infected individuals off ART reported marijuana use, whereby significant proportions of HIV-infected participants on ART reported marijuana use (37%) ($p = 0.008$, Fisher's exact test).

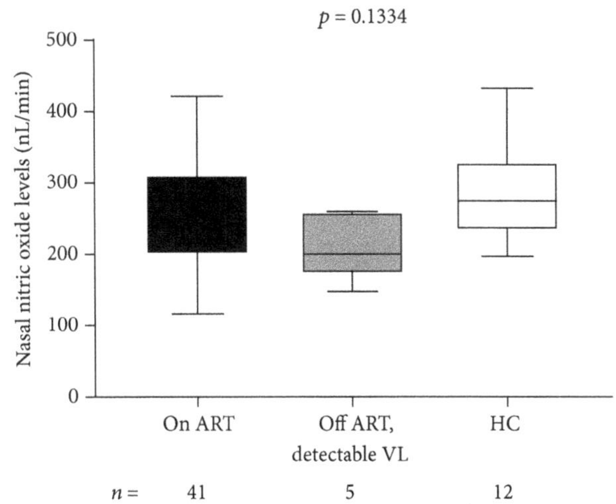


FIGURE 1: *Nasal NO levels across the 3 groups of participants.* Mean nasal NO levels in HIV-infected individuals with suppressed viral load on ART (black bar), HIV-infected individuals with detectable viral loads (VLs) off antiretroviral therapy (ART) (grey bar), and healthy controls (HC, white bar). The differences of mean nasal NO levels among groups did not reach statistical significance.

Figure 1 depicts mean nasal NO levels between the 3 groups. Healthy controls had the highest mean nasal NO levels (289 ± 68 nL/min), followed by HIV-infected ART-treated patients (253 ± 77 nL/min) and HIV-infected viremic individuals not on ART (213 ± 48 nL/min). However, the overall differences of mean nasal NO levels among the groups did not reach statistical significance (ANOVA, $p = 0.133$) despite a trend towards decreased nasal NO levels in viremic individuals off ART. In post hoc analysis, decreased nasal NO levels in viremic individuals off ART compared to healthy controls were nearly significant ($p = 0.057$). However, multivariate analysis confirmed no difference of nasal NO levels in untreated versus ART-treated HIV-infected persons adjusting for clinical factors such as age, sex, time of NO measurement, BMI, and absolute eosinophil count. The multivariate analysis could not include healthy controls owing to missing information in several variables such as body mass index and absolute eosinophil count.

We did not find any associations between nasal NO levels and age, current CD4 counts, CD4/CD8 ratio, CD4 nadir, duration of HIV seropositivity, smoking status, ART regimen, or SNOT-20 score (all $p > 0.05$). Similar correlation analyses

TABLE 1: Characteristics of study participants.

| *Characteristics or outcome* | HIV+ with suppressed VL on ART (*n* = 41) | HIV+ with detectable VL off ART (*n* = 5) | Healthy controls (*n* = 12) | *p* |
|---|---|---|---|---|
| Age, years [mean (std)][#] | 48 (10) | 45 (9) | 43 (12) | 0.327 |
| Male sex [*n* (%)][$] | 28 (68%) | 3 (60%) | 5 (42%) | 0.297 |
| Duration of HIV infection, years [mean (std)][~] | 16 (9) | 10 (8) | - - | 0.209 |
| Antiretroviral regimen [number (%)][1]; NRTIs and | | | | |
| PI | 11 (27%) | NA | NA | NA |
| NNRTI | 10 (24%) | | | |
| Integrase inhibitor | 27 (66%) | | | |
| Cell-entry inhibitor | 1 (2%) | | | |
| Duration of viral load suppression, years [mean (std)] | 6 (3) | NA | NA | NA |
| Duration of detectable viral load years [mean (std)] | NA | 3 (3) | NA | NA |
| CD4 count (cells/$\mu$l) | | | | |
| All patients [mean (std)][~] | 543 (301) | 496 (195) | - - | 0.737 |
| Patients with CD4 ≤350 [*n* (%)][$] | 16 (39%) | 1 (20%) | | 0.674 |
| Patients with CD4 351–499 [*n* (%)] | 5 (12%) | 1 (20%) | | |
| Patients with CD4 ≥500 [*n* (%)] | 20 (49%) | 3 (60%) | | |
| CD4% [mean (std)][~] | 31 (12) | 25 (6%) | | 0.256 |
| CD8 count (cells/$\mu$l), [mean (std)][~] | 809 (452) | 1041 (331) | | 0.275 |
| CD4/CD8 ratio [mean (std)][~] | 0.817 (0.509) | 052 (0.278) | | 0.210 |
| Nadir CD4 count (cells/$\mu$l) [mean (std)] | 203 (147) | 280 (166) | - - | 0.329 |

Viral load, VL; standard deviation, std; nucleoside reverse transcriptase inhibitor, NRTI; protease inhibitor, PI; nonnucleoside reverse transcriptase inhibitor, NNRTI; integrase inhibitor, II; not applicable, NA; [1]percentages surpass 100% as some individuals were on more than 1 drug class in addition to a NRTI backbone; statistical tests used for comparison: [#]ANOVA; [$]Fisher's exact test; [~]independent sample *t*-test.

of NO levels by group categories also showed insignificant results. Furthermore, the difference in mean nasal NO levels between participants tested between 11 am and 5 pm versus 5.01 pm and 10.59 pm did not significantly differ ($t$-test, $p$ = 0.543).

As shown in Table 2, mean SNOT-20 scores significantly differed among groups (ANOVA, $p$ = 0.013). HIV-infected individuals on ART had significantly higher (indicating worse sinonasal disease symptoms) mean SNOT-20 scores than healthy controls (19 ± 16/100 versus 4 ± 4/100, LSD post hoc test $p$ = 0.004). There were significantly higher proportions of individuals with ≥15 points on the SNOT-20, indicative of moderate-to-severe symptoms, in HIV-infected individuals on ART (54%) and HIV-infected individuals off ART (40%) versus healthy controls (0%, $p$ = 0.001; Fisher's exact test). Furthermore, a greater proportion of individuals on ART with suppressed VL reported experiencing at least 2 symptoms together ≥7 times per year, which is more often than individuals with detectable VL off ART versus healthy controls ($p < 0.001$; Fisher's exact test, Table 2).

Figure 2 depicts SNOT-20 scores for the 3 groups broken down by domain and expressed as a percentage for the possible total score in that domain (i.e., a score of 5 out of possible 25 points was expressed as 20%). For all domains, HIV+ participants had higher scores than the healthy control group, although the higher SNOT-20 scores observed in the HIV groups were driven more by sleep and psychological symptoms than by rhinosinusitis or ear and facial symptoms. HIV+ participants both on and off ART also had high scores in the "Others" category which asks about cough and whether the individual wakes up tired.

## 4. Discussion

For the first time in the modern ART era, we examined nasal NO levels in HIV-infected individuals on ART with suppressed VLs and HIV-infected individuals off ART with detectable VLs. We did not find statistically significant differences in nasal NO levels between these groups and age/sex-matched healthy controls. However, participants with HIV infection have increased clinical symptoms from chronic rhinosinusitis as measured by the SNOT-20 questionnaire.

In the cross-sectional study by Palm and colleagues from 2001, nasal NO levels were measured in 31 HIV-infected individuals and 26 controls [3]. Of the persons with HIV, 28 were on ART and 7 previously had an AIDS-defining illness. The average CD4 count was 320 ± 40 cells/mm$^3$ (CD4% 20 ± 1.8) and average viral load was 26,300 ± 14,560 copies/ml. Nasal NO was 21% lower in HIV patients than controls (152 ± 11.4 in HIV patients versus 193 ± 16.7 nL/min in controls, $p$ = 0.004). In our study, HIV-infected individuals on ART and off ART had much higher mean NO values (253 ± 77 nL/min and 231 ± 48, resp.) than found by Palm et al. This variation may result from our nasal NO measurement technique, which

TABLE 2: Nasal nitric oxide levels and responses to items on the impact of Sinonasal Outcomes Test-20 (SNOT-20) questionnaire.

| *Characteristics or outcome* | HIV+ with suppressed VL on ART (*n* = 41) | HIV+ with detectable VL off ART (*n* = 5) | Healthy Controls (*n* = 12) | *p* |
|---|---|---|---|---|
| Nasal nitric oxide levels (nL/min) [mean (std)][#] | 253 (77) | 213 (48) | 289 (68) | 0.133 |
| Nasal nitric oxide levels (nl/min) [median (IQR)] | 251 (200, 311) | 200 (172, 259) | 274 (233, 330) | |
| Range in nitric oxide levels (nL/min) | 116–421 | 147–264 | 197–432 | |
| Participants with levels ≤300 nL/min, [*n*(%)][$] | 29 (71%) | 5 (100%) | 7 (58%) | 0.291 |
| Total points on the SNOT-20 questionnaire (100 possible) [mean (std)][#] | 19 (16) | 18 (26) | 4 (4) | **0.013** |
| Participants with total points 0–14[$] (no problem to mild problem) [*n* (%)] | 19 (46%) | 3 (60%) | 12 (100%) | **0.001** |
| Participants with ≥15 points (moderate to severe) [*n* (%)] | 22 (54%) | 2 (40%) | 0 (0%) | **0.001** |
| Range in points | 0–59 | 0–60 | 0–13 | |
| Number of times per year a person experiences ≥2 symptoms in the SNOT-20 together [*n*(%)][$] | | | | |
| Never | 9 (24%) | 2 (40%) | 7 (58%) | <**0.001** |
| 1-2 times | 4 (11%) | 1 (20%) | 1 (8%) | |
| 3-4 times | 1 (2%) | 0 (%) | 4 (33%) | |
| ≥7 | 24 (63.2%) | 2 (40%) | 0 (0%) | |
| Question left blank | 3 (7%) | 0 (0%) | 0 (0%) | |

Statistical tests used for comparison: [#]ANOVA and [$]Fisher's exact test.

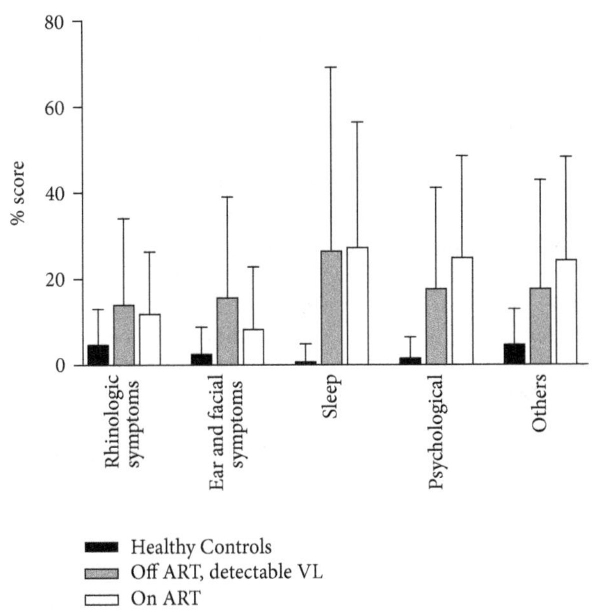


FIGURE 2: *SNOT-20 questionnaire scores across the 3 groups of participants.* Participants with HIV infection both on and off ART had higher total scores on the questionnaire ($p = 0.013$). This difference was observed in all domains, although higher scores among HIV groups were driven by sleep and psychological symptoms more than rhinologic or ear and facial symptoms.

was slightly different from the technique used by Palm and colleagues, as even modest changes in nasal NO measurement protocols can result in significantly different final values [9]. However, our higher nasal NO values are more likely from baseline immunologic differences and data analysis schema in the studied populations. First, Palm and colleagues analyzed nasal NO values from individuals with detectable and undetectable VL as one single group, which may have masked the differences we observed between these two populations. Additionally, the mean CD4 count in our study population was higher at 546 and 496 cells/mm$^3$ in persons on and off ART, respectively, and 50% of participants in both of our groups had CD4 ≥500 cells/mm$^3$. Furthermore, our HIV study populations had significantly higher CD4/CD8 ratios (mean ± std 0.817 ± 0.51 in individuals on ART and 0.52 ± 0.280 in individuals off ART) compared with the participants in Palm et al. (0.41 ± 0.05), which is indicative of greater immune reconstitution in our population. These differences between CD4/CD8 ratios of our HIV participants both on and off ART versus those in the Palm et al. study were statistically significant ($p < 0.001$ and $p = 0.040$, resp.). The higher CD4 and CD4/CD8 ratios in our study may reflect the current practice to initiate ART sooner in the course of HIV than was done in the past years. The average viral load in our HIV+ participants off ART was 27,752 ± 24,477 copies/ml, which is similar to that of the patients in the study by Palm et al. Overall, our findings suggest that HIV suppression mediated through ART is associated with improvements in the immune system including nasal NO production, although differences observed between our groups on and off ART were not statistically significant. We did not observe any significant correlations between various patient characteristics and nasal NO levels in HIV-infected individuals. Our lack of ability to detect correlations between nasal NO levels and various clinical parameters, such as CD4 count, may be due to our small sample size or due to the fact that there truly is no correlation between these parameters and nasal NO levels in HIV-infected adults.

Like other studies performed in HIV-infected populations, we noted a high proportion of individuals who reported tobacco and/or marijuana smoking [10–12], but we did not find any significant correlation between smoking and nasal NO levels, nor did we find a correlation between marijuana smoking and nasal NO levels in our study. In HIV-uninfected populations, tobacco smoking has been associated with increased nasal NO levels [13, 14]. Zhou et al. found that active smokers with high urine cotinine levels had significantly increased nasal NO levels compared to both nonsmokers and nonsmokers exposed to second-hand smoke [14]. In an observational cohort study of individuals undergoing functional endoscopic sinus surgery for management of persistent chronic rhinosinusitis, both smokers and nonsmokers had similar preoperative SNOT-20 scores [15]. However, prior smoking history was associated with smaller improvements in postsurgical quality-of-life SNOT-20 scores than in nonsmokers [15]. In another study examining the effect of smoking on outcomes after endoscopic sinus surgery, average SNOT-16 scores were significantly higher (indicating worse disease symptoms) in smokers versus nonsmokers [16]. In patients undergoing endoscopic sinus surgery for chronic sinusitis, additional studies have also shown that tobacco smoking negatively impacts patient-reported outcomes and quality-of-life measures in smokers versus nonsmokers, although not all of these studies employed the SNOT questionnaire [17–19]. In our study, we observed similar SNOT-20 scores in never, past, and current smokers.

To our knowledge the association between marijuana smoking and nasal NO levels has never been previously examined. In a study examining illicit drug use and various health conditions, marijuana smoking was associated with bronchitis but not sinusitis [20]. Whether marijuana smoking could have artificially increased nasal NO levels in our HIV-infected population on ART, who had significantly higher rates of marijuana smoking than the other two groups, is a matter of speculation. Studying the associations between smoked marijuana and nasal NO levels may also be confounded by the fact that individuals who smoke marijuana may also smoke tobacco and possibly other substances.

A major limitation of our study is our small sample size of 5 individuals off ART. Given the awareness of the benefits of treating HIV as early as possible in the course of infection [21], very few individuals off ART presented to our clinic. Furthermore, when patients who were lost to follow-up did return to clinic after a period of absence with ART noncompliance, they often had major psychosocial stressors prohibiting participation in a research protocol. Many other patients who presented to the clinic after a long period of absence were quickly reinitiated on ART during that same visit. We also did not examine participants for nasal polyps or deviated septum. However, a deviated septum should not matter for this study as we averaged the values for the 2 nostrils together to obtain a final nasal NO level. Furthermore, for healthy controls we were missing information such as body mass index, eosinophil count, CD4 count, and CD4/CD8 ratio. Therefore, the multivariate analysis could not include healthy controls owing to the missing information.

Our reliance on a retrospective chart review for clinical and laboratory data is another limitation. For many patients diagnosed in the 1990s and early 2000s, it was not clear if the lowest CD4 counts found in the charts were truly the nadir CD4 counts. Finally, ideally we would have measured inflammatory markers and associations with nasal NO levels; however, resource constraints precluded this additional testing. Despite these limitations, this study provides insight into a relatively unexplored area of immunology in people living with HIV both on and off effective ART in the modern ART era.

## 5. Conclusion

Respiratory tract immunity is important for preserving health and quality of life in HIV patients. Though previously thought to have decreased nasal NO values, HIV-infected patients on ART, as well as a small population of HIV-infected viremic individuals off ART, have nasal NO levels similar to healthy controls. Despite this, HIV-infected individuals have increased clinical symptoms from chronic rhinosinusitis as measured by the SNOT-20 questionnaire. Further investigation into immune disturbances of the respiratory tract in individuals on and off ART is needed to elucidate reasons for increased rhinosinusitis in this population and targets amenable to intervention.

## Disclosure

Cecilia T. Costiniuk is the recipient of an FRQ-S chercheur-boursier-clinicien Junior 1 salary award. Mohammad-Ali Jenabian is the holder of the Canada chair tier 2 in immunovirology. A portion of the preliminary work was presented at the Canadian Association for HIV Research (CAHR) conference held this April 2017 in Montreal, Canada.

## Conflicts of Interest

The authors declare no conflicts of interest with regard to the publication of this paper.

## Acknowledgments

Funds to support this study were obtained from the McGill Department of Medicine and Fondation du Recherche du Québec—Santé (FRQ-S).

## References

[1] A. R. Shah, J. A. Hairston, and T. A. Tami, "Sinusitis in HIV: microbiology and therapy," *Current Infectious Disease Reports*, vol. 7, no. 3, pp. 165–169, 2005.

[2] A. Predonzani, B. Calì, A. H. Agnellini, and B. Molon, "Spotlights on immunological effects of reactive nitrogen species: when inflammation says nitric oxide," *World Journal of Experimental Medicine*, vol. 5, no. 2, pp. 64–76, 2015.

[3] J. Palm, C. Lidman, P. Graf, K. Alving, and J. Lundberg, "Nasal nitric oxide is reduced in patients with HIV," *Acta Oto-Laryngologica*, vol. 120, no. 3, pp. 420–423, 2000.

[4] J. F. Piccirillo, M. G. Merritt Jr., and M. L. Richards, "Psychometric and clinimetric validity of the 20-Item Sino-Nasal Outcome Test (SNOT-20)," *Otolaryngology—Head and Neck Surgery*, vol. 126, no. 1, pp. 41–47, 2002.

[5] M. W. Leigh, M. J. Hazucha, K. K. Chawla et al., "Standardizing nasal nitric oxide measurement as a test for primary ciliary dyskinesia," *Annals of the American Thoracic Society*, vol. 10, no. 6, pp. 574–581, 2013.

[6] A. J. Shapiro, M. A. Chilvers, S. D. Davis, and M. W. Leigh, "Nasal Nitric Oxide and Ciliary Videomicroscopy: Tests Used for Diagnosing Primary Ciliary Dyskinesia," in *Diagnostic Tests in Pediatric Pulmonology*, Respiratory Medicine, pp. 55–72, Springer New York, New York, NY, 2015.

[7] "ATS/ERS recommendations for standardized procedures for the online and offline measurement of exhaled lower respiratory nitric oxide and nasal nitric oxide, 2005," *American Journal of Respiratory and Critical Care Medicine*, vol. 171, no. 8, pp. 912–930, 2005.

[8] H. Dressel, A. Bihler, F. Jund et al., "Diurnal variation of nasal nitric oxide levels in healthy subjects," *Journal of Investigational Allergology and Clinical Immunology*, vol. 18, no. 4, pp. 316-317, 2008.

[9] A. R. Deschamp, L. Schornick, C. Clem, M. Hazucha, A. J. Shapiro, and S. D. Davis, "A comparison of nasal nitric oxide measurement modes," *Pediatric Pulmonology*, vol. 52, no. 11, pp. 1381-1382, 2017.

[10] C. T. Costiniuk, L. Brunet, K. C. Rollet-Kurhajec et al., "Tobacco smoking is not associated with accelerated liver disease in human immunodeficiency virus-hepatitis C coinfection: A longitudinal cohort analysis," *Open Forum Infectious Diseases*, vol. 3, article ofw050, no. 2, 2016.

[11] L. Balfour, S. A. Wiebe, W. D. Cameron et al., "An HIV-tailored quit-smoking counselling pilot intervention targeting depressive symptoms plus Nicotine Replacement Therapy," *AIDS Care Psychological and Socio-medical Aspects of AIDS/HIV*, vol. 29, no. 1, pp. 24–31, 2017.

[12] M. Helleberg, M. T. May, S. M. Ingle et al., "Smoking and life expectancy among HIV-infected individuals on antiretroviral therapy in Europe and North America," *AIDS*, vol. 29, no. 2, pp. 221–229, 2015.

[13] H. Zhou, X. Wang, L. Brighton, M. Hazucha, I. Jaspers, and J. L. Carson, "Increased nasal epithelial ciliary beat frequency associated with lifestyle tobacco smoke exposure," *Inhalation Toxicology*, vol. 21, no. 10, pp. 875–881, 2009.

[14] H. Zhou, B. Zou, M. Hazucha, and J. L. Carson, "Nasal nitric oxide and lifestyle exposure to tobacco smoke," *Annals of Otology, Rhinology & Laryngology*, vol. 120, no. 7, pp. 455–459, 2011.

[15] S. Das, S. S. Khichi, H. Perakis, T. Woodard, and S. E. Kountakis, "Effects of smoking on quality of life following sinus surgery: 4-year follow-up," *The Laryngoscope*, vol. 119, no. 11, pp. 2284–2287, 2009.

[16] R. D. Briggs, S. T. Wright, S. Cordes, and K. H. Calhoun, "Smoking in chronic rhinosinusitis: a predictor of poor long-term outcome after endoscopic sinus surgery," *The Laryngoscope*, vol. 114, no. 1, pp. 126–128, 2004.

[17] B. R. Harrow and P. S. Batra, "Sinonasal quality of life outcomes after minimally invasive resection of sinonasal and skull-base tumors," *International Forum of Allergy & Rhinology*, vol. 3, no. 12, pp. 1013–1020, 2013.

[18] D. D. Reh, T. S. Higgins, and T. L. Smith, "Impact of tobacco smoke on chronic rhinosinusitis: a review of the literature," *International Forum of Allergy & Rhinology*, vol. 2, no. 5, pp. 362–369, 2012.

[19] E. Tamashiro, N. A. Cohen, J. N. Palmer, and W. T. A. Lima, "Effects of cigarette smoking on the respiratory epithelium and its role in the pathogenesis of chronic rhinosinusitis.," *Brazilian Journal of Otorhinolaryngology*, vol. 75, no. 6, pp. 903–907, 2009.

[20] B. Han, J. C. Gfroerer, and J. D. Colliver, "Associations Between Duration of Illicit Drug Use and Health Conditions: Results from the 2005-2007 National Surveys on Drug Use and Health," *Annals of Epidemiology*, vol. 20, no. 4, pp. 289–297, 2010.

[21] R. A. Franco and M. S. Saag, "When to start antiretroviral therapy: As soon as possible," *BMC Medicine*, vol. 11, no. 1, article no. 147, 2013.

6

# Socioeconomic Status and Vulnerability to HIV Infection in Uganda: Evidence from Multilevel Modelling of AIDS Indicator Survey Data

**Patrick Igulot**[1] **and Monica A. Magadi**[2]

[1] *University of Sunderland in London, UK*
[2] *University of Hull, UK*

Correspondence should be addressed to Patrick Igulot; patrick.igulot@sunderland.ac.uk

Academic Editor: David Katzenstein

*Background.* There is controversy on the association between socioeconomic status (SES) and HIV infection. Some evidence claims higher SES is negatively associated with HIV infection while others report the reverse. *Objectives.* To examine the association between SES and HIV infection in Uganda and to examine whether the SES-HIV relationship varies by gender, rural-urban place of residence, and time (2004-2005 and 2011) in Uganda. *Methods.* Multilevel analysis was applied to 39,766 individual cases obtained in 887 clusters of Uganda HIV/AIDS Indicators Survey conducted in 2004-2005 and 2011. *Results.* Household wealth is associated with increased vulnerability in the general population and in rural areas. Compared with no educational attainment, secondary or higher education is associated with reduced vulnerability to the risk of HIV infection by 37% in the general population. However, this effect was stronger in urban than rural areas. Besides individual-level factors, unobserved community factors too play an important role and account for 9% of unexplained variance after individual-level factors are considered. *Conclusion.* Household wealth increases vulnerability but education reduces it. The social environment influences vulnerability to HIV infection independent of individual-level factors. HIV/AIDS awareness targeting sexual practices of wealthy individuals and those with primary-level educational attainment together with improving educational attainment and addressing contextual factors influencing vulnerability to HIV infection are necessary strategies to reduce HIV infections in Uganda.

## 1. Introduction

The association between socioeconomic status (SES) and HIV infection in sub-Saharan Africa (SSA) is controversial. Considerable research attention has been given to the relationship between SES and HIV in SSA, a region that suffers a disproportionate higher burden of HIV/AIDS. Some studies suggest that people with low, while others suggest that those with high SES are more vulnerable to HIV infection [1–3]. More studies have demonstrated the positive relationship between SES and vulnerability to HIV infection in SSA [4–6]. Previous studies have used diverse measures of SES, including employment. However, in this paper, wealth and education are used as the main measures of SES because they are consistently defined and measured in the AIDS Indicator Survey (AIS).

*1.1. Household Wealth Status.* Wealth status is linked to HIV infection through complex pathways. The first link is through the income effect [7] that may be in the opposite direction. People with high income tend to lead lifestyles associated with increased number of sexual partners which increases their vulnerability to HIV, while those with low income may be unable to access HIV services also leading to increased vulnerability [4, 6, 7]. Poverty makes people vulnerable to HIV in diverse ways including dropping out of school; marrying early; loss of livelihood; and being homeless due to displacement by war, all of which have been linked to increased HIV vulnerability (e.g., [4, 8]).

*1.2. Educational Attainment.* The education-HIV evidence is also mixed. Some studies indicate that education is negatively associated with HIV infection [9, 10] while others report a positive association [1, 11–14]. There is more convincing argument in support of the former; for example, education may be associated with HIV infection through schooling. Schooling keeps young people away from environments which would increase their vulnerability to HIV infection and inspires students to develop long term goals. These contribute to delaying sex, which makes young people avoid HIV infection [15, 16]. Higher educational attainment (defined here as complete secondary or higher education) provides knowledge, which individuals use to avoid HIV infection [6, 17], and provides employment, which enhances the capacity of people to act on their plans to reduce vulnerability [4, 15, 16].

The SES-HIV evidence is controversial and context specific. However, one study [2] examined changes in HIV prevalence over time, and as much as the role of rural-urban residential area and gender in the construction of vulnerability has been addressed in the previous research (e.g., [14, 18, 19]) there is none about Uganda. Besides the controversy on SES, majority of previous research has focused on the influence of individual characteristics (demographic factors) on their risk of being infected with HIV [20–23]. Scholars, including Clarke et al. [24], argue that the personal characteristics of the individual do not fully explain their risk of HIV infection. In this research, we use multilevel modelling, a method that simultaneously measures the effect of individual characteristics (observed effects) and the effects of community characteristics (unobserved effects) [24, 25]. Understanding social context is important because these factors cause social practices [26]; they increase vulnerability to HIV infection and curtail the success of proven HIV/AIDS interventions (e.g., [27, 28]), while others protect individuals from HIV risk.

This study contributes to these debates by providing evidence from Uganda, a country which was previously a global model in the response to HIV/AIDS [29] but where prevalence has been rising from 6.2% in early 2000s, to 6.4% in the 2005 to 7.3% in 2012 [30]. As much as this may be due to increased survival rates because of antiretroviral treatment [31–33] or other remedies [34], this worrying trend in HIV/AIDS epidemic has occurred in the context of grim socioeconomic development, with 65 percent of the population being classified as being poor [35, 36] and the majority having only primary or no education [37].

The objectives of this research are as follows:

(1) To examine the association between socioeconomic status and HIV infection in Uganda.

(2) To examine whether the SES-HIV relationship varies by gender, rural-urban place of residence, and time (2004-5 and 2011) in Uganda.

## 2. Data and Methods of Analysis

*2.1. The Data.* This research is based on a nationally representative sample of 22,979 women and 18,418 men of reproductive age from 20,869 households with 33,692 rural and 7,705 urban respondents obtained from the 2004-2005 and 2011 Uganda AIS. AIDS Indicator Survey is a global research programme that collects data to inform national policies and facilitate international comparison [38]. All adults aged 15–59 years interviewed were also requested to voluntarily give blood for HIV testing. A two-stage sampling strategy was applied, starting with the selection of clusters in each region and then sampling 25 households in every cluster [39]. In this research, a cluster is synonymous with a community, which is defined as 50–500 households clustered within the same geographical area. This classification is based on the country's census sampling frame, which classifies these households into primary sampling units (i.e., clusters) or communities. This is the standard definition of community in the Demographic and Health Survey (DHS) data for measuring community effects [40].

The survey protocols were approved by the Science and Ethics Committee of Uganda Virus Research Institute, ICF Macro Institutional Review Board, Ethics Review Committee at CDC, Atlanta, and the Ethics Committee of Uganda Council for Science and Technology [38].

*2.2. Sample Characteristics.* This research is based on 39,766 individual cases aged 15–49 years (women) and 15–59 (men). Sixty-five percent of the respondents were under 35 years of age with an average age of 30.5 years for females and males. There were 82.7% rural residents in the surveys, with the remaining 17.3% being urban residents. Women respondents comprised 55.6% of the sample. Most respondents did not have secondary or higher education. Respondents with primary or no educational attainment comprised 72.9%; more women had less education than men. Among rural residents, 89.6% had primary or no education at all. The mean years of education for men and women were 5.7. These sample characteristics reflect the structure of the general Ugandan population (e.g., [37]).

*2.3. Methods of Analysis.* Multilevel logistic regression was used to predict the probability of having HIV infection, represented by 1, against the probability of not having, which was represented by 0 [5]. To create the wealth index, DHS uses a subset of indicators common to rural and urban areas to create wealth scores for households in both areas. Some of the indicators used are those that measure access to the mass media, access to efficient means of communication, household's capacity to afford pricy items and to hygienically store food, and access to public services, markets, and exposure to other development areas. Other indicators used are those that measure access of households to means of production and social standing seen through characteristics of the dwelling (floor, wall, and roofing materials used), type of drinking water source, type of energy used, and type of toilet facilities that a household uses.

In the second step, separate component scores are produced for households in urban and rural areas using area-specific indicators. The third step entails combining the separate area-specific scores to produce a nationally applicable combined wealth index, by adjusting the area-specific score through regression on the common component score [41, 42]. Because of the compositional nature of the wealth index and

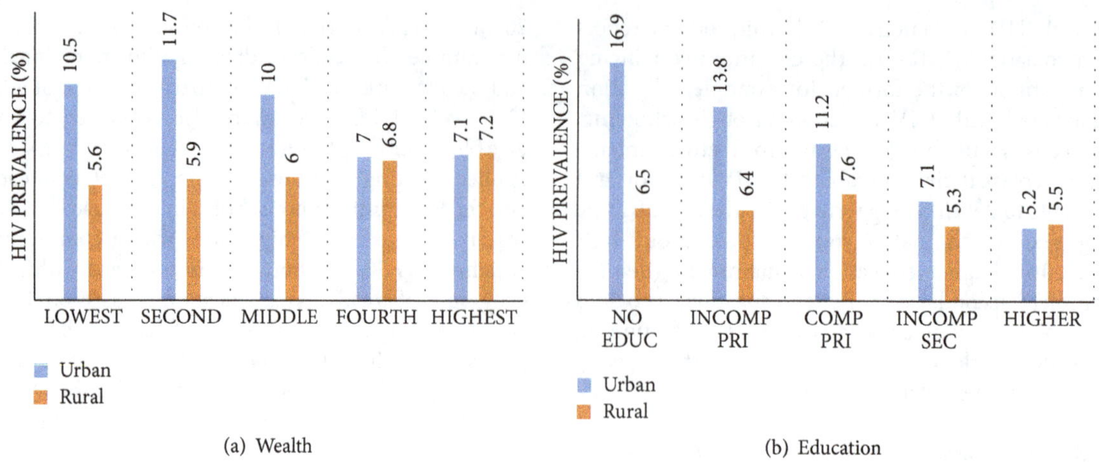


FIGURE 1: HIV prevalence by household wealth status (a) and educational attainment (b) in rural and urban areas, UAIS, 2004-2005 and 2011 ($n$ = 39,767).

difference in country contexts, we measure SES using this survey/country specific wealth/poverty index [42] classified into five quintiles: lowest; second; middle; fourth; and highest [41]. Educational attainment is categorized into five ordinal levels: no education; incomplete primary; complete primary; incomplete secondary; and complete secondary and higher education.

Analysis started with bivariate analysis of HIV status by wealth and education. We control for SES factors first for 2 main reasons: first, as an independent variable(s) of interest, we want to know the size of its effect; and second, given its known correlation with many other variables, controlling for SES first allows us to know its contribution to the overall model. This was then extended to multivariate analysis which used the logit model to sequentially fit two-level nested models. The analysis first controlled for potential confounders before adding sexual behavior factors in the final model to identify potential pathways through which SES is associated with HIV prevalence.

During modelling, analysis started by obtaining general models based on pooled data. After analysis of pooled data, interactions between SES and gender, rural-urban residence, and time were obtained to explore potential variations in the effect of SES by these factors. This was necessary to investigate whether evidence of heterogeneity in the SES-HIV relationship regarding gender and urban/rural residence that has been observed in other SSA settings [19, 43–45] is applicable in Uganda and to explore whether the nature of the relationship has changed over time. Every step started by running a model with wealth and education only and then adding other covariates to establish potential pathways of the link between SES and HIV vulnerability, using MLwiN [46].

This research focuses on gender and rural-urban residential areas because these concepts are important dimensions of SES and are significant in the construction of HIV vulnerability and yet they are less explored in SSA [5]. This analysis focused on residential areas because they represent physical spaces and networks for the spread of HIV and present different conditions with influence on HIV vulnerability [7]. Change in vulnerability to risk over 2 time periods, i.e., 2004-2005 and 2011, was considered important given its relevance to changes in policies and programmes [47] which are likely to influence HIV vulnerability.

## 3. Descriptive Findings

*3.1. HIV Prevalence by Sample Characteristics.* The overall prevalence of HIV was 6.4% in 2004-2005 but it increased to 7.3% in 2011 and was higher among women than in men (Table 1). With respect to SES, there was no evidence of a significant association between wealth status and HIV prevalence for both males and females in 2004-2005 and 2011. For education, men with no educational attainment had the highest prevalence in 2004-2005 and 2011. It is interesting to note that in 2004-2005 while men with the highest educational attainment had the lowest HIV prevalence, for women, HIV prevalence was lowest among those with no education. In 2011, there was evidence of higher educational attainment beyond primary level being associated with reduced HIV prevalence for both males and females.

Interesting patterns in HIV prevalence were observed by other key factors, besides SES. The overall rise in HIV prevalence between 2004-2005 and 2011 was mainly driven by a rise in prevalence among older men and women aged 35 years and above, rural residents, and never married men. HIV prevalence was particularly high among widowed men in 2004-2005 at 27%. In terms of age, HIV prevalence in 2004-2005 was highest among women aged 25–34 years and men aged 35–44 years. In 2011, prevalence was highest among both men and women aged 35–44. The HIV prevalence among women in female headed households is about twice that in male headed households in 2004-2005 and 2011. However, prevalence among women in male headed households was lower than men in the same household. These patterns suggest that the observed higher prevalence among women than men is driven by heightened vulnerability among women in women headed households.

Figure 1 shows further how HIV prevalence varies by SES characteristics and by urban/rural residence. In Figure 1(a),

TABLE 1: Weighted HIV prevalence by key characteristics, Uganda AIDS Indicator Survey (UAIS), 2004-2005 and 2011.

| Characteristic | UAIS, 2004-5 | | | | UAIS, 2011 | | | |
|---|---|---|---|---|---|---|---|---|
| | Women | | Men | | Women | | Men | |
| | % HIV+ | Cases | % HIV+ | Cases | % HIV+ | Cases | % HIV+ | Cases |
| *Age Group* | * | | * | | * | | * | |
| 15–24 | 4.3 | 3842 | 1.1 | 3089 | 4.9 | 4504 | 2.1 | 3450 |
| 25–34 | 10.3 | 3035 | 7.0 | 2248 | 10.3 | 3331 | 6.3 | 2493 |
| 35–44 | 9.3 | 1741 | 9.3 | 1603 | 11.5 | 2247 | 11.1 | 2006 |
| 45–59 | 6.6 | 1448 | 6.6 | 1295 | 8.5 | 1760 | 8.1 | 1574 |
| *Wealth/poverty Status* | *ns* | | *ns* | | *ns* | | *ns* | |
| Lowest | 6.4 | 1767 | 4.3 | 1360 | 8.1 | 2278 | 6.9 | 1677 |
| Second | 7.4 | 1948 | 5.4 | 1583 | 9.2 | 2358 | 5.1 | 1933 |
| Middle | 7.5 | 2070 | 5.2 | 1688 | 7.4 | 2303 | 6.2 | 1901 |
| Fourth | 7.3 | 2145 | 5.7 | 1692 | 7.4 | 2407 | 6.5 | 2012 |
| Highest | 7.9 | 2236 | 5.2 | 1914 | 8.9 | 2495 | 6.0 | 2001 |
| *Educational Attainment* | * | | * | | * | | * | |
| No education | 5.6 | 2531 | 7.2 | 741 | 8.6 | 1923 | 7.5 | 597 |
| Incomplete primary | 7.6 | 4657 | 4.8 | 3862 | 8.7 | 5481 | 6.6 | 4055 |
| Complete primary | 9.9 | 1100 | 6.2 | 1178 | 9.4 | 1441 | 7.0 | 1390 |
| Incomplete secondary | 7.3 | 1579 | 4.8 | 1919 | 6.7 | 2334 | 5.2 | 2493 |
| Complete sec & higher | 8.6 | 279 | 4.4 | 524 | 5.4 | 662 | 4.6 | 989 |
| *Area of Residence* | * | | * | | *ns* | | * | |
| Rural | 6.4 | 8672 | 4.9 | 7087 | 7.6 | 9407 | 6.1 | 7711 |
| Urban | 12.6 | 1493 | 7.0 | 1151 | 10.8 | 2436 | 6.3 | 1813 |
| *Current Marital Status* | * | | * | | * | | * | |
| Never been in union | 2.8 | 2084 | 0.8 | 2915 | 2.0 | 3204 | 3.9 | 2604 |
| Married/living together | 5.7 | 6428 | 6.6 | 4624 | 7.4 | 5710 | 7.0 | 7430 |
| Widowed | 24.0 | 803 | 27.0 | 141 | 22.7 | 75 | 24.0 | 692 |
| Divorced/separated | 14.0 | 850 | 11.1 | 557 | 15.0 | 534 | 16.4 | 1117 |
| *Sex of Household Head* | * | | * | | * | | * | |
| Male headed household | 5.4 | 6864 | 5.6 | 7073 | 6.1 | 7264 | 6.4 | 7992 |
| Female headed household | 11.4 | 3301 | 2.9 | 1165 | 11.6 | 4578 | 4.7 | 1532 |
| Total | 7.3 | 10165 | 5.2 | 8238 | 8.2 | 11842 | 6.1 | 9524 |

*Statistically significant at 5% significance level, chi-square $P < 0.05$, ns: not significant at 5% level, $P > 0.05$.

there is a positive wealth-HIV gradient in rural areas, steadily rising from a prevalence of 5.6% among the lowest to 7.1% among the highest. However, in the urban areas, the trend is reversed. HIV prevalence declines from 11.7% among people in the second wealth category to 7.2% among those in the highest. In Figure 1(b), education is negatively associated with HIV in urban areas but in rural areas, a negative but somewhat consistent trend can be observed only after complete primary education.

## 4. Multilevel Findings

In the multilevel modelling, four models were fitted, starting with wealth and education in the first model and then controlling for other characteristics. In the final model, evidence in Table 2 shows that there is a general positive association between wealth and HIV prevalence, with prevalence in the highest wealth households being 20% higher than in the lowest wealth quintile households after controlling for background characteristics. The higher HIV prevalence among those in the highest wealth quintile becomes evident when socioeconomic and demographic factors were controlled for in Model 3. However, this ceased to be significant in Model 4 when sexual behavior factors were controlled for, suggesting that the higher HIV vulnerability among wealthy individuals was partly explained by sexual behavior factors, which is consistent with existing literature.

For education, secondary or higher educational attainment was associated with reduced odds of HIV infection, while primary education was associated with increased odds, compared to no education. However, the higher HIV vulnerability associated with primary-level education only became apparent in Model 3 when background socioeconomic and demographic factors, especially, current marital status, were controlled for and ceased to be significant when sexual behavior factors were controlled for. Overall,

TABLE 2: Odds ratios (OR) of being HIV positive for women and men, Uganda AIS, 2004-2005 and 2011 ($n$ = 39,766).

| Parameters | Model 1 | | Model 3 | | Model 4 | |
|---|---|---|---|---|---|---|
| | OR | 95% CI | OR | 95% CI | OR | 95% CI |
| *Fixed effects* | | | | | | |
| Constant | 0.06 | [0.06–0.08]* | 0.02 | [0.02–0.03]* | 0.01 | [0.00–0.01]* |
| *Model 1: Socio-economic factors* | | | | | | |
| *Wealth status (Ref: Lowest)* | | | | | | |
| Second | 1.04 | [0.90–1.20] | 1.07 | [0.93–1.24] | 1.04 | [0.90–1.20] |
| Middle | 1.00 | [0.86–1.15] | 1.06 | [0.91–1.23] | 1.02 | [0.88–1.19] |
| Fourth | 1.02 | [0.88–1.18] | 1.09 | [0.93–1.27] | 1.05 | [0.90–1.22] |
| Highest | 1.05 | [0.90–1.22] | 1.20 | [1.02–1.40]* | 1.15 | [0.98–1.35] |
| *Education (Ref: No)* | | | | | | |
| Incomplete primary | 0.91 | [0.80–1.04] | 1.23 | [1.08–1.41]* | 1.12 | [0.98–1.28] |
| Complete primary | 1.00 | [0.86–1.18] | 1.32 | [1.12–1.56]* | 1.17 | [0.99–1.39] |
| Incomplete secondary | 0.67 | [0.57–0.78]* | 1.10 | [0.93–1.30] | 0.95 | [0.80–1.13] |
| Complete secondary & higher | 0.54 | [0.43–0.68]* | 0.74 | [0.58–0.94]* | 0.63 | [0.49–0.81]* |
| Missing | 1.20 | [0.34–4.23] | 1.70 | [0.47–6.10] | 1.58 | [0.44–5.65] |
| *Model 2: Other socio-economic factors* | | | | | | |
| *Place of residence (Ref: Urban)* | | | | | | |
| Rural | | | 0.52 | [0.44–0.60]* | 0.60 | [0.51–0.70]* |
| *Ethnicity (Ref: Baganda)* | | | | | | |
| Banyankole/Bakiga | | | 1.18 | [0.99–1.40] | 1.43 | [1.21–1.70]* |
| Iteso/Karimojong | | | 0.75 | [0.60–0.93]* | 0.86 | [0.69–1.07] |
| Lubgbara/Madi | | | 0.48 | [0.36–0.62]* | 0.61 | [0.47–0.80]* |
| Basoga | | | 0.79 | [0.63–0.98]* | 0.76 | [0.62–0.95]* |
| Langi/Acholi | | | 1.22 | [0.99–1.50] | 1.42 | [1.16–1.75]* |
| Bagisu/Sabiny | | | 0.80 | [0.61–1.05] | 0.73 | [0.56–0.95]* |
| Alur/Japadhola | | | 0.79 | [0.61–1.03] | 0.83 | [0.64–1.08] |
| Banyoro/Batoro | | | 1.36 | [1.11–1.67]* | 1.33 | [1.08–1.64]* |
| All others | | | 0.87 | [0.72–1.04] | 0.95 | [0.80–1.14] |
| *Time in years (Ref: 2004-05)* | | | | | | |
| 2011 | | | 1.23 | [1.09–1.39]* | 1.23 | [1.09–1.38]* |
| *Model 3: Socio-demographic factors* | | | | | | |
| *Age of respondent (Ref: 45–59 years)* | | | | | | |
| 15–24 years | | | 0.82 | [0.69–0.97]* | 1.08 | [0.91–1.29] |
| 25–34 years | | | 1.53 | [1.34–1.75]* | 1.71 | [1.49–1.96]* |
| 35–44 years | | | 1.69 | [1.48–1.93]* | 1.77 | [1.54–2.03]* |
| *Marital status (Ref: Never been married)* | | | | | | |
| Married/living together | | | 2.32 | [1.94–2.77]* | 2.22 | [1.81–2.73]* |
| Widowed | | | 11.12 | [8.88–13.93]* | 7.94 | [6.24–10.11]* |
| Divorced/separated | | | 5.22 | [4.28–6.36]* | 3.60 | [2.90–4.47]* |
| *Sex of respondent (Ref: Men)* | | | | | | |
| Women | | | 1.13 | [1.03–1.24]* | 1.72 | [1.54–1.91]* |
| *Model 4: Sexual practices* | | | | | | |
| *Drunk with alcohol (Ref: No)* | | | | | | |
| Drunk | | | | | 1.25 | [1.12–1.40]* |
| Not applicable | | | | | 0.27 | [0.02–4.84] |
| *Condom use during risky sex (Ref: No)* | | | | | | |
| Used condom | | | | | 2.31 | [2.00–2.67]* |
| Not applicable | | | | | 5.83 | [0.33–103.37] |
| *Multiple sexual partners (Ref: 1 partner)* | | | | | | |
| 2–4 partners | | | | | 2.13 | [1.86–2.44]* |
| >4 partners | | | | | 3.87 | [3.29–4.54]* |
| Not applicable | | | | | 0.82 | [0.58–1.14] |

TABLE 2: Continued.

| Parameters | Model 1 | | Model 3 | | Model 4 | |
|---|---|---|---|---|---|---|
| | OR | 95% CI | OR | 95% CI | OR | 95% CI |
| *HIV/AIDS knowledge (Ref: No knowledge)* | | | | | | |
| Lowest knowledge | | | | | 1.13 | [0.80–1.59] |
| Medium knowledge | | | | | 1.12 | [0.82–1.52] |
| Highest knowledge | | | | | 1.39 | [1.03–1.89]* |
| *Random effects* | | | | | | |
| Cluster variance | 0.566 | 0.049* | 0.363 | 0.039* | 0.313 | 0.036* |
| Clusters | 887 | | 887 | | 887 | |
| Individual | 39766 | | 39766 | | 39766 | |

OR: odds ratios; 95% CI: confidence intervals. *Statistical significance at 5%, $P < 0.05$.

complete secondary education was associated with lower HIV prevalence, conditional on background characteristics and sexual behaviors. For instance, if those with complete secondary or higher education had the same background characteristics and sexual behavior (to the extent measured in our model) as those with no education, their HIV prevalence would still be 37% lower.

To check the robustness of the findings in this research, we rerun the analysis that controlled for age in single-year dummies in Models 3 and 4 instead of 10-year age categories/dummies (Table 3). Using 39,766 cases used to produce results in Table 2 with age of 59 years having the least number of cases (203), we wanted to find out if the SES-HIV association would substantially change with this approach. The results in Table 3 did not show any substantial difference with those in Table 2 that are based on the analysis that controlled for age in broad 10-year age group categories.

*4.1. Determinants of HIV Vulnerability by Urban/Rural Residence.* The SES determinants of HIV prevalence in Uganda by urban/rural residence (Table 4) were further explored. HIV prevalence was negatively associated with incomplete secondary and complete secondary and higher educational attainment in urban areas. People with incomplete secondary were 36% less likely to be infected while those with complete secondary or higher were 57% less likely to have HIV compared to people with no education in urban areas with similar other characteristics. There was no evidence of a significant education effect in rural areas once sociodemographic factors and sexual practices were controlled for in the final model; when age was controlled for, the effects of higher education reduced from odds ratio 0.63 [0.46–0.87] to 0.93 [0.67–1.29] and when marital status was controlled for, the effects reduced further to 0.96 [0.79–1.17]. This indicates that these factors, especially age, confound the association between education and HIV vulnerability in rural areas.

Compared to men with the same other social characteristics, women were significantly more likely to be HIV-positive than men (average OR = 1.61 in rural and 2.13 in urban areas), suggesting that all other factors being equal, women were more vulnerable than men and the gender gap was greater in urban than rural areas. In relation to trends, there was evidence of significantly higher HIV prevalence in 2011 than 2004-2005 and in rural but not in urban areas.

*4.2. Interaction Effects.* To check the robustness of our results further, we investigated whether there were significant differences in association between SES and HIV prevalence by gender, rural-urban residential area, and across 2 surveys, 2004-2005 and 2011, interaction modelling was performed [48]. Wealth and education were separately interacted with residential area, gender, and time. There was no evidence of significant interactions between wealth status and rural/rural residence, gender, or time. However, secondary or higher education was associated with increased odds of being HIV-positive among rural residents (Table 5). This may point to the possible influence of social and sexual practices in increasing vulnerability among people with higher educational attainment in rural areas.

*4.3. Effect of Unobserved Community-Level Factors.* Random effects were used to calculate the effects of community-level factors on HIV vulnerability based on the following formula [49].

$$p = \frac{uoj}{(uoj + eij)}, \quad (1)$$

where $p$ is the intracluster correlation, $eij$ is variation at level 1 (individual), which is represented by 3.29 [46, 49] (for Logistic Regression) and $uoj$ is variation at level 2 (Cluster). Community random variance estimates were used to calculate the intracluster correlation coefficient. Overall, after accounting for individual-level factors included in the model, 9% of the residual variance occurs at the cluster level. This community effect is notably stronger in rural (ICC = 0.13) than in urban (ICC = 0.05) areas.

## 5. Discussion

*5.1. Household Wealth Status.* There is an association between wealth status and HIV infection in the pooled 2004-2005 and 2011 data (Table 2), and in rural areas (Table 4). These findings were consistent with a previous Ugandan research [2] and those of other previous researches (e.g., [50]) showing higher HIV prevalence among individuals in wealthy households, especially rural residents. Interactions between wealth and gender, residential areas, and across two surveys (2004-2005 and 2011) were also examined but did not find any significant interactions.

TABLE 3: Odds ratios (OR) of being HIV positive for women and men, Uganda AIS, 2004-2005 and 2011 ($n$ = 39,766) controlling for age in single-year dummy variables.

| Parameter | Model 1 | | Model 2 | | Model 3 | | Model 4 | |
|---|---|---|---|---|---|---|---|---|
| | OR | 95% CI | OR | 95% CI | OR | 95% CI | OR | 95% CI |
| *Fixed Effect* | | | | | | | | |
| Constant | 0.06 | [0.06–0.08]* | 0.13 | [0.10–0.16]* | 0.01 | [0.01–0.02]* | 0.00 | [0.00–0.01]* |
| *Model 1: SES factors* | | | | | | | | |
| *Wealth (Ref: Lowest)* | | | | | | | | |
| Second | 1.04 | [0.90–1.20] | 1.03 | [0.89–1.18] | 1.07 | [0.92–1.23] | 1.03 | [0.89–1.19] |
| Middle | 1.00 | [0.86–1.15] | 0.98 | [0.85–1.13] | 1.06 | [0.91–1.23] | 1.02 | [0.88–1.18] |
| Fourth | 1.02 | [0.88–1.18] | 1.00 | [0.86–1.16] | 1.08 | [0.93–1.26] | 1.04 | [0.89–1.21] |
| Highest | 1.05 | [0.90–1.22] | 1.06 | [0.91–1.24] | 1.18 | [1.00–1.38] | 1.13 | [0.96–1.33] |
| *Education (Ref: No education)* | | | | | | | | |
| Incomplete primary | 0.91 | [0.80–1.04] | 0.87 | [0.76–0.99]* | 1.23 | [1.08–1.41]* | 1.12 | [0.97–1.28] |
| Complete primary | 1.00 | [0.86–1.18] | 0.92 | [0.78–1.08] | 1.31 | [1.11–1.54]* | 1.16 | [0.98–1.37] |
| Incomplete secondary | 0.67 | [0.57–0.78]* | 0.58 | [0.49–0.68]* | 1.09 | [0.92–1.29] | 0.95 | [0.80–1.12] |
| Complete secondary & higher | 0.54 | [0.43–0.68]* | 0.43 | [0.34–0.55]* | 0.69 | [0.54–0.89]* | 0.61 | [0.48–0.79]* |
| Missing | 1.20 | [0.34–4.23] | 1.22 | [0.35–4.27] | 1.83 | [0.51–6.60] | 1.71 | [0.47–6.15] |
| *Model 2: Other SES factors* | | | | | | | | |
| *Place of residence (Ref: Urban)* | | | | | | | | |
| Rural | | | 0.51 | [0.43–0.59]* | 0.52 | [0.45–0.61]* | 0.60 | [0.52–0.70]* |
| *Ethnicity (Ref: Baganda)* | | | | | | | | |
| Banyankole/Bakiga | | | 1.13 | [0.95–1.34] | 1.17 | [0.98–1.39] | 1.42 | [1.19–1.68]* |
| Iteso/Karimojong | | | 0.67 | [0.54–0.84]* | 0.74 | [0.59–0.93]* | 0.85 | [0.68–1.06] |
| Lubgbara/Madi | | | 0.45 | [0.35–0.60]* | 0.47 | [0.36–0.62]* | 0.60 | [0.46–0.79]* |
| Basoga | | | 0.77 | [0.62–0.95]* | 0.78 | [0.63–0.97]* | 0.76 | [0.61–0.94]* |
| Langi/Acholi | | | 1.13 | [0.92–1.39] | 1.22 | [0.99–1.50] | 1.42 | [1.16–1.75]* |
| Bagisu/Sabiny | | | 0.75 | [0.57–0.98]* | 0.80 | [0.61–1.04] | 0.73 | [0.56–0.95]* |
| Alur/Japadhola | | | 0.72 | [0.56–0.94]* | 0.80 | [0.62–1.05] | 0.84 | [0.64–1.09] |
| Banyoro/Batoro | | | 1.28 | [1.04–1.58] | 1.35 | [1.09–1.66]* | 1.33 | [1.08–1.63]* |
| All others | | | 0.82 | [0.69–0.98]* | 0.86 | [0.72–1.04] | 0.95 | [0.79–1.14] |
| *Time in years (Ref: 2005-05)* | | | | | | | | |
| UG6 | | | 1.22 | [1.08–1.38]* | 1.23 | [1.08–1.39]* | 1.22 | [1.08–1.37]* |
| *Model 3: socio-demographics* | | | | | | | | |
| *Age of respondent (Ref: 15 years)* | | | | | | | | |
| Age 16 | | | | | 0.94 | [0.50–1.75] | 0.86 | [0.46–1.61] |
| Age 17 | | | | | 1.04 | [0.57–1.90] | 0.88 | [0.48–1.64] |
| Age 18 | | | | | 1.66 | [0.97–2.84] | 1.24 | [0.70–2.18] |
| Age 19 | | | | | 1.85 | [1.07–3.19]* | 1.33 | [0.74–2.37] |
| Age 20 | | | | | 1.89 | [1.11–3.22]* | 1.27 | [0.72–2.24] |
| Age 21 | | | | | 2.95 | [1.74–5.01]* | 1.86 | [1.05–3.30]* |
| Age 22 | | | | | 2.74 | [1.63–4.63]* | 1.75 | [1.00–3.08]* |
| Age 23 | | | | | 2.84 | [1.67–4.83]* | 1.75 | [0.98–3.11] |
| Age 24 | | | | | 2.51 | [1.48–4.26]* | 1.51 | [0.85–2.67] |
| Age 25 | | | | | 2.90 | [1.73–4.86]* | 1.73 | [0.99–3.02] |
| Age 26 | | | | | 3.36 | [1.97–5.71]* | 1.98 | [1.12–3.51]* |
| Age 27 | | | | | 3.33 | [1.96–5.65]* | 1.89 | [1.07–3.35]* |
| Age 28 | | | | | 3.81 | [2.28–6.35]* | 2.24 | [1.29–3.90]* |
| Age 29 | | | | | 5.01 | [2.98–8.42]* | 2.80 | [1.60–4.92]* |
| Age 30 | | | | | 4.41 | [2.66–7.29]* | 2.55 | [1.48–4.41]* |
| Age 31 | | | | | 4.60 | [2.72–7.77]* | 2.45 | [1.39–4.33]* |
| Age 32 | | | | | 4.73 | [2.83–7.92]* | 2.67 | [1.53–4.66]* |

Table 3: Continued.

| Parameter | Model 1 | | Model 2 | | Model 3 | | Model 4 | |
|---|---|---|---|---|---|---|---|---|
| | OR | 95% CI | OR | 95% CI | OR | 95% CI | OR | 95% CI |
| Age 33 | | | | | 5.91 | [3.49–9.99]* | 3.20 | [1.81–5.64]* |
| Age 34 | | | | | 4.96 | [2.91–8.43]* | 2.76 | [1.56–4.89]* |
| Age 35 | | | | | 4.90 | [2.94–8.17]* | 2.64 | [1.52–4.60]* |
| Age 36 | | | | | 4.29 | [2.51–7.33]* | 2.33 | [1.31–4.15]* |
| Age 37 | | | | | 5.37 | [3.15–9.15]* | 2.93 | [1.65–5.22]* |
| Age 38 | | | | | 4.29 | [2.54–7.25]* | 2.25 | [1.27–3.96]* |
| Age 39 | | | | | 5.37 | [3.13–9.23]* | 2.84 | [1.59–5.08]* |
| Age 40 | | | | | 3.96 | [2.35–6.67]* | 2.17 | [1.24–3.82]* |
| Age 41 | | | | | 5.26 | [3.05–9.07]* | 2.79 | [1.55–5.01]* |
| Age 42 | | | | | 4.21 | [2.45–7.21]* | 2.14 | [1.20–3.83]* |
| Age 43 | | | | | 4.64 | [2.58–8.34]* | 2.38 | [1.28–4.46]* |
| Age 44 | | | | | 4.57 | [2.58–8.10]* | 2.38 | [1.29–4.38]* |
| Age 45 | | | | | 3.66 | [2.13–6.27]* | 1.82 | [1.02–3.25]* |
| Age 46 | | | | | 3.26 | [1.80–5.89]* | 1.64 | [0.88–3.08] |
| Age 47 | | | | | 3.57 | [1.97–6.45]* | 1.84 | [0.98–3.46] |
| Age 48 | | | | | 3.18 | [1.80–5.63]* | 1.60 | [0.87–2.96] |
| Age 49 | | | | | 4.62 | [2.57–8.30]* | 2.34 | [1.25–4.37]* |
| Age 50 | | | | | 1.69 | [0.92–3.11] | 0.85 | [0.44–1.62] |
| Age 51 | | | | | 2.87 | [1.52–5.39]* | 1.44 | [0.74–2.81] |
| Age 52 | | | | | 3.03 | [1.67–5.51]* | 1.54 | [0.82–2.92] |
| Age 53 | | | | | 2.75 | [1.39–5.47]* | 1.41 | [0.69–2.90] |
| Age 54 | | | | | 2.07 | [1.06–4.04]* | 1.11 | [0.55–2.24] |
| Age 55 | | | | | 1.50 | [0.72–3.11] | 0.77 | [0.36–1.65] |
| Age 56 | | | | | 1.67 | [0.82–3.43] | 0.81 | [0.38–1.72] |
| Age 57 | | | | | 2.20 | [1.06–4.58]* | 1.13 | [0.53–2.44] |
| Age 58 | | | | | 1.93 | [0.95–3.92] | 0.99 | [0.47–2.09] |
| Age 59 | | | | | 1.51 | [0.66–3.47] | 0.74 | [0.31–1.75] |
| *Marital status (Ref: Never)* | | | | | | | | |
| Married/living together | | | | | 1.65 | [1.36–2.00]* | 2.00 | [1.61–2.47]* |
| Widowed | | | | | 8.12 | [6.39–10.31]* | 7.18 | [5.61–9.19]* |
| Divorced/separated | | | | | 3.74 | [3.02–4.63]* | 3.22 | [2.58–4.02]* |
| *Sex of respondent (Ref: Men)* | | | | | | | | |
| Women | | | | | 1.16 | [1.05–1.27]* | 1.73 | [1.55–1.93]* |
| *Model 4: Sexual Practices* | | | | | | | | |
| *Drunk alcohol (Ref: No)* | | | | | | | | |
| Drunk | | | | | | | 1.23 | [1.10–1.37]* |
| Not applicable | | | | | | | 0.26 | [0.01–4.89] |
| *Used condom (Ref: No)* | | | | | | | | |
| Used condom | | | | | | | 2.34 | [2.02–2.71]* |
| Not applicable | | | | | | | 6.22 | [0.34–115.28] |
| *Sexual partners (Ref: 1 partner)* | | | | | | | | |
| 2–4 partners | | | | | | | 2.08 | [1.82–2.38]* |
| >4 partners | | | | | | | 3.76 | [3.19–4.42]* |
| Not applicable | | | | | | | 0.99 | [0.68–1.44] |
| *HIV/AIDS Knowledge (Ref: No)* | | | | | | | | |
| Lowest knowledge | | | | | | | 1.12 | [0.79–1.58] |
| Medium knowledge | | | | | | | 1.11 | [0.82–1.52] |
| Highest knowledge | | | | | | | 1.38 | [1.02–1.87]* |

TABLE 3: Continued.

| Parameter | Model 1 | | Model 2 | | Model 3 | | Model 4 | |
|---|---|---|---|---|---|---|---|---|
| | OR | 95% CI | OR | 95% CI | OR | 95% CI | OR | 95% CI |
| *Random Effects* | | | | | | | | |
| Cluster variance | 0.566 | 0.049* | 0.385 | 0.039* | 0.365 | 0.039* | 0.318 | 0.036* |
| Units: Cluster | 887 | | 887 | | 887 | | 887 | |
| Units: Individual | 39766 | | 39766 | | 39766 | | 39766 | |
| Estimation: | IGLS (MQL1) | | IGLS (PQL2) | | IGLS (PQL2) | | IGLS (PQL2) | |

OR: odds ratios; 95% CI: confidence intervals. *Statistical significance at 5% level, $P < 0.05$.

TABLE 4: Odds ratios (OR) of HIV prevalence in rural and urban areas, UAIS, 2004-2005 and 2011.

| Parameter | Rural | | | | Urban | | | |
|---|---|---|---|---|---|---|---|---|
| | Model 1 | | Model 2 | | Model 1 | | Model 2 | |
| | OR | 95% CI | OR | 95% CI | OR | 95% CI | OR | 95% CI |
| *Fixed effects* | | | | | | | | |
| Constant | 0.05 | [0.04–0.06]* | 0.00 | [0.00-0.00]* | 0.21 | [0.15–0.29]* | 0.02 | [0.01–0.03]* |
| *Model 1: Socio-economic factors* | | | | | | | | |
| *Wealth status (Ref: Lowest quintile)* | | | | | | | | |
| Second | 1.04 | [0.88–1.23] | 1.06 | [0.89–1.26] | 1.18 | [0.92–1.52] | 1.13 | [0.87–1.46] |
| Middle | 1.01 | [0.85–1.20] | 1.05 | [0.88–1.25] | 1.15 | [0.88–1.50] | 1.18 | [0.89–1.55] |
| Fourth | 1.13 | [0.95–1.34] | 1.17 | [0.98–1.39] | 0.88 | [0.66–1.18] | 0.89 | [0.66–1.21] |
| Highest | 1.17 | [0.98–1.40] | 1.23 | [1.02–1.47]* | 0.87 | [0.64–1.19] | 0.99 | [0.71–1.36] |
| *Education (Ref: No education)* | | | | | | | | |
| Incomplete primary | 0.91 | [0.79–1.04] | 1.15 | [0.99–1.33] | 0.67 | [0.48–0.92]* | 0.93 | [0.66–1.32] |
| Complete primary | 1.04 | [0.87–1.24] | 1.30 | [1.08–1.57]* | 0.54 | [0.37–0.78]* | 0.73 | [0.49–1.07] |
| Incomplete secondary | 0.68 | [0.57–0.82]* | 1.07 | [0.88–1.30] | 0.35 | [0.25–0.49]* | 0.64 | [0.45–0.93]* |
| Complete secondary & higher | 0.63 | [0.45–0.87]* | 0.83 | [0.59–1.17] | 0.25 | [0.17–0.38]* | 0.43 | [0.28–0.67]* |
| Missing | 1.05 | [0.23–4.84] | 1.21 | [0.26–5.71] | 1.27 | [0.12–13.37] | 2.49 | [0.21–29.13] |
| *Model 2: Socio-demographic factors* | | | | | | | | |
| *Age of respondents (Ref: 45–59 years)* | | | | | | | | |
| 15–24 years | | | 1.12 | [0.91–1.37] | | | 0.89 | [0.63–1.27] |
| 25–34 years | | | 1.80 | [1.54–2.12]* | | | 1.46 | [1.08–1.96]* |
| 35–44 years | | | 1.90 | [1.62–2.22]* | | | 1.53 | [1.13–2.07]* |
| *Current marital status (Ref: Never been in union)* | | | | | | | | |
| Married/living together | | | 2.28 | [1.75–2.97]* | | | 2.03 | [1.45–2.83]* |
| Widowed | | | 8.75 | [6.47–11.83]* | | | 6.14 | [3.97–9.49]* |
| Divorced/separated | | | 3.92 | [2.97–5.16]* | | | 2.97 | [2.09–4.21]* |
| *Sex of respondent (Ref: Men)* | | | | | | | | |
| Women | | | 1.61 | [1.42–1.82]* | | | 2.13 | [1.71–2.64]* |
| *Time in years (Ref: 2004-05)* | | | | | | | | |
| 2011 | | | 1.33 | [1.14–1.54]* | | | 0.97 | [0.78–1.21] |
| *Random effects* | | | | | | | | |
| Cluster variance | 0.584 | 0.058* | 0.487 | 0.053* | 0.175 | 0.052* | 0.162 | 0.052* |
| Clusters | 719 | | 719 | | 168 | | 168 | |
| Individuals | 32506 | | 32506 | | 7260 | | 7260 | |

OR: odds ratios; 95% CI: confidence intervals. *Statistical significance at 5% level, $P < 0.05$.

The association between household wealth status and HIV infection was explained by current marital status. For example, when education, ethnicity, rural-urban place of residence, time (2004-2005 and 2011), and age were controlled for, the odds ratio for the highest wealth quintile was not significant. However, when current marital status was considered, the odds ratio for the highest wealth quintile increased to 1.21 [1.03–1.42], suggesting marital practices of wealthy people influence their vulnerability to HIV infection. This is consistent with the literature showing that relatively

TABLE 5: Odds ratios of HIV prevalence showing significant interactions with place of residence, UAIS, 2004-2005 and 2011.

| Parameter | Model 1 | | Model 2 | | Model 3 | |
|---|---|---|---|---|---|---|
| | OR | 95% CI | OR | 95% CI | OR | 95% CI |
| *Fixed effects* | | | | | | |
| Constant | 0.09 | [0.08–0.10]* | 0.20 | [0.13–0.29]* | 0.01 | [0.00–0.03]* |
| *Model 1: Place of residence* | | | | | | |
| *Place of residence (Ref: Urban)* | | | | | | |
| Rural | 0.58 | [0.50–0.68]* | 0.45 | [0.28–0.71]* | 0.30 | [0.10–0.90]* |
| *Model 2: Socio-economic factors* | | | | | | |
| *Wealth status (Ref: Lowest)* | | | | | | |
| Second | | | 1.14 | [0.88–1.47] | 1.20 | [0.91–1.57] |
| Middle | | | 1.12 | [0.85–1.46] | 1.27 | [0.95–1.69] |
| Fourth | | | 0.86 | [0.64–1.16] | 0.98 | [0.71–1.34] |
| Highest | | | 0.85 | [0.62–1.17] | 1.05 | [0.75–1.47] |
| Second. Rural | | | 0.88 | [0.65–1.18] | 0.84 | [0.61–1.16] |
| Middle. Rural | | | 0.85 | [0.62–1.17] | 0.77 | [0.55–1.07] |
| Fourth. Rural | | | 1.22 | [0.87–1.70] | 1.10 | [0.77–1.58] |
| Highest. Rural | | | 1.28 | [0.89–1.83] | 1.08 | [0.73–1.59] |
| *Education (Ref: No education)* | | | | | | |
| Incomplete primary | | | 0.68 | [0.49–0.93]* | 0.95 | [0.67–1.35] |
| Complete primary | | | 0.54 | [0.38–0.78]* | 0.75 | [0.50–1.11] |
| Incomplete secondary | | | 0.36 | [0.26–0.50]* | 0.66 | [0.45–0.95]* |
| Complete secondary & higher | | | 0.26 | [0.17–0.38]* | 0.42 | [0.27–0.65]* |
| Missing | | | 1.11 | [0.10–12.23] | 3.04 | [0.27–34.38] |
| Incomplete primary. Rural | | | 1.30 | [0.92–1.84] | 1.15 | [0.79–1.70] |
| Complete primary. Rural | | | 1.83 | [1.22–2.73]* | 1.64 | [1.06–2.55]* |
| Incomplete secondary. Rural | | | 1.85 | [1.27–2.69]* | 1.55 | [1.02–2.37]* |
| Complete secondary & higher. Rural | | | 2.41 | [1.46–3.99]* | 1.91 | [1.10–3.33]* |
| Missing. Rural | | | 1.00 | [0.06–16.57] | 0.43 | [0.02–7.63] |
| *Ethnicity (Ref: Baganda)* | | | | | | |
| Banyankole/Bakiga | | | 1.43 | [1.07–1.91]* | 1.64 | [1.21–2.24]* |
| Iteso/Karimojong | | | 1.41 | [0.94–2.12] | 1.74 | [1.14–2.67]* |
| Lubgbara/Madi | | | 1.17 | [0.75–1.82] | 1.53 | [0.94–2.48] |
| Basoga | | | 1.11 | [0.79–1.57] | 1.14 | [0.79–1.64] |
| Langi/Acholi | | | 1.52 | [1.02–2.27]* | 2.03 | [1.33–3.08]* |
| Bagisu/Sabiny | | | 1.19 | [0.71–1.98] | 1.02 | [0.59–1.77] |
| Alur/Japadhola | | | 0.79 | [0.46–1.35] | 1.00 | [0.57–1.74] |
| Banyoro/Batoro | | | 1.60 | [1.12–2.27]* | 1.62 | [1.11–2.37]* |
| All others | | | 0.94 | [0.68–1.29] | 1.16 | [0.83–1.62] |
| Banyankole/Bakiga. Rural | | | 0.62 | [0.44–0.89]* | 0.71 | [0.49–1.04] |
| Iteso/Karimojong. Rural | | | 0.35 | [0.22–0.56]* | 0.36 | [0.22–0.59]* |
| Lubgbara/Madi. Rural | | | 0.26 | [0.15–0.44]* | 0.26 | [0.14–0.46]* |
| Basoga.Rural | | | 0.51 | [0.33–0.79]* | 0.50 | [0.32–0.78]* |
| Langi/Acholi. Rural | | | 0.60 | [0.38–0.96]* | 0.55 | [0.34–0.90]* |
| Bagisu/Sabiny. Rural | | | 0.48 | [0.27–0.87]* | 0.56 | [0.30–1.05] |
| Alur/Japadhola. Rural | | | 0.80 | [0.44–1.48] | 0.68 | [0.36–1.29] |
| Banyoro/Batoro. Rural | | | 0.64 | [0.42–1.00] | 0.66 | [0.42–1.04] |
| All others. Rural | | | 0.74 | [0.51–1.09] | 0.67 | [0.45–1.00] |
| *Time in years (Ref: 2004-05)* | | | | | | |
| UG6 (2011) | | | 0.96 | [0.75–1.23] | 1.00 | [0.78–1.29] |
| UG6.Rural | | | 1.29 | [0.98–1.71] | 1.26 | [0.95–1.67] |

TABLE 5: Continued.

| Parameter | Model 1 | | Model 2 | | Model 3 | |
|---|---|---|---|---|---|---|
| | OR | 95% CI | OR | 95% CI | OR | 95% CI |
| *Model 3: Socio-demographic factors* | | | | | | |
| *Age of respondent (45–59 years)* | | | | | | |
| 15–24 years | | | | | 0.89 | [0.62–1.28] |
| 25–34 years | | | | | 1.42 | [1.05–1.92]* |
| 35–44 years | | | | | 1.50 | [1.10–2.04]* |
| 15–24 years. Rural | | | | | 1.27 | [0.84–1.91] |
| 25–34 years. Rural | | | | | 1.27 | [0.90–1.78] |
| 35–44 years. Rural | | | | | 1.24 | [0.88–1.76] |
| *Sex of respondent (Ref: Men)* | | | | | | |
| Women | | | | | 2.18 | [1.75–2.71]* |
| Women. Rural | | | | | 0.74 | [0.57–0.95]* |
| *Marital status (Ref: Never been married)* | | | | | | |
| Married/living together | | | | | 2.02 | [1.44–2.84]* |
| Widowed | | | | | 6.22 | [3.99–9.68]* |
| Divorced/separated | | | | | 2.99 | [2.09–4.27]* |
| Married/living together. Rural | | | | | 1.14 | [0.75–1.75] |
| Widowed. Rural | | | | | 1.36 | [0.80–2.32] |
| Divorced/separated. Rural | | | | | 1.29 | [0.82–2.02] |
| *Drunk with alcohol before risky sex (Ref: No)* | | | | | | |
| Drunk | | | | | 1.54 | [1.22–1.95]* |
| Not applicable | | | | | 0.69 | [0.03–14.80] |
| Drunk. Rural | | | | | 0.78 | [0.60–1.02] |
| Not applicable. Rural | | | | | 0.32 | [0.00–24.69] |
| *Condom use during risky sex (Ref: No)* | | | | | | |
| Used condom | | | | | 1.91 | [1.48–2.47]* |
| Not applicable | | | | | 1.99 | [0.09–42.92] |
| Used condom. Rural | | | | | 1.34 | [0.98–1.83] |
| Not applicable. Rural | | | | | 3.78 | [0.05–291.30] |
| *Multiple sexual partners (Ref: 1 sex partner)* | | | | | | |
| 2–4 partners | | | | | 1.97 | [1.47–2.64]* |
| >4 partners | | | | | 3.55 | [2.54–4.95]* |
| Not applicable | | | | | 0.50 | [0.25–1.02] |
| 2–4 partners.Rural | | | | | 1.09 | [0.78–1.51] |
| >4 partners. Rural | | | | | 1.10 | [0.75–1.61] |
| Not applicable. Rural | | | | | 1.89 | [0.84–4.25] |
| *AIDS knowledge (Ref: No knowledge)* | | | | | | |
| Lowest knowledge | | | | | 0.66 | [0.29–1.52] |
| Medium knowledge | | | | | 0.77 | [0.37–1.61] |
| Highest knowledge | | | | | 0.89 | [0.43–1.83] |
| Lowest knowledge. Rural | | | | | 1.82 | [0.73–4.54] |
| Medium knowledge. Rural | | | | | 1.47 | [0.65–3.31] |
| Highest knowledge. Rural | | | | | 1.61 | [0.73–3.57] |
| *Random effects* | | | | | | |
| Constant | 0.478 | 0.044* | 0.363 | 0.035* | 0.293 | 0.035* |
| Cluster | 887 | | 887 | | 887 | |
| Individual | 39766 | | 39766 | | 39766 | |

OR: odds ratios; 95% CI: confidence intervals. *Statistical significance at 5% level, $P < 0.05$.

rich people or those living in wealthy households and having a higher rate of partner change, a phenomenon associated with relative autonomy and mobility, increased the vulnerability of such individuals to HIV infection [4, 5, 51].

Patterns from bivariate analysis provide no evidence of a significant association between wealth and HIV infection (Table 1), but the analysis by urban rural residence (Figure 1) suggests a positive gradient in rural areas and a negative one in urban areas. Although there was no evidence that the effect of wealth on vulnerability to HIV infection varied significantly by time, gender, or urban/rural residence based on interaction effects (Table 5), the analysis by urban/rural residence (Table 4) provides evidence of a positive association between wealth and HIV prevalence only in rural areas, consistent with patterns observed in other SSA settings (e.g., [44, 45]).

The positive wealth-HIV gradient observed in this research supports recent evidence by (e.g., [50]) using DHS data from 8 sub-Saharan African countries demonstrating wealth as an important driver of HIV infections in SSA. This reenforcement of evidence necessitates a shift in thinking and action aimed at preventing HIV infections. It is important to create HIV/AIDS awareness based on identified social and sexual practices that increase the vulnerability of wealthy people or those who live in wealthy households to HIV infections. Strategies for creating awareness targeting marital practices, multiple sexual partnership practices of, alcoholism, among other practices, by wealthy people, may specifically need to be prioritized. Nevertheless, it is important to recognize that since HIV prevalence depends on both HIV incidence and survival rates of those infected, the higher prevalence among those who are wealthier could be partly attributable to them living longer with the condition.

*5.2. Educational Attainment.* Higher educational attainment was consistently negatively associated with HIV prevalence. Overall, people with higher education were 37% less likely to be HIV-positive compared to those of similar other characteristics with no education. The education effect was stronger for those in urban than rural areas (Table 4). These findings (i.e., that people who had higher education were generally less likely to be infected) are in line with previous research (e.g., [9, 10, 48, 52, 53]).

The protective benefits of educational attainment were greater for people in urban areas than those in rural areas which had nonsignificant findings (Table 4). The greater benefit urbanites derive from education may be due to several factors. Kelly has suggested that education reduces vulnerability to HIV infection by enhancing self-protection, fostering the development of a value system, and adoption and promotion of behaviors that lower vulnerability to HIV risk [54]. For gender, the effect of educational attainment in reducing vulnerability was not significantly different between women and men (interaction effect not significant) once other significant factors were controlled for, but bivariate analysis showed interesting patterns. While men with secondary or higher education had the lowest HIV prevalence, for women, HIV prevalence was lowest among those with no education in 2004-2005 (Table 1). The apparent edge educated men enjoy over women is possibly due to their better access to other resources resulting from their "privileged" status in society [5].

*5.3. Community Effects.* The 9% residual variance apportioned to the community-level could be due to several factors. First, the improved road transport networks and the development of trading centres or urbanization. Proximity to a centre of development has been linked to increased vulnerability to HIV infection in SSA [18, 20, 55]. The community effect was observed to be stronger in rural than urban areas, consistent with patterns observed elsewhere [45]. In Uganda, rural residents with higher SES are more likely to frequent trading centres (periurban areas) to drink alcohol, to shop, and generally to socialize.

The unobserved community-level effects on vulnerability to HIV infection implies that, besides individual and household level characteristics, contextual factors also influence vulnerability to HIV infection (e.g., [20, 21]). It is thus pertinent that efforts to prevent HIV focus on the wider contextual factors that shape household factors and individual-level practices (e.g., [22, 23]). Community factors such cultural practices, health infrastructure, poverty and wealth, education, sexual violence and gender issues, and legal-policy and other institutional issues merit attention in this regard.

## 6. Conclusion

This research set out to examine the association between SES and HIV infection in Uganda. This research found significant positive associations between household wealth status and HIV infection at the population level, in rural areas, and among women. However, higher educational attainment was negatively associated with being infected with HIV at the population level, among women and men, in urban areas, and in 2011. Overall, secondary or higher education was associated with reduced vulnerability to HIV infection by 37%, compared to no education.

The second objective was to examine whether the SES-HIV relationship varies by gender, rural-urban place of residence, and time (2004-5 and 2011) in Uganda. This research found no evidence of significant interaction between wealth and gender and rural/urban residence. There was also no significant interaction between wealth and time in 2004-2005 and 2011. For education, there was a significant interaction with rural/urban residence which showed that secondary or higher education was less protective among rural compared to urban residents.

The general lessons from this study with respect to the relationship between wealth and HIV prevalence relate to the complex and context specific nature of the relationship. While studies elsewhere in sub-Saharan Africa have highlighted clear gender differences, suggesting increased vulnerability of poor women, the analysis for Uganda presented here provides no evidence of significant gender differences in the relationship between SES and HIV prevalence. This may be attributable to the fact that some of the factors responsible for an apparent relationship are already considered (e.g., increased vulnerability among women in women headed households accounting for the disadvantaged socioeconomic status of women) or may indeed reflect the context specific nature of the relationship.

The research also examined the effect of community-level factors on vulnerability to HIV infection. This research found that 9% of the residual variance could be attributable to the community environment, with the effect being substantially higher in rural than urban areas. About 5% of the total unexplained variance in HIV infection in urban areas was attributable to unobserved community-level factors, compared to 13% of unexplained variance in rural areas.

These findings call for policies to support people to attain higher education as a strategy to effectively prevent HIV infections; attainment of secondary or higher education provides prospects for multiple benefits ranging from knowledge, attitudes and capabilities, aspects that are transformable into economic resources. Education is also an avenue to achieve general social transformation that would influence a range of development aspects linked to health. Focusing attention on Uganda's education is particularly urgent given astounding evidence showing its gradual decline at primary level [56, 57]. Development attention also needs to be paid to the rural social environments, areas which substantially account for the greatest social influence in the construction of HIV vulnerability and which account for the increasing HIV prevalence in Uganda.

Further, these findings show that there are factors at the community level that influence vulnerability to the risk of HIV infection, evidence which justifies a focus of interventions on both individual and community factors such as sexual relationships, cultural norms, beliefs, and attitudes, socioeconomic status, availability of good health services, and religious values, among others. The findings validate and reenforce the need for community-level programme interventions including community HIV/AIDS education and making health services including those for HIV/AIDS accessible. Given the limited success of individually oriented HIV programme interventions in preventing HIV infection, an appreciation of the need to change approach is overdue.

These findings need to be interpreted bearing in mind the fact these were cross-sectional surveys which make it inappropriate to infer causality. This is because these surveys use prevalence estimates which do not reveal whether observed associations existed before infection or infection preceded the observations. Since antiretroviral therapy became widely available in SSA, people living with HIV can live longer for up to 10 or more years following the progression of HIV to AIDS (e.g., [33]). The increased survival rates and decreased mortality rates have thus contributed to increased HIV prevalence [31–33, 58].

Nevertheless, by testing respondents for HIV, these surveys establish objective measures of HIV prevalence which allow for an accurate measurement of associations with HIV. Further, higher HIV prevalence among people in wealthy households could be due to longer survival, a phenomenon known to influence prevalence. This research used data from Uganda's only 2 AIS, which limited the ability of the research to determine the trend of these associations over a longer period. Future research needs to track these trends over a longer period. As much as associations based on residential areas were observed, there was limited data to determine spatial distribution of cases, an aspect which future research also needs to address.

Notwithstanding the above limitations, this research, which was part of a bigger research for PhD in Sociology [59], supports research evidence reported elsewhere in SSA and it is the first multilevel modelling to demonstrate the effect of community factors and vulnerability to HIV infection in Uganda. Besides individual and household factors, community factors also influence vulnerability to the risk of HIV in Uganda. HIV/AIDS awareness targeting sexual practices of individuals in wealthy households and those with primary educational attainment together with improving educational attainment in Uganda and addressing contextual factors influencing vulnerability to HIV infection are necessary strategies to prevent HIV infections in Uganda. Given that these surveys are nationally representative; these findings are generalizable to the whole of Uganda and perhaps beyond.

## Disclosure

Patrick Igulot is a Lecturer in Health and Social Care at the University of Sunderland in London, UK. Monica A. Magadi is a Professor of Social Research at the University of Hull, UK.

## Authors' Contributions

Patrick Igulot conceptualized the study, performed analysis, and drafted the article. Monica A. Magadi provided technical guidance to the conceptualization and analysis and revised the draft paper. Both authors approved the final draft of the article.

## Conflicts of Interest

The authors have no conflicts of interest to declare.

## Acknowledgments

MEASURE DHS and Ministry of Health, Uganda, are acknowledged for providing access to the data analysed in this research and City, University of London is acknowledged for providing a 3-year full Ph.D. studentship to the primary author. Lastly, the authors thank participants at the Annual Conference of British Society for Population Studies, University of Winchester, 2014, who gave feedback to the initial draft of this manuscript.

## References

[1] J. G. Fortson, "The gradient in sub-saharan Africa: socioeconomic status and HIV/AIDS," *Demography*, vol. 45, no. 2, pp. 303–322, 2008.

[2] J. O. Parkhurst, "Understanding the correlations between wealth, poverty and human immunodeficiency virus infection in African countries," *Bulletin of the World Health Organization*, vol. 88, no. 7, pp. 519–526, 2010.

[3] A. M. Fox, "The HIV-poverty thesis RE-examined: Poverty, wealth or inequality as a social determinant of hiv infection in sub-Saharan Africa?" *Journal of Biosocial Science*, vol. 44, no. 4, pp. 459–480, 2012.

[4] S. Gillespie, R. Greener, A. Whiteside, and J. Whitworth, "Investigating the empirical evidence for understanding vulnerability and the associations between poverty, HIV infection and AIDS impact," *AIDS*, vol. 21, p. S1, 2007.

[5] W. M. Msisha, S. H. Kapiga, F. Earls, and S. V. Subramanian, "Socioeconomic status and HIV seroprevalence in Tanzania: a counterintuitive relationship," *International Journal of Epidemiology*, vol. 37, no. 6, pp. 1297–1303, 2008.

[6] D. Durevall and A. Lindskog, "Economic Inequality and HIV in Malawi," *World Development*, vol. 40, no. 7, pp. 1435–1451, 2012.

[7] J.-C. Fotso and B. Kuate-Defo, "Measuring socioeconomic status in health research in developing countries: should we be focusing on households, communities or both?" *Social Indicators Research*, vol. 72, no. 2, pp. 189–237, 2005.

[8] A. Whiteside, "Poverty and HIV/AIDS in Africa," *Third World Quarterly*, vol. 23, no. 2, pp. 313–332, 2002.

[9] N. Gupta and M. Mahy, "Sexual initiation among adolescent girls and boys: trends and differentials in sub-saharan Africa," *Archives of Sexual Behavior*, vol. 32, no. 1, pp. 41–53, 2003.

[10] J. R. Glynn, M. Carael, A. Buvé et al., "Does increased general schooling protect against HIV infection? A study in four African cities," *Tropical Medicine & International Health*, vol. 9, no. 1, pp. 4–14, 2004.

[11] D. Meekers and G. Ahmed, "Contemporary patterns of adolescent sexuality in urban Botswana," *Journal of Biosocial Science*, vol. 32, no. 4, pp. 467–485, 2000.

[12] T. Dinkelman, D. Lam, and M. Leibbrandt, "Household and community income, economic shocks and risky sexual behavior of young adults: Evidence from the Cape Area Panel Study 2002 and 2005," *AIDS*, vol. 21, no. 7, pp. S49–S56, 2007.

[13] L. Marteleto, D. Lam, and V. Ranchhod, "Sexual behavior, pregnancy, and schooling among young people in Urban South Africa," *Studies in Family Planning*, vol. 39, no. 4, pp. 351–368, 2008.

[14] M. A. Magadi, "Understanding the gender disparity in HIV infection across countries in sub-Saharan Africa: evidence from the demographic and Health Surveys," *Sociology of Health and Illness*, vol. 33, no. 4, pp. 522–539, 2011.

[15] D. de Walque, "How does the impact of an HIV/AIDS information campaign vary with educational attainment? Evidence from rural Uganda," *Journal of Development Economics*, vol. 84, no. 2, pp. 686–714, 2007.

[16] S. S. Zuilkowski and M. C. H. Jukes, "The impact of education on sexual behavior in sub-Saharan Africa: a review of the evidence," *AIDS Care*, vol. 24, no. 5, pp. 562–576, 2012.

[17] H. Bradley, A. Bedada, H. Brahmbhatt, A. Kidanu, D. Gillespie, and A. Tsui, "Educational attainment and HIV status among Ethiopian voluntary counseling and testing clients," *AIDS and Behavior*, vol. 11, no. 5, pp. 736–742, 2007.

[18] J. P. Messina, M. Emch, J. Muwonga et al., "Spatial and socio-behavioral patterns of HIV prevalence in the Democratic Republic of Congo," *Social Science & Medicine*, vol. 71, no. 8, pp. 1428–1435, 2010.

[19] N. J. Madise, A. K. Ziraba, J. Inungu et al., "Are slum dwellers at heightened risk of HIV infection than other urban residents? Evidence from population-based HIV prevalence surveys in Kenya," *Health & Place*, vol. 18, no. 5, pp. 1144–1152, 2012.

[20] S. S. Bloom, M. Urassa, R. Isingo, J. Ng'weshemi, and J. T. Boerma, "Community effects on the risk of HIV infection in rural Tanzania," *Sexually Transmitted Infections*, vol. 78, no. 4, pp. 261–266, 2002.

[21] M. M. Hillemeier, J. Lynch, S. Harper, and M. Casper, "Measuring contextual characteristics for community health," *Health Services Research*, vol. 38, no. 6p2, pp. 1645–1718, 2003.

[22] R. Stephenson, "Community factors shaping HIV-related stigma among young people in three African countries," *AIDS Care Psychological and Socio-medical Aspects of AIDS/HIV*, vol. 21, no. 4, pp. 403–410, 2009.

[23] F. N. Tiruneh, K.-Y. Chuang, P. A. M. Ntenda, and Y.-C. Chuang, "Individual-level and community-level determinants of cervical cancer screening among Kenyan women: A multilevel analysis of a Nationwide survey," *BMC Women's Health*, vol. 17, no. 1, article no. 109, 2017.

[24] P. Clarke, C. Crawford, F. Steele, and A. F. Vignoles, "The choice between fixed and random effects models: some considerations for educational research," 2010.

[25] P. Clarke, C. Crawford, F. Steele, and A. Vignoles, "Revisiting fixed- and random-effects models: some considerations for policy-relevant education research," *Education Economics*, vol. 23, no. 3, pp. 259–277, 2015.

[26] B. G. Link and J. Phelan, "Social conditions as fundamental causes of disease," *Journal of Health and Social Behavior*, vol. 35, pp. 80–94, 1995, Extra Issue: Forty Years of Medical Sociology: The State of the Art and Directions for the Future.

[27] D. M. Tuller, D. R. Bangsberg, J. Senkungu, N. C. Ware, N. Emenyonu, and S. D. Weiser, "Transportation costs impede sustained adherence and access to HAART in a clinic population in Southwestern Uganda: a qualitative study," *AIDS and Behavior*, vol. 14, no. 4, pp. 778–784, 2010.

[28] P. Duff, W. Kipp, T. C. Wild, T. Rubaale, and J. Okech-Ojony, "Barriers to accessing highly active antiretroviral therapy by HIV-positive women attending an antenatal clinic in a regional hospital in western Uganda," *Journal of the International AIDS Society*, vol. 13, no. 1, article 37, 2010.

[29] J. O. Parkhurst, "The Ugandan success story? Evidence and claims of HIV-1 prevention," *The Lancet*, vol. 360, no. 9326, pp. 78–80, 2002.

[30] Joint United Nations Programme on HIV/AIDS (UNAIDS), *Global Report: UNAIDS Report on the Global AIDS Epidemic 2013*, vol. 3, UNAIDS, Geneva, Switzerland, 2014.

[31] J. M. S. Granados, J. T. R. Amador, S. F. De Miguel et al., "Impact of highly active antiretroviral therapy on the morbidity and mortality in Spanish human immunodeficiency virus-infected children," *The Pediatric Infectious Disease Journal*, vol. 22, no. 10, pp. 863–868, 2003.

[32] T. C. Quinn, "HIV epidemiology and the effects of antiviral therapy on long-term consequences," *AIDS*, vol. 22, supplement 3, pp. S7–S12, 2008.

[33] J. Poorolajal, E. Hooshmand, H. Mahjub, N. Esmailnasab, and E. Jenabi, "Survival rate of AIDS disease and mortality in HIV-infected patients: a meta-analysis," *Public Health*, vol. 139, pp. 3–12, 2016.

[34] Y. Wang, F. Jin, Q. Wang, and Z. Suo, "Long-Term Survival of AIDS Patients Treated with only Traditional Chinese Medicine," *AIDS Research and Human Retroviruses*, vol. 33, no. 2, pp. 90–92, 2017.

[35] World Bank (WB), "The World Bank Annual Report," 2010.

[36] National Planning Authority [Uganda], "National development report 2010-2011 financial year," 2012.

[37] Uganda Bureau of Statistics (UBOS) and Macro International Inc, "Uganda Demographic and Health Survey, 2006," 2007.

[38] V. Mishra, M. Vaessen, J. T. Boerma et al., "HIV testing in national population-based surveys: experience from the demographic and health surveys," *Bulletin of the World Health Organization*, vol. 84, no. 7, pp. 537–545, 2006.

[39] Ministry of Health [Uganda] and ICF International, *Uganda AIDS Indicator Survey*, 2012.

[40] O. A. Uthman, T. Moradi, and S. Lawoko, "The independent contribution of individual-, neighbourhood-, and country-level socioeconomic position on attitudes towards intimate partner violence against women in sub-Saharan Africa: A multilevel model of direct and moderating effects," *Social Science & Medicine*, vol. 68, no. 10, pp. 1801–1809, 2009.

[41] S. O. Rutstein, K. Johnson, and O. Macro, "The DHS wealth index , ORC Macro," *MEASURE DHS*, 2004.

[42] S. Rutstein and S. Staveteig, "Making the demographic and health surveys wealth index comparable," Tech. Rep. 9, ICF International, Maryland, Md, USA, 2014.

[43] C. Rodrigo and S. Rajapakse, "HIV, poverty and women," *International Health*, vol. 2, no. 1, pp. 9–16, 2010.

[44] M. A. Magadi, "The disproportionate high risk of HIV infection among the urban poor in sub-Saharan Africa," *AIDS and Behavior*, vol. 17, no. 5, pp. 1645–1654, 2013.

[45] M. A. Magadi, "Understanding the urban–rural disparity in HIV and poverty nexus: the case of Kenya," *Journal of Public Health*, pp. 1–10, 2016.

[46] J. Rasbash, F. Steele, W. Browne, and H. Goldstein, *A User's Guide to MLwiN, v2. 10*, Centre for Multilevel Modelling, University of Bristol, Bristol, UK, 2009.

[47] P. Obalenskaya, *Attitudes towards family and marriage in time and context: using two British birth cohorts for comparison [Ph.D. in Sociology]*, City University, London, UK, 2012.

[48] C. Asiedu, E. Asiedu, and F. Owusu, "The socio-economic determinants of HIV/AIDS infection rates in Lesotho, Malawi, Swaziland and Zimbabwe," *Development Policy Review*, vol. 30, no. 3, pp. 305–326, 2012.

[49] R. Tarling, "Statistical modelling for social researchers: principles and practice, Taylor and Francis," 2008.

[50] V. Mishra, S. B.-V. Assche, R. Greener et al., "HIV infection does not disproportionately affect the poorer in sub-Saharan Africa," *AIDS*, vol. 21, no. 7, pp. S17–S28, 2007.

[51] S. N. Mavedzenge, R. Olson, A. M. Doyle, J. Changalucha, and D. A. Ross, "The epidemiology of HIV among young people in sub-Saharan Africa: know your local epidemic and its implications for prevention," *Journal of Adolescent Health*, vol. 49, no. 6, pp. 559–567, 2011.

[52] R. J. Magnani, A. M. Karim, L. A. Weiss, K. C. Bond, M. Lemba, and G. T. Morgan, "Reproductive health risk and protective factors among youth in Lusaka, Zambia," *Journal of Adolescent Health*, vol. 30, no. 1, pp. 76–86, 2002.

[53] T. Barnighausen, V. Hosegood, I. M. Timaeus, and M. L. Newell, "The socioeconomic determinants of HIV incidence: evidence from a longitudinal, population-based study in rural South Africa," *AIDS*, vol. 21, pp. S29–S38, 2007.

[54] M. J. Kelly, "What HIV/AIDS Can Do to Education, and what Education Can Do to HIV/AIDS, UN AIDS," 2000.

[55] C. Feldacker, S. T. Ennett, and I. Speizer, "It's not just who you are but where you live: an exploration of community influences on individual HIV status in rural Malawi," *Social Science & Medicine*, vol. 72, no. 5, pp. 717–725, 2011.

[56] S. Sumra and J. Mugo, "Are our children learning? Assessment of learning outcomes among children in Tanzania, Kenya and Uganda," 2012.

[57] S. Jones, Y. Schipper, S. Ruto, and R. Rajani, "Can your child read and count? Measuring learning outcomes in East Africa," *Journal of African Economies*, vol. 23, no. 5, pp. 643–672, 2014.

[58] A. Edmonds, M. Yotebieng, J. Lusiama et al., "The effect of highly active antiretroviral therapy on the survival of HIV-infected children in a resource-deprived setting: a cohort study," *PLoS Medicine*, vol. 8, no. 6, Article ID e1001044, 2011.

[59] P. Igulot, Vulnerability and risk to HIV infection in Uganda: multilevel modelling of Uganda AIDS Indicator Survey Data, (Unpublished Doctoral thesis), 2017.

# Mortality and Its Predictors among HIV Infected Patients Taking Antiretroviral Treatment in Ethiopia

**Mohammed Biset Ayalew**

*Department of Clinical Pharmacy, School of Pharmacy, College of Medicine and Health Sciences, University of Gondar, Gondar, Ethiopia*

Correspondence should be addressed to Mohammed Biset Ayalew; mb6767@gmail.com

Academic Editor: Patrice K. Nicholas

*Background.* Even though the benefit of antiretroviral therapy (ART) is well established, there is a regional variation in the extent of its benefit. The aim of this review is to highlight mortality and its predictors in Ethiopian adult HIV patients who were on ART. *Methods.* Relevant articles were searched on PubMed and Google Scholar databases. The search terms used in different combinations were predictor/determinant/factors, mortality/death/survival, HIV, ART/HAART, and Ethiopia. *Result.* 5–40.8% of the patients died during the follow-up period. More than half (50–68.8%) of the deaths occurred within 6 months of initiating ART. Advanced stage disease (stage III and stage IV), nonworking functional status (bedridden and ambulatory), low baseline CD4 count, low baseline hemoglobin level, TB coinfection, lower baseline weight, and poor treatment adherence were commonly identified as predictors of death in HIV patients. *Conclusion.* 5–40.8% of HIV patients in Ethiopia die in 2–5 years of initiating antiretroviral treatment. Most of the deaths in HIV patients occur early in the course of treatment. Special emphasis should be given for patients with advanced stage disease, nonworking functional status, low baseline CD4 count, low baseline hemoglobin level, TB coinfection, lower baseline weight, and poor treatment adherence.

## 1. Introduction

HIV/AIDS is among the primary public health challenges that have affected the world's social, economic, and political system in the recent past. During the last three decades, millions of people died due to HIV infection. In the year 2012, more than 1.6 million AIDS deaths were recorded [1]. The burden of the disease is very high in the sub-Saharan African region. Even though only 12.5% of the world's population is living in this region, about 68% of the world's HIV infected population is found there [2]. According to a 2013 report, the sub-Saharan African region covers 74% of HIV-related deaths [3]. Ethiopia, as one of the sub-Saharan region countries, has one of the largest populations of HIV infected people in the world [4]. There are about 1.2 million HIV infected people in Ethiopia. An estimated prevalence of HIV/AIDS in the adult Ethiopian population is 2.4% with the incidence rate of 0.29% [5].

The introduction of antiretroviral therapy (ART) significantly improved the survival of HIV patients [6] and changed HIV infection from a fatal illness to a manageable chronic disease [7]. ART suppresses viral replication, restores immune function, reduces HIV associated morbidity and mortality, increases quality of life, and prolongs survival [1]. Because of these benefits of ART, there is a high effort globally to increase its coverage. As a result, access to ART was improved even in resource constrained countries. Ethiopia has been also struggling on the scale-up of ART in order to increase its access to all people with HIV/AIDS. ART was introduced in Ethiopia as a subsidized, fee-based scheme in 2003 and two years later (in 2005) it was made freely available. Furthermore, in 2006, the service was decentralized to health centers which facilitated the rapid expansion of the ART program throughout the country [8].

Even though the benefit of ART for people living with HIV/AIDS in terms of improving quality of life and reducing morbidity and mortality is well established, there is a regional variation in the extent of its benefit. A significant number of mortalities in HIV patients were also recorded within a few years of starting ART. This early mortality is higher in resource constrained settings. A high rate of early mortality was reported from a number of sub-Saharan African ART programs [9–11]. Different factors were attributed in various studies to the occurrence of death in patients who already started their ART. There are various studies conducted in Ethiopia to determine the mortality rate and its determinants in HIV patients who started ART. Summarizing the findings from these studies will show the overall picture of mortality in HIV patients who are on ART in Ethiopia and the main contributing factors to death. Better knowledge of factors/predictors of mortality is essential as it allows closer follow-up and facilitates targeted interventions in patients who have a higher risk; as a result, mortality will be reduced [11–13]. So, the aim of this study is to determine the overall mortality rate in adult HIV patients who were already on ART and summarize the main predictors of mortality in these patient groups in Ethiopia.

## 2. Methods

*2.1. Search Strategy.* Studies conducted on mortality and its predictors among HIV patients who had started ART were searched on PubMed and Google Scholar databases. Additional articles were also obtained from the reference lists of retrieved articles and manual Google search. Retrospective cohort studies conducted on adult HIV patients in Ethiopia and written in English language were included. No restriction was applied on the year of publication. The following search terms were used in different combinations: mortality/death/survival, HIV, ART/HAART, predictor/determinant/factors, and Ethiopia.

*2.2. Article Selection.* Studies were included in this review if they assess mortality and factors associated with it among HIV infected patients taking antiretroviral treatment in Ethiopia. Studies which were conducted on pediatric populations and those studies which include HIV patients who did not start ART were excluded.

*2.3. Assessment of Methodological Quality.* Included studies were critically appraised by using the "STROBE Checklist" [14]. The checklist has 22 items which state the standards to be included in the cohort study. Values of 0, 1, and 2 were given for each study against each item: 0 means the study did not satisfy the criteria mentioned by that particular item, 1 means it partially fulfilled the criteria, and 2 means the study completely addresses the issue mentioned by the item. So, a single study was scored out of the maximum total value of 44 and expressed in terms of percentage. An article with a total score of 90% and more was considered to be of high quality, 75–89% indicated medium quality, and below 75% was considered as low quality.

*2.4. Data Abstraction.* Relevant information was obtained from the 17 studies by using a data extraction form. Author, year of publication, study area, study subjects, sample size, study design, median follow-up period, mortality incidence density/100 person-years (PY), mortality during the full follow-up period and at 3, 6, and 12 months, and factors affecting mortality with respective odds ratio (OR) were recorded in data abstraction format.

## 3. Result

*3.1. Literature Search Results.* A total of 217 articles were obtained from database (PubMed and Google Scholar) search, out of which 132 were duplicates. After screening the titles and abstracts of 85 studies, 69 were excluded. Two additional articles were obtained from reference lists of retrieved articles and one article was found to be of no importance after its full text was assessed. Finally, 17 articles were selected to be included in this review. The details of the article selection process are indicated in Figure 1.

*3.2. Methodological Quality of Included Studies.* After evaluation of each study against STROBE Checklist [14], fourteen studies were found to be of high quality and the remaining 3 were of medium quality. There was no significant difference in the mortality rate between the high and medium quality studies.

*3.3. Study Characteristics.* All of the studies included in this review were retrospective cohort studies conducted on adult HIV patients. A total of 19321 (range = 272–4210) study participants were included in the 17 studies reviewed. The detailed description of individual study characteristics is shown in Table 1.

*3.4. Mortality.* The included studies followed up patients for a median of 25–60 months with an average of 38.8 months of follow-up. As indicated in Table 2, 5%–40.8% of the patients died during the follow-up period. Most of the studies (82%) reported that 5–15% of the patients died within the follow-up period. The highest death rate recorded was 40.8% from Debremarkos General Hospital, while the minimum was 5% from South Gondar Zone. All of the studies which reported death rates at different points of follow-up indicated that more than half of the deaths occurred within 6 months of initiating ART. The mortality incidence density ranged from 0.2 to 10.74 per 100 person-years. Majority of the studies reported an incidence density of 1.89–5.3 per 100 person-years.

*3.5. Predictors of Mortality.* Among the demographic and clinical characteristics mentioned as a predictor for death in the reviewed studies, the most frequently mentioned were advanced stage disease (stage III and stage IV), nonworking functional status (bedridden and ambulatory), low CD4

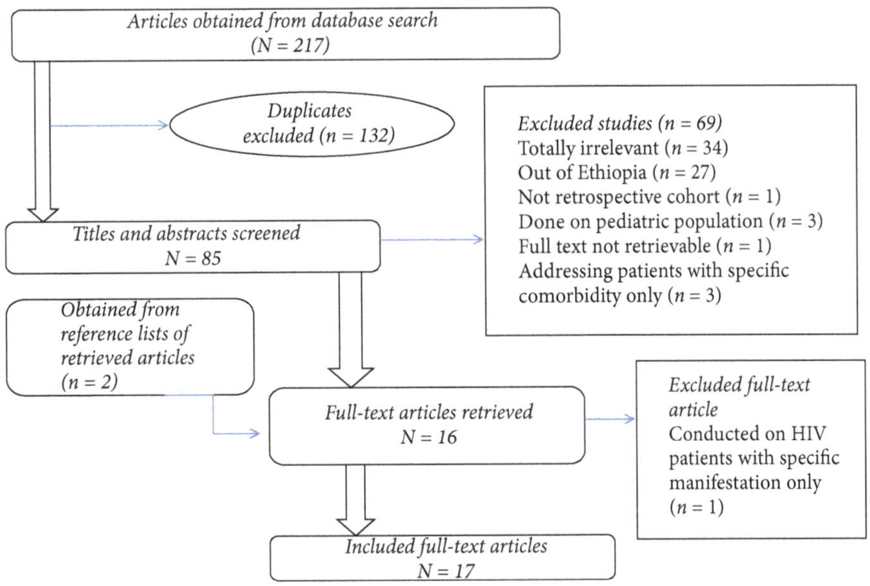


FIGURE 1: Article selection process.

count, low hemoglobin level, TB coinfection, poor adherence to ART, older age, lower weight, and lower baseline BMI. A detailed description of factors that predict mortality is indicated in Table 3.

Patients who started ART after they developed advanced stage disease are 1.4–11.2 times more likely to die than patients who started ART while they are in stage I or II. Patients who are bedridden and ambulatory are 2.4–6.9 and 1.4–4.2 times more likely to die than those who have a working functional status, respectively. Some studies express the effect of CD4 count as a continuous variable and demonstrated that the risk of death decreases by 1%–22% as the CD4 at initiation of ART rises by one unit. Other studies reported that CD4 < 50 cells/microliter at ART initiation increases the risk of death by 1.8–4.5 times. Lower hemoglobin level has 1.9–5.5 times increased risk of death. TB-HIV coinfection increases the risk of mortality 1.3–4.5-fold.

## 4. Discussion

Most of the studies (82%) included in the current review reported that 5–15% of the patients died within the respective follow-up periods. These rates of mortality were higher than what was reported in Uganda (4.5%) [15] and lower than the finding in Tanzania (29.7%) [13], Cameron (23%) [12], Berhampur (21.3%) [16], and Korea (20.8) [17]. The mortality incidence densities reported in the reviewed articles ranged from 0.2 to 10.74 per 100 person-years. Majority of the studies reported an incidence density of 1.89–5.3 per 100 person-years. This is in close agreement with the result of the study conducted in Ruanda which reported 3.7 per 100 person-years [18]. The mortality incidence density reported in this study is lower than the report from South Africa (12/100 PY and 17/100 PY) and Cameron (21.2/100 PY) [19]. The lower rate found in the current reviewed articles may be because of the absence of active search for patients who were lost to follow-up, and real case scenarios (only confirmed dead cases) were used as events in most of the studies reviewed.

All of the studies which reported death rates at different points of follow-up indicated that more than half (50%–68.8%) of the deaths occurred within 6 months of initiating ART. This indicated that most of the deaths in HIV patients occur early in the course of treatment. The reports that compare early mortality in HIV patients of low income and high income countries indicated that patients starting ART in resource constrained settings have increased mortality rates in the first months of therapy compared to those in developed countries [13, 20–22]. Several other studies in developing countries also demonstrated that mortality in the first few months of initiating ART was high [11, 23, 24]. The high early mortality rate observed in this review may be due to the fact that most of the patients included in most of the studies reviewed had either advanced stage disease or low CD4 cell count or both at initiation of their antiretroviral treatment so that they have higher probability of death due to serious opportunistic infections.

Many factors were found as a determinant of death. Among these, advanced stage disease, nonworking (bedridden and ambulatory) functional status, lower baseline CD4 count, lower baseline weight, lower baseline hemoglobin, TB coinfection, and poor adherence were frequently mentioned.

WHO clinical stage of the disease is the most important predictor of mortality reported by many of the studies included in this review. Many other studies conducted outside Ethiopia also reported the same result [11, 12, 25–28]. The higher mortality recorded in patients with advanced stage disease indicated that starting ART treatment earlier before the advancement of the disease is beneficial. But this needs an effort to early diagnose HIV infection by improving the counseling and testing practices. According to the result of this review, patients with bedridden and ambulatory baseline

Table 1: Individual study characteristics.

| Sr. number | Author, year of publication | Study area | Study subjects | Study design | Sample size |
|---|---|---|---|---|---|
| (1) | Hambisa MT et al., 2013 | Nekemte Referral Hospital, East Wollega | Adult HIV patients (age > 14) | Retrospective cohort study | 416 |
| (2) | Tsehaineh B. et al., unpublished | JUSH, SW Ethiopia | Adult HIV patients | Retrospective cohort study | 832 |
| (3) | Setegn et al., 2015 | Goba Hospital, Bale Zone | Adult HIV patients (age >15) | Retrospective cohort study | 2036 |
| (4) | Biadgilign S. et al., 2012 | Hiwot Fana, Jugal and Dil Chora Hospitals, Eastern Ethiopia | Adult HIV patients | Retrospective cohort study | 1537 |
| (5) | Kassa A. et al., 2012 | Zewditu Memorial Hospital | Adult HIV patients (aged 15 or more) | Retrospective cohort study | 4210 |
| (6) | Seyoum D. et al., 2017 | JUSH | Adult HIV patients (age ≥ 18) | Retrospective cohort study | 456 |
| (7) | Damtew B. et al., 2015 | Kharamara Hospital, Jijiga Town, Eastern Ethiopia | Adult HIV patients (age ≥ 15) | Retrospective cohort study | 784 |
| (8) | Alemu AW and Sebastian MS, 2010 | Shashemene and Assela Hospitals, Arsi Zone | Adult HIV patients (age ≥ 15) | Retrospective cohort study | 272 |
| (9) | Ayalew et al., 2014 | Boru Meda and Dessie Referral Hospitals and Kombolcha Health Center | Adult HIV patients (age ≥ 15) | Retrospective cohort study | 654 |
| (10) | Ahunie MA and Ebrahim EA, 2017 | Debre Tabor General Hospital and Woreta Health Center | Adult HIV patients (age ≥ 15) | Retrospective cohort study | 698 |
| (11) | Abebe N et al., 2014 | Debremarkos Referral Hospital, NW Ethiopia | Adult HIV patients (age ≥15) | Retrospective cohort study | 640 |
| (12) | Tadesse K et al., 2014 | Aksum Hospital | Adult HIV patients (age ≥ 15) | Retrospective cohort study | 520 |
| (13) | Bedru A. and worku A, unpublished | Zewditu Hospital | Adult HIV patients (age ≥14) | Retrospective cohort study | 1070 |
| (14) | Mengesha S et al., 2014 | Zewditu Memorial Hospital | Adult HIV patients (age ≥14) | Retrospective cohort study | 416 |
| (15) | Moshago T et al., 2012 | Mizan Aman Hospital | Adult HIV patients | Retrospective cohort study | 2655 |
| (16) | Sapa et al., 2016 | Dilla Hospital | Adult HIV patients (age ≥15) | Retrospective cohort study | 1391 |
| (17) | Kebebew K and wencheko E, 2012 | Armed Forces Teaching and General Hospital | Adult HIV patients (age >15) | Retrospective cohort study | 734 |

TABLE 2: Mortality indicators.

| Sr. number | Author, year of publication | Median follow-up period | Death, $n$ (%) | Mortality incidence density/100 PY | Mean survival time (95% CI) | Mortality at each period | | |
|---|---|---|---|---|---|---|---|---|
| | | | | | | First 3 months | First 6 months | First 12 months |
| (1) | Hambisa MT et al., 2013 | 47 months | 30 (7.2%) | 1.89 | NR | NR | 17 (56.7%) | 21 (70%) |
| (2) | Tsehaineh B. et al., unpublished | 40 months | 144 (17.3%) | NR | 63.7 months (61.1–66.3) | 70 (48.6%) | 99 (68.8%) | NR |
| (3) | Setegn et al., 2015 | NR | 120 (5.9%) | 2.03 | 34.9 months (33.8–35.9) | NR | NR | 78 (65%) |
| (4) | Biadgilign S. et al., 2012 | NR | 86 (5.6%) | 2.03 | NR | NR | NR | 63 (73.3%) |
| (5) | Kassa A. et al., 2012 | NR | 291 (6.9%) | 2.8 | NR | NR | 166 (57%) | NR |
| (6) | Seyoum D. et al., 2017 | NR | 66 (14.5%) | 5.3 | 34 months (22.8–42.0) | NR | NR | 40 (60.6%) |
| (7) | Damtew B. et al., 2015 | 60 months | 87 (11.1) | 5.15 | 20.7 months | 49 (56.3%) | NR | NR |
| (8) | Alemu AW and Sebastian MS, 2010 | | 28 (10.3%) | 7 | NR | NR | NR | NR |
| (9) | Ayalew et al., 2014 | NR | 92 (14.1%) | NR | 41.8 months (40.61–43.00) | NR | NR | NR |
| (10) | Ahunie MA and Ebrahim EA | NR | 35 (5.0%) | 1.5 | NR | NR | NR | NR |
| (11) | Abebe N et al., 2014 | NR | 261 (40.8%) | 10.74 | NR | NR | NR | NR |
| (12) | Tadesse K et al., 2014 | 32 months | 46 (8.9%) | 3.2 | NR | NR | NR | 27 (59%) |
| (13) | Bedru A. and worku A, unpublished | 34 months | 360 (33.6%) | NR | NR | 200 (55.6%) | NR | NR |
| (14) | Mengesha S et al., 2014 | 34 months | 37 (9%) | 3.8 | 39 months | 22 (59.5%) | NR | NR |
| (15) | Moshago T et al., 2012 | NR | 159 (5.9%) | 0.2 | 89 months | NR | NR | NR |
| (16) | Sapa et al., 2016 | 25 months | 128 (9.2%) | 3.5 | NR | 33 (26%) | NR | 66 (52%) |
| (17) | Kebebew K and wencheko E, 2012 | 38.5 months | 86 (11.7%) | NR | NR | 28 (32.6%) | 43 (50%) | 86 (100%) |

NR: not reported.

functional status were more likely to die than patients with working functional status. In this regard, many studies documented supporting evidence that poor performance status at the initiation of ART was a predictor of death during ART care [28–30].

Furthermore, the risk of death is higher for patients with low baseline CD4 count. The CD4 count is a reflection of the patients' immune status, so when it becomes low, the risk of developing opportunistic infections will increase, which may finally lead to death. Low CD4 count at initiation of ART was mentioned as the main predictor of death in HIV patients in various studies [11, 12, 31, 32]. Lower baseline hemoglobin level is also another very important predictor of mortality in HIV patients, which is reported by eight of the reviewed studies. Many other studies also support this finding [13, 25–27, 31, 33]. The possible explanation for increased mortality with low hemoglobin count may be due to the fact that the incidence of anemia increases with progression of HIV disease and most of the patients with low hemoglobin count had advanced stage disease which is a strong predictor of mortality in HIV patients.

Presence of TB coinfection is another important risk factor for death in HIV patients. According to Suchindran et al., the risk of death in TB-HIV coinfected individuals

TABLE 3: Predictors of mortality.

| Sr. number | Author, year of publication | Predictor variable | AHR | 95% CI (upper limit, lower limit) |
|---|---|---|---|---|
| (1) | Hambisa MT et al., 2013 | Age ≥ 40 | 3.055 | 1.292–7.223 |
| | | Baseline hemoglobin level | 0.523 | 0.335–0.816 |
| | | Poor ART adherence | 27.848 | 8.928–86.863 |
| (2) | Tsehaineh B. et al., unpublished | Old age | 1.03 | 1.01–1.051 |
| | | CD4 count at baseline | 0.994 | 0.992–0.996 |
| | | Weight at baseline | 0.902 | 0.816–0.996 |
| | | Bedridden functional status | 6.904 | 4.005–11.902 |
| | | Ambulatory functional status | 2.877 | 1.899–4.360 |
| | | Coinfection with TB | 1.906 | 1.305–2.784 |
| | | Substance use | 1.42 | 1.016–1.985 |
| (3) | Setegn et al., 2015 | Male | 2.67 | 1.74–4.10 |
| | | Bedridden clients | 4.4 | 1.55–12.36 |
| | | TB coinfected at ART initiation | 4.51 | 2.86–7.11 |
| | | Primary education | 0.28 | 0.11–0.70 |
| | | Secondary education | 0.34 | 0.154–0.728 |
| | | WHO stage 1 | 0.16 | 0.08–0.33 |
| | | WHO stage 2 | 0.34 | 0.16–0.73 |
| | | WHO stage 3 | 0.24 | 0.13–0.43 |
| (4) | Biadgilign S. et al., 2012 | WHO stage IV | 3.19 | 1.51–6.76 |
| | | Bedridden | 4.09 | 2.12–7.90 |
| | | >10% weight loss from baseline | 4.93 | 1.20–20.41 |
| | | CD4 | 0.40 | 0.17–0.93 |
| | | Education | 2.79 | 1.26–6.16 |
| (5) | Kassa A. et al., 2012 | CD4 < 50 cells/$\mu$l | 1.80 | 1.17–2.83 |
| | | WHO stage III | 1.46 | 1.03–2.08 |
| | | WHO stage IV | 2.72 | 1.91–3.88 |
| | | Those who developed TB after ART | 1.60 | 1.19–2.15 |
| | | Ambulatory functional status | 1.44 | 1.07–1.93 |
| | | Bedridden functional status | 2.95 | 2.10–4.13 |
| (6) | Seyoum D. et al., 2017 | Age > 35 | 3.8 | 1.6–9.1 |
| | | Baseline weight | 0.93 | 0.90–0.97 |
| | | Baseline WHO stage IV | 6.2 | 2.2–14.2 |
| | | Low adherence to ART | 4.2 | 2.5–7.1 |
| (7) | Damtew B. et al., 2015 | Single marital status | 2.31 | 1.18–4.50 |
| | | Bedridden functional status | 5.91 | 2.87–12.16 |
| | | Advanced WHO stage | 7.36 | 3.17–17.12 |
| | | BMI < 18.5 kg/m$^2$ | 2.20 | 1.18–4.09 |
| | | CD4 count < 50 cells/$\mu$L | 2.70 | 1.26–5.80 |
| | | Severe anemia | 4.57 | 2.30–9.10 |
| | | TB coinfection | 2.30 | 1.28–4.11 |
| (8) | Alemu AW and Sebastian MS, 2010 | Hemoglobin < 10 g/dL | 2.56 | 1.11–5.88 |
| | | WHO stage IV | 5.13 | 2.33–11.33 |
| | | Not on cotrimoxazole prophylaxis | 7.14 | 2.7–20.00 |
| (9) | Ayalew et al., 2014 | Age 30–40 | 0.49 | 0.28–0.85 |
| | | Rural residency | 1.74 | 1.11–2.74 |
| | | CD4 count | 0.998 | 0.996–0.999 |
| | | Weight | 0.968 | 0.943–0.993 |
| | | Not working functional status | 3.62 | 1.96–6.68 |
| | | Lymphocyte count | 0.969 | 0.945–0.994 |
| | | WHO stage IV | 2.38 | 1.21–4.63 |
| | | TB positive | 1.87 | 1.03–3.40 |

TABLE 3: Continued.

| Sr. number | Author, year of publication | Predictor variable | AHR | 95% CI (upper limit, lower limit) |
|---|---|---|---|---|
| (10) | Ahunie MA and Ebrahim EA | Ambulatory functional status | 4.2 | 1.7–10.7 |
| | | Bedridden functional status | 6.5 | 2.0–20.7 |
| | | Poor antiretroviral drug adherence | 5.1 | 1.6–16.3 |
| (11) | Abebe N et al., 2014 | Baseline hemoglobin < 10 g/mm$^3$ | 1.86 | 1.39–2.64 |
| | | Ambulatory functional status | 2.72 | 1.90–3.90 |
| | | Bedridden functional status | 2.38 | 1.32–4.27 |
| | | WHO stages III and IV | 2.16 | 1.10–4.25 |
| | | Poor adherence | 2.16 | 1.03–4.56 |
| | | Fair adherence | 1.88 | 1.08–3.29 |
| | | Unexplained chronic diarrhea | 1.53 | 1.09–2.15 |
| | | Not on TB prophylaxis | 3.98 | 1.87–8.44 |
| (12) | Tadesse K et al., 2014 | Hemoglobin level < 11 mg/dl | 1.9 | 1.01–3.52 |
| | | CD4 cell count < 50 cells/$\mu$l | 2.1 | 1.13–3.89 |
| | | Male gender | 1.9 | 1.01–3.52 |
| | | Weight < 40 kg | 2.3 | 1.24–4.55 |
| | | Primary and lower level of education | 2.6 | 1.29–5.55 |
| (13) | Bedru A. and worku A, unpublished | Poor ART adherence | 3.92 | 3.13–4.90 |
| | | Advanced WHO staging | 2.47 | 1.58–3.81 |
| | | Being unemployed | 1.87 | 1.49–2.34 |
| | | Moderate anemia | 1.86 | 1.35–2.56 |
| | | Low CD4 count | 1.85 | 1.35–2.52 |
| (14) | Mengesha S et al., 2014 | WHO clinical stage | 2.99 | 1.26–5.31 |
| | | Anemia | 5.54 | 2.58–11.86 |
| | | Having past TB coinfection | 4.13 | 1.79–9.51 |
| (15) | Moshago T et al., 2012 | WHO clinical stage IV | 4.5 | 1.36–14.88 |
| | | WHO clinical stage III | 3.2 | 1.06–10.24 |
| | | History of TB coinfection | 1.25 | 1.03–1.53 |
| | | Bedridden functional status | 2.63 | 2.05–3.37 |
| | | Ambulatory functional status | 1.56 | 1.31–1.86 |
| (16) | Sapa et al., 2016 | BMI < 18.5 kg/m$^2$ | 3.12 | 1.39–7.76 |
| | | CD4 cell count < 50 cells/mm$^3$ | 4.55 | 1.19–8.44 |
| | | Drug addiction | 2.03 | 1.11–4.56 |
| | | WHO stages III and IV | 11.25 | 8.67–17.96 |
| | | Severe anemia | 5.14 | 3.12–9.65 |
| (17) | Kebebew K and Wencheko E, 2012 | CD4 cell count at baseline | 0.78 | 0.64–0.95 |
| | | Employment status | 2.31 | 1.25–4.28 |
| | | Ambulatory functional status | 2.01 | 1.02–3.98 |
| | | Bedridden functional status | 3.36 | 1.73–6.50 |
| | | WHO clinical stage III | 7.05 | 1.68–29.66 |
| | | WHO clinical stage IV | 12.64 | 3.00–53.20 |
| | | TB coinfection | 1.73 | 1.04–2.89 |
| | | Presence of opportunistic infections | 8.99 | 1.24–65.09 |

is double as compared to HIV infected individuals without TB [34]. Other studies also report that the presence of TB coinfection is significantly associated with higher odds of mortality among HIV patients taking ART [28, 35, 36]. This may be because TB by itself is a deadly disease worldwide, and the virulence of the organism is high in patients that have a suppressed immune system and are able to establish infection easily [37]. Low baseline weight and BMI of less than 18.5 was also found to be a predictor of mortality in many of the studies reviewed. This is in line with the result of studies conducted outside Ethiopia [11, 23, 38]. BMI is an indicator of patients' nutritional status. Patients with BMI less than

18.5 and lower weight are mostly malnourished and unable to cope with the disease and will have a high chance of death due to opportunistic infections.

Medication adherence is very important to get the full benefit of antiretroviral drugs. Nonadherence to ART will result in treatment failure by increasing the chance of mutation that could lead to a drug resistant virus and finally death. Even though a self-reported adherence assessment method was used in all of the reviewed studies, which is not as such reliable to measure adherence, some of the studies revealed that poor adherence is significantly associated with mortality. Those who did not have proper adherence to their ART medication were 2.2–27.8 times at greater risk of death than those who adhered to their medication. This was also reported in different studies conducted in various parts of the world [16, 31].

Age of patients was found to affect survival in HIV patients who are on ART. Four of the studies included in this review found significant association between age and death due to HIV after starting ART. Other studies also confirmed that most of the patients of older age were more likely to die [15, 39–41]. This may be due to the fact that as the patient gets older, there will be a decline in the body's physiologic function, and the patient will have an incompetent immune status and become at a high risk of complication and respond poorly to ART.

In addition to the above factors, lower level of education, male sex, substance abuse, and unemployment were also mentioned as a significant predictor of mortality by some of the studies included in this review. Another study also reported negative influence of low level of education on mortality among ART users [42]. The more educated patients will have a better understanding of the disease, its treatment, and the instructions given by healthcare providers; as a result, he/she will have enhanced health outcome [43]. The higher rate of mortality in males than females reported in some of the studies reviewed may be because of the males' higher tendency for drug abuse than females in Ethiopia. Earlier health seeking behavior of females might also be a reason for lesser mortality among females than males [44]. This finding was also supported by other studies [11, 25, 26, 28–30, 45].

Even though the inclusion of many homogeneous studies is the strength of this review, there are also some limitations that should be considered in the interpretation of the result of this study. The retrospective nature of the included studies limits the cause and effect relation between death and the different factors reported in the individual studies. Mortality might also be underestimated, since individuals dying at home without being reported were considered as lost to follow-up. On the other hand, HIV-related mortality might also be overestimated since the exact cause of death was not determined and every recorded death in HIV patients was considered as HIV-related.

## 5. Conclusion

5%–40.8% of HIV patients in Ethiopia die in 2–5 years of initiating antiretroviral treatment. Most of the deaths in HIV patients occur early in the course of treatment. The main predictors for death were advanced stage disease, nonworking (bedridden and ambulatory) functional status, lower baseline CD4 count, lower baseline hemoglobin, TB coinfection, lower baseline weight, and poor treatment adherence. Special emphasis and closer follow-up should be given for patients with such characteristics.

## Abbreviations

AIDS: Acquired immune deficiency syndrome
ART: Antiretroviral therapy
BMI: Body mass index
HAART: Highly active antiretroviral therapy
HIV: Human immunodeficiency virus
PY: Person-years
TB: Tuberculosis.

## Disclosure

This research did not receive any specific grant from funding agencies in the public, commercial, or not-for-profit sectors.

## Conflicts of Interest

The author declares that he has no conflicts of interest.

## Acknowledgments

The author would like to express his thanks to the University of Gondar for granting him Internet access.

## References

[1] UNAIDS, "UNAIDS report on the global AIDS epidemic," Tech. Rep., UNAIDS, Geneva, Switzerland, 2013.

[2] S. O. Muhula, M. Peter, B. Sibhatu, N. Meshack, and K. Lennie, "Effects of highly active antiretroviral therapy on the survival of hiv-infected adult patients in urban slums of kenya," *Pan African Medical Journal*, vol. 20, no. 1, 2015.

[3] WHO, "Consolidated guidelines on the use of antiretroviral drugs for treating and preventing HIV infection: summary of key features and recommendations," Tech. Rep., WHO, Geneva, Switzerland, 2013.

[4] HAPCOF, "Report on progress towards implementation of the UN declaration of commitment on HIV/AIDS," Tech. Rep., 2010.

[5] W. B. Sapa, N. T. Negassi, and A. H. Chofore, "Survival pattern and its determinants among adult HIV-infected patients after initiation of HAART in Dilla hospital Ethiopia," *Journal of AIDS & Clinical Research*, vol. 1, no. 1, pp. 1–6, 2016.

[6] "Five year survival probabilities after ART start at 3 hospitals in Guyana," in *Proceedings of the Caribbean HIV Conference*, I. Wanyeki, D. Cole, G. Sills, and P. Bass, Eds., Nassau, The Bahamas, November 2011.

[7] J. Ayalew, H. Moges, and A. Worku, "Identifying factors related to the survival of AIDS patients under the follow-up of Antiretroviral Therapy (ART): the case of South Wollo," *International Journal of Data Envelopment Analysis and Operations Research*, vol. 1, no. 2, pp. 21–27, 2014.

[8] T. Setegn, A. Takele, T. Gizaw, D. Nigatu, and D. Haile, "Predictors of mortality among adult antiretroviral therapy users in southeastern Ethiopia: retrospective cohort study," *AIDS Research and Treatment*, vol. 2015, Article ID 148769, 8 pages, 2015.

[9] P. MacPherson, M. Moshabela, N. Martinson, and P. Pronyk, "Mortality and loss to follow-up among HAART initiators in rural South Africa," *Transactions of the Royal Society of Tropical Medicine and Hygiene*, vol. 103, no. 6, pp. 588–593, 2009.

[10] Z. Mulissa, D. Jerene, and B. Lindtjørn, "Patients present earlier and survival has improved, but pre-ART attrition is high in a six-year HIV cohort data from Ethiopia," *PLoS ONE*, vol. 5, no. 10, Article ID e13268, 2010.

[11] S. D. Lawn, A. D. Harries, X. Anglaret, L. Myer, and R. Wood, "Early mortality among adults accessing antiretroviral treatment programmes in sub-Saharan Africa," *AIDS*, vol. 22, no. 15, pp. 1897–1908, 2008.

[12] I. Sieleunou, M. Souleymanou, A.-M. Schönenberger, J. Menten, and M. Boelaert, "Determinants of survival in AIDS patients on antiretroviral therapy in a rural centre in the Far-North Province, Cameroon," *Tropical Medicine & International Health*, vol. 14, no. 1, pp. 36–43, 2009.

[13] A. Johannessen, E. Naman, B. J. Ngowi et al., "Predictors of mortality in HIV-infected patients starting antiretroviral therapy in a rural hospital in Tanzania," *BMC Infectious Diseases*, vol. 8, no. 1, article 52, 2008.

[14] E. Von Elm, G. Altman, and M. Egger, "The Strengthening the Reporting of Observational Studies in Epidemiology [STROBE] statement: guidelines for reporting observational studies," *Gaceta Sanitaria*, vol. 22, no. 2, pp. 144–150, 2008.

[15] J. Rubaihayo, N. M. Tumwesigye, J. Konde-Lule et al., "Trends and predictors of mortality among HIV positive patients in the era of highly active antiretroviral therapy in Uganda," *Infectious Disease Reports*, vol. 7, no. 3, pp. 66–73, 2015.

[16] Y. Ramani Roja, P. Benu, S. H. Rao, R. M V, P. Simanchal, and K. Prasanna, "Predictors of mortality among HIV patients on HAART in an ART centre—a retrospective study," *International Journal of Medicine and Public Health*, vol. 6, no. 4, pp. 175–179, 2016.

[17] S. H. Lee, K.-H. Kim, S. G. Lee et al., "Causes of death and risk factors for mortality among HIV-infected patients receiving antiretroviral therapy in korea," *Journal of Korean Medical Science*, vol. 28, no. 7, pp. 990–997, 2013.

[18] D. W. Lowrance, F. Ndamage, E. Kayirangwa et al., "Adult clinical and immunologic outcomes of the national antiretroviral treatment program in Rwanda during 2004-2005," *Journal of Acquired Immune Deficiency Syndromes*, vol. 52, no. 1, pp. 49–55, 2009.

[19] M. Rougemont, B. E. Stoll, N. Elia, and P. Ngang, "Antiretroviral treatment adherence and its determinants in Sub-Saharan Africa: a prospective study at Yaounde Central Hospital, Cameroon," *AIDS Research and Therapy*, vol. 6, article 21, 2009.

[20] P. Braitstein, M. W. Brinkhof, F. Dabis, and M. Schechter, "Mortality of HIV-1-infected patients in the first year of antiretroviral therapy: comparison between low-income and high-income countries," *The Lancet*, vol. 367, no. 9513, pp. 817–824, 2006.

[21] D. Bachani, R. Garg, B. B. Rewari et al., "Two-year treatment outcomes of patients enrolled in India's national first-line antiretroviral therapy programme," *National Medical Journal of India*, vol. 23, no. 1, pp. 7–12, 2010.

[22] N. I. Paton, S. Sangeetha, A. Earnest, and R. Bellamy, "The impact of malnutrition on survival and the CD4 count response in HIV-infected patients starting antiretroviral therapy," *HIV Medicine*, vol. 7, no. 5, pp. 323–330, 2006.

[23] R. Zachariah, M. Fitzgerald, M. Massaquoi et al., "Risk factors for high early mortality in patients on antiretroviral treatment in a rural district of Malawi," *AIDS*, vol. 20, no. 18, pp. 2355–2360, 2006.

[24] J. S. A. Stringer, I. Zulu, J. Levy et al., "Rapid scale-up of antiretroviral therapy at primary care sites in Zambia: feasibility and early outcomes," *Journal of the American Medical Association*, vol. 296, no. 7, pp. 782–793, 2006.

[25] V. Poka-Mayap, E. W. Pefura-Yone, A. P. Kengne, and C. Kuaban, "Mortality and its determinants among patients infected with HIV-1 on antiretroviral therapy in a referral centre in Yaounde, Cameroon: a retrospective cohort study," *British Medical Journal*, vol. 3, no. 7, Article ID e003210, 2013.

[26] A. Gupta, G. Nadkarni, W.-T. Yang et al., "Early mortality in adults initiating antiretroviral therapy (ART) in low- and middle-income countries (LMIC): a systematic review and meta-analysis," *PLoS ONE*, vol. 6, no. 12, Article ID e28691, 2011.

[27] G. Chalamilla, C. Hawkins, J. Okuma et al., "Mortality and treatment failure among HIV-infected adults in Dar Es Salaam, Tanzania," *Journal of the International Association of Physicians in AIDS Care*, vol. 11, no. 5, pp. 296–304, 2012.

[28] B. Amuron, J. Levin, J. Birunghi et al., "Mortality in an antiretroviral therapy programme in Jinja, south-east Uganda: a prospective cohort study," *AIDS Research and Therapy*, vol. 8, article 39, 2011.

[29] L. Bhatta, E. Klouman, K. Deuba et al., "Survival on antiretroviral treatment among adult HIV-infected patients in Nepal: a retrospective cohort study in far-western Region, 2006–2011," *BMC Infectious Diseases*, vol. 13, no. 1, article 604, 2013.

[30] K. Mageda, G. H. Leyna, and E. J. Mmbaga, "High initial HIV/AIDS-Related mortality and—its predictors among patients on antiretroviral therapy in the kagera region of Tanzania: a five-year retrospective cohort study," *AIDS Research and Treatment*, vol. 2012, Article ID 843598, 7 pages, 2012.

[31] B. O. Ojikutu, H. Zheng, R. P. Walensky et al., "Predictors of mortality in patients initiating antiretroviral therapy in Durban, South Africa," *South African Medical Journal*, vol. 98, no. 3, pp. 204–208, 2008.

[32] G. P. Bisson, T. Gaolathe, R. Gross et al., "Overestimates of survival after HAART: implications for global scale-up efforts," *PLoS ONE*, vol. 3, no. 3, Article ID e1725, 2008.

[33] D. D. Cuong, A. Thorson, A. Sönnerborg et al., "Survival and causes of death among HIV-infected patients starting antiretroviral therapy in north-eastern Vietnam," *Infectious Diseases*, vol. 44, no. 3, pp. 201–208, 2012.

[34] S. Suchindran, E. S. Brouwer, and A. Van Rie, "Is HIV infection a risk factor for multi-drug resistant tuberculosis? A systematic review," *PLoS ONE*, vol. 4, no. 5, Article ID e5561, 2009.

[35] M. Ghate, S. Deshpande, S. Tripathy et al., "Mortality in HIV infected individuals in Pune, India," *Indian Journal of Medical Research*, vol. 133, no. 4, pp. 414–420, 2011.

[36] B. K. Kigozi, S. Sumba, P. Mudyope et al., "The effect of AIDS defining conditions on immunological recovery among patients initiating antiretroviral therapy at Joint Clinical Research Centre, Uganda," *AIDS Research and Therapy*, vol. 6, article 17, 2009.

[37] F. A. Khan, J. Minion, M. Pai et al., "Treatment of active tuberculosis in HIV-coinfected patients: a systematic review and meta-analysis," *Clinical Infectious Diseases*, vol. 50, no. 9, pp. 1288–1299, 2010.

[38] E. Mossdorf, M. Stoeckle, E. G. Mwaigomole et al., "Improved antiretroviral treatment outcome in a rural African setting is associated with cART initiation at higher CD4 cell counts and better general health condition," *BMC Infectious Diseases*, vol. 11, article 98, 2011.

[39] S. Grabar, L. Weiss, and D. Costagliola, "HIV infection in older patients in the HAART era," *Journal of Antimicrobial Chemotherapy*, vol. 57, no. 1, pp. 4–7, 2005.

[40] S. Kouanda, I. B. Meda, L. Nikiema et al., "Determinants and causes of mortality in HIV-infected patients receiving antiretroviral therapy in Burkina Faso: a five-year retrospective cohort study," *AIDS Care Psychological and Socio-medical Aspects of AIDS/HIV*, vol. 24, no. 4, pp. 478–490, 2012.

[41] R. Lubis, A. Bulgiba, A. Kamarulzaman, N. N. Hairi, M. Dahlui, and D. Peramalah, "Predictors of death in Malaysian HIV-infected patients on anti-retroviral therapy," *Preventive Medicine*, vol. 57, pp. S54–S56, 2013.

[42] I. Jarrin, B. Lumbreras, I. Ferreros, S. Pérez-Hoyos, I. Hurtado, and I. Hernández-Aguado, "Effect of education on overall and cause-specific mortality in injecting drug users, according to HIV and introduction of HAART," *International Journal of Epidemiology*, vol. 36, no. 1, pp. 187–194, 2006.

[43] S. I. Bello and O. A. Itiola, "Drug adherence amongst tuberculosis patients in the university of ilorin teaching hospital, ilorin, nigeria," *African Journal of Pharmacy and Pharmacology*, vol. 4, no. 3, pp. 109–114, 2010.

[44] K. Deribe, A. Yami, A. Deribew et al., "Predictors of mortality among tuberculosis/HIV-coinfected persons in southwest ethiopia: a case-control study," *Journal of the International Association of Providers of AIDS Care*, vol. 14, no. 3, pp. 269–273, 2015.

[45] K. Taylor-Smith, H. Tweya, A. Harries, E. Schoutene, and A. Jahn, "Gender differences in retention and survival on antiretroviral therapy of HIV-1 infected adults in Malawi," *Malawi Medical Journal*, vol. 22, no. 2, pp. 49–56, 2010.

8

# Prevalence and Associated Factors of Depression among PLHIV in Ethiopia

**Tadele Amare, Wondale Getinet, Shegaye Shumet, and Biksegn Asrat**

*Department of Psychiatry, College of Medicine and Health Science, University of Gondar, Gondar, Ethiopia*

Correspondence should be addressed to Tadele Amare; tadeleamare@ymail.com

Academic Editor: Krishna Mohan

*Background.* Depression is a substantial contributor to the global burden of disease and affects people in all communities across the globe. Depression is the most common psychiatric problem associated with HIV/AIDS and half of all PLWHIV with depression go underdiagnosed and untreated. Psychiatric complications of HIVAIDS delay mental health services in less affluent countries. However, there is lack of study with regard to the pooled estimation prevalence of depression in PLWHIV in Ethiopia. *Objectives.* The aim of this systematic review and meta-analysis is to summarize the most current available evidence from 2010 to March 2017 among adult PLWHIV in Ethiopia. *Methods.* The team explored multiple databases searching methods including MEDLINE/PubMed, PsycINFO, Google Advance Scholar, and Google Scholar to find studies published with the data on the prevalence of depression among PLWHIV. We searched 150 research articles; of these 143 articles were excluded. Subsequently, thirteen articles were used for synthesis prevalence and four studies were included in the synthesis effect of sex on depression among PLWHIV. *Results.* The total of pooled estimated prevalence of depression in PLWHIV was 36.65. Estimated prevalence of depression in three studies by using CES-D was 31.19% and in six studies by using PHQ-9 was 37.91%. The remaining four studies used a single tool: Kessler-6 Scale (15.5%), HADS (41.2%), HDSQ (43.9%), and BDI (55.8%). Factors such as age, marital status, living alone, poor medication adherence, poor social support, clinical stages II and III of HIV, stigma, income, and occupation were significantly associated with depression. *Conclusions and Recommendation.* The pooled estimate prevalence of depression among PLWHIV was higher than that in the general population. It is better to offer special attention to these populations.

## 1. Introduction

Depression is the most common psychiatric problem associated with HIV disease. The large meta-analysis of 10 studies found that people living with HIV had twice the risk for depression than those who were at risk for HIV but were not actually infected [1]. According to the Joint United Nations Programme on HIV/AIDS (UNAIDS), as of December 1999, globally, more than 33 million people were estimated to be living with HIV/AIDS; among these, 95% were living in the developing world [2]. Depression rates for HIV-positive people are about 60%; but half of all PLWHIV with depression go underdiagnosed and untreated [3]. Depression is a substantial contributor to the global burden of disease and affects people in all communities across the globe. Nowadays, depression is estimated to affect 350 million people. The World Mental Health Survey conducted in seventeen countries found that about 1 in 20 people reported having an episode of depression in the preceding year [4]. Many people living with HIV have depression [5, 6]. About 90% of people who die by suicide have at least one psychiatric diagnosis; of these, depressive disorders are the most commonly associated with suicidal behavior [7]. Undetected mental health problems such as depression, personality disorders, cognitive disorders, and cooccurring conditions such as substance-related disorders can affect drug adherence, clinic attendance, and quality of life and can influence the outcome of disease and high-risk behaviors that increase risk of HIV transmission [8, 9]. Globally, by 2030, depression will be the leading cause of disease burden. In low- and middle-income countries, about 76% and 85% of people with severe mental disorders do not get treatment for their mental health problem [10]. The prevalence of mental problems in HIV-infected individuals is significantly higher than that

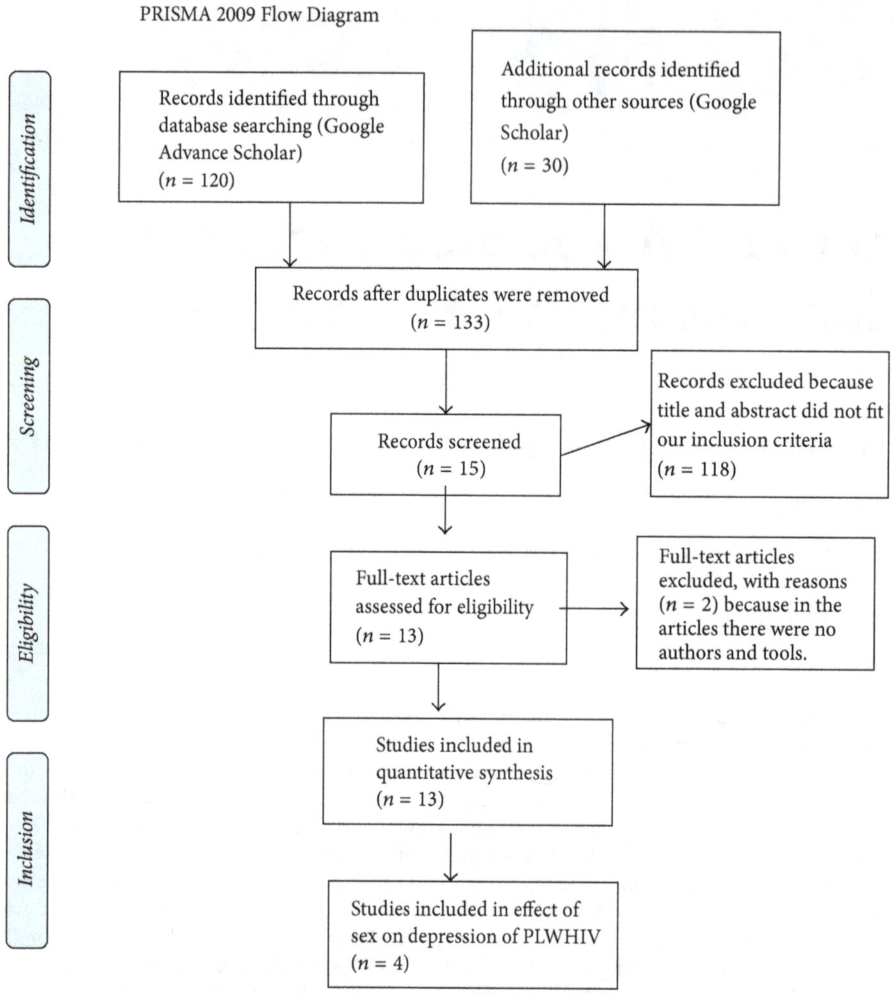


FIGURE 1: Flow chart showing how the research articles were searched (2017) [24].

in the general population [8]. Psychiatric complications of HIV/AIDS signify a significant additional burden for mental health services and professionals in less affluent countries with high HIV prevalence rates [6]. In India, the prevalence of depression among the HIV/AIDS patients was 40% [11]. The pooled prevalence of depression in PLWHIV in sub-Saharan Africa was 9 to 32% [12]. The prevalence of depression among the HIV/AIDS patients in Nigeria was 56.7% [13], in Uganda it was 47% [14], and in South Africa it was 37.6% [15]; and in Uganda, depressive symptoms in cognitive function impaired advanced HIV (53.9%) [16]. In systematic review and meta-analysis in low-, middle-, and high-income countries, the prevalence was 12.8 to 78% [17]. In France, it was 28.1% [18]; in three African countries (Kenya, Namibia, and Tanzania), it was 28% [19]; and in Black Americans it was 58% [20]. In Ethiopia, the prevalence of HIV is unevenly distributed in the geographical locations due to varying social, structural, and economic dynamics. The prevalence of HIV was 1.6% in Amhara, 1% in Oromia, 1.1% in Somalia, 1.8% in Tigray, 0.9% in SNNP, 5.2% in Addis Ababa, and 2.8% in Harari [21]. In another study, the prevalence of HIV was 1% in Harari, 5.8% in Gambela, 0.3% in SNNP, 0.6% in Oromia, 1.1% in Amhara, 0.9% in Afar, and 1.3% in Tigray (1.3%) [22]. When there is a variation in HIV prevalence, there is also a variation of depression prevalence. In Africa, the systematic review showed that factors that associated with depression among PLWHIV were receiving poor-quality health services, being female, and lack of emotional support from friends and family [23]. In Uganda, age above 50 years and being female were associated factors for depression [14].

The aim of this systematic review and meta-analysis is to condense the most current available evidence to March 2017 among adult PLWHIV in Ethiopia: (1) prevalence of depression (defined based on screening tools) and (2) factors that affect depression in PLWHIV.

## 2. Methods

*2.1. Eligibility Criteria.* The PRISMA guidelines protocol was used to write the systematic review [24]. The studies were searched in Google advance search: "depression ([MeSH Terms]) OR mental illnesses ([MeSH Terms]) AND associated factors ([MeSH Terms]) OR factors associated ([MeSH Terms]) AND HIV ([MeSH Terms]) OR PLWHIV AND Ethiopia ([MeSH Terms])" (Figure 1). The date of publication from 2010 to March 2017 and age greater than or equal to 18 years were included. Cross-sectional and longitudinal study designs were included. A comprehensive literature search was done by the terms "prevalence and associated factors of depression among PLWHIV in Ethiopia." Mental illness and associated factors among PLWHIV in Ethiopia by Cochrane review database library and PsycINFO search strategies were also used. Figures were extracted from published reports and any lost information was gotten from investigators through email and phone.

*2.1.1. Inclusion and Exclusion Criteria.* Literatures not written in the English language and literatures without tool to screen depression and author were excluded.

*2.1.2. Data Extraction and Synthesis.* The assessment of each of the studies in accordance with the checklist revealed that almost all of the reports were of acceptable quality; there are eight points used to screen articles; out of these, this review document was scored 7.77 out of eight points [25]. Data were primarily appraised for quality and then extraction was made by using data extraction method. Data were analyzed using STATA V.14 statistical software. Due to the possibility of heterogeneity among the studies, random-effects meta-analysis models were preferentially reported. We developed the data extraction form that outfits the specific objective of the systematic review. It included a date of publication, the name of an author, setting, study methods, and results. Meta-analysis package was accustomed reason the pooled prevalence of depression among PLWHIV supported the tool distinction. The 1st six studies were assessed with PHQ-9 [26–31] and 3 different studies were used (CES-D) [32–34]. The remainder of studies used HADS [35], HDSQ [36], and BDI [37] and Kessler 6 scale was used to identify depression [38].

*2.1.3. Search Outcomes.* The electronic searching of literature produced 150 articles. Among 150 research articles, 17 were excluded due to duplication and our inclusion criteria and 118 articles were excluded because title and abstract did not fit our inclusion criteria. Finally, two articles were excluded after reading full texts due to the absence of tool and author. Thirteen research articles were included to quantify the pooled estimation of depression among PLWHIV and four studies were included in effect of sex on depression (meta-analysis) (Figure 1).

*2.1.4. Features of Studies.* All studies were conducted in Ethiopia. Eleven of them were cross-sectional surveys and the remaining two were cohort and prospective studies (Table 1).

## 3. Result

Thirteen studies were included in this study. According to different literatures in Ethiopia, the prevalence of depression ranged from 7.3% to 73.3%. The pooled estimated prevalence of depression among PLWHIV was 36.65% (95% CI: 25.48–47.82). Six regions were incorporated in this study. In Hara and Southern Nation and Nationalities of People (SNNP), a single study of each was conducted. In subgroup analysis related to region, the prevalence ranged from 15.5% (SNNP) to 64.6% (Oromia region) (Figure 2).

The subgroup analysis of pooled estimated prevalence of depression in PLWHIV in Ethiopia according to the tool used ranged from 15.5% (Kessler) to 55.8% (BDI) (Figure 3).

## 4. Associated Factors for Depression

The factors that affect depression were different according to different studies (Table 2).

Is being female a risk factor for depression among PLWHIV? In four studies, being female had no significant association with depression when compared to being male (Figure 4).

## 5. Discussion

The pooled prevalence of depression symptoms in Ethiopia from 2010 to March 2017 was 36.65% (95% CI: 25.48, 47.82). The current systematic review result was almost in line with the pooled prevalence of depression in sub-Saharan African countries, 9 to 32% [12]. Our finding was similar to the finding of countries in Sub-Saharan Africa; this is due to Ethiopia being one of the countries in the Sub-Saharan Africa. The Ethiopian pooled prevalence of depressive symptoms was lower than that in the study done in Nigeria (56.7%) [13]. The difference might be due to the fact that the study done in Nigeria had a single finding, but in Ethiopia the finding was pooled. This finding was in line with the researches done in Uganda (47%) [14], South Africa (37.6%) [15], three African countries (Kenya, Namibia, and Tanzania) (28%) [19], and France (28.1%) [18]. The finding was in line with the research done in India (40%) [11]. However, this finding was lower than the result of Uganda (53.9%) [16] and Black Americans (58%) [20]. The difference might be that in Uganda the study was conducted among advanced HIV stage population and in Black Americans there are sociodemographic and tool differences. The prevalence of depression among PLWHIV in low-, middle-, and high-income countries ranged from 12.8% to 78% [17]. Our finding was also in line with this result because Ethiopia is one of the low-income countries. Based on the tool, six studies were screened by using PHQ-9 and the pooled prevalence was 37.91%, which was similar to studies that screened patients by using Center for Epidemiological Studies Depression Scale (CES-D) (31.19%) [32–34]. The reason might be that when the number of studies increases, the consistency also increases. One study indicated that the prevalence of depression in PLWHIV was 43.9% by using Hamilton's Depression Scale Questionnaire. By using Beck Depression Inventory (BDI) [37], HADS [35], and Kessler-6 Scale [38], the prevalence of depression was 55.8%, 41.2%, and 15%, respectively. In relation to regions, in Addis Ababa, three studies were conducted and the pooled prevalence was 22.87% (10.55, 35.19) [34, 35, 38], which was in line with the study done in Amhara region, 28.42% (11.96, 44.88) [27–29, 33]. This might be due to equivalent number of studies

TABLE 1: The prevalence of depression and the tool used in each study among PLWHIV in Ethiopia, 2017.

| First author | Study year | Region | Study design | Outcome | Sample size | Number of cases | Prevalence | Age (years) | Tool |
|---|---|---|---|---|---|---|---|---|---|
| Tesfaw [35] | 2016 | Addis Ababa | Cross-sectional | Depression | 417 | 172 | 41.2 | ≥18 | HADS |
| Tolasa [32] | 2012 | Oromia | Cross-sectional | Depression | 390 | 299 | 73.3 | ≥18 | CES-D |
| Mohhamed [26] | 2013 | Harar | Cross-sectional | Depression | 740 | 339 | 45.8 | ≥18 | PHQ-9 |
| Berhe [36] | 2012 | Tigray | Cross-sectional | Depression | 269 | 118 | 43.9 | ≥18 | HDSQ |
| Dejenu [27] | 2014 | Amhara | Cross-sectional | Depression | 412 | 48 | 11.7 | ≥18 | PHQ-9 |
| Asmare Eshetu [28] | 2013 | Amhara | Cross-sectional | Depression | 416 | 162 | 38.94 | ≥18 | PHQ-9 |
| Amberbir [37] | 2006-2007 | Oromia | Prospective | Depression | 400 | 223 | 55.8 | ≥18 | BDI |
| Endeshaw [29] | 2011 | Amhara | Cross-sectional | Depression | 55 | 33 | 60 | ≥18 | PHQ-9 |
| Bezabhe [33] | 2012-2013 | Amhara | Cohort | Depression | 246 | 18 | 7.3 | ≥18 | CES-D |
| Alemu [34] | 2010 | Addis Ababa | Cross-sectional | Depression | 1815 | 238 | 13.1 | ≥18 | CES-D |
| Woldehawaria [30] | 2014 | Tigray | Cross-sectional | Depression | 340 | 197 | 57.9 | ≥18 | PHQ-9 |
| Yakob [31] | 2015 | SNNP* | Cross-sectional | Depression | 485 | 75 | 15.5 | ≥18 | PHQ-9 |
| Mekuria [38] | 2013 | Addis Ababa | Cross-sectional | Depression | 664 | 99 | 15 | ≥18 | Kessler-6 Scale |

*Southern Nation and Nationalities of People. HADS: Hospital Anxiety and Depression Scale; PHQ-9: Patient Health Questionnaire-9; CES-D: Center for Epidemiological Studies Depression Scale; BDI: Beck Depression Inventory; HDSQ: Hamilton's Depression Scale Questionnaire.

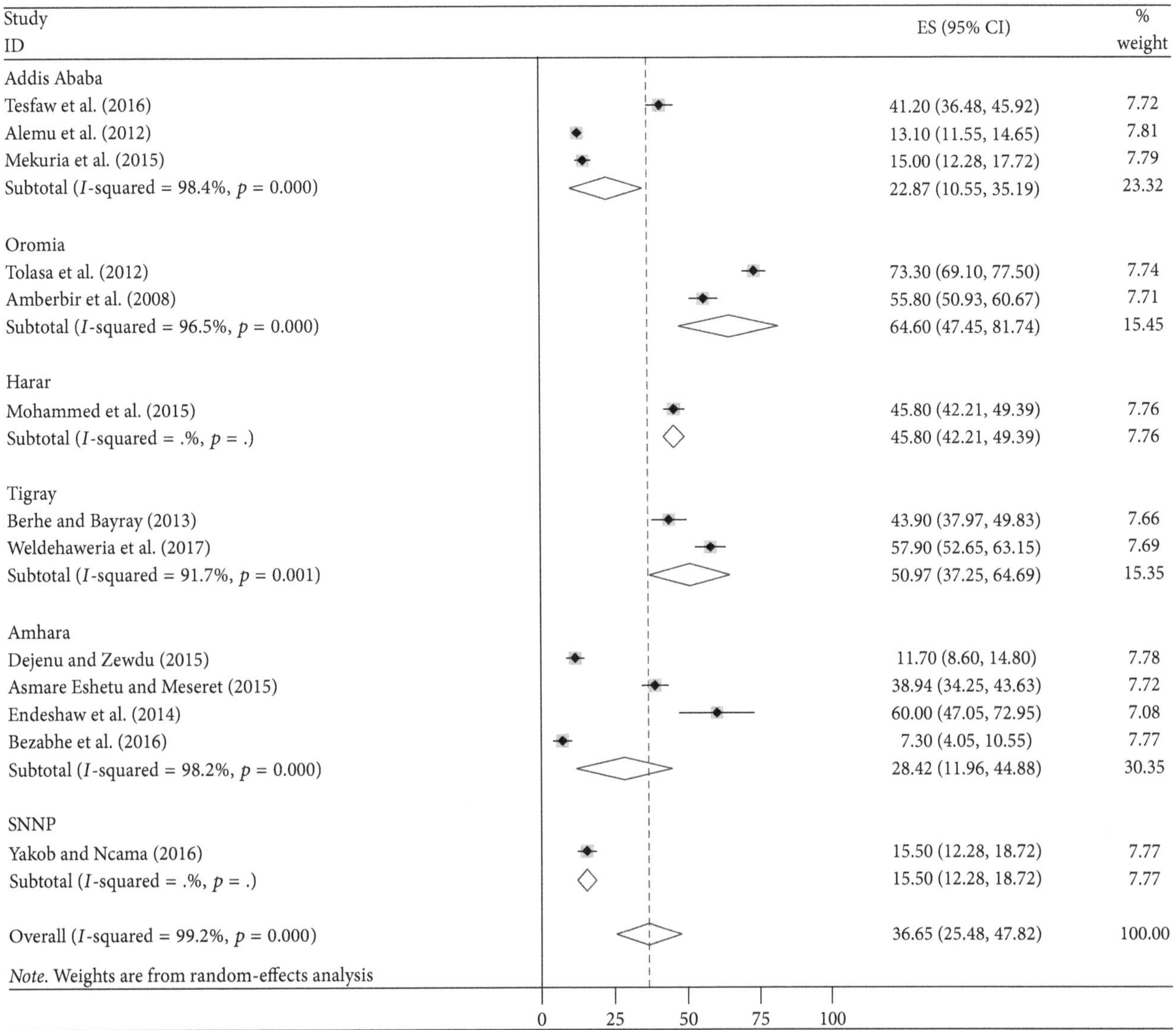


FIGURE 2: The pooled estimated prevalence of depression by region among PLWHIV in Ethiopia, 2017.

(Addis Abba = 3 studies; Amhara = 4 studies). The finding of Addis Ababa was lower than that of Oromia (64.6%) [32, 37] and Tigray region (50.97%) (37.25, 64.69) [30, 36]. The reason might be due to the fact that, in Oromia and Tigray region, two studies of each were conducted but in Addis Ababa three studies were incorporated, which means that when the number of studies increases, the precision of the study increases. The pooled prevalence of depressive symptoms in Amhara region was lower than that in the study done in Oromia and Tigray region. The possible reason might be that in Amhara four studies were included but not in the counterparts (Oromia and Tigray) and three of the Amhara region studies were assessed by PHQ-9 [27–29]. The prevalence of depression in Harar [26] and SNNP [31] was 45.8% and 15.5%, respectively. However, the finding of these two regions could not be comparable to other findings because a single study was conducted in each region.

Perceived HIV stigma and feeling stigmatized [27, 28, 35] were predictors for depression. The justification might be due to the fact that those who isolated themselves from others lead to worsening the depression. Poor social support and living alone [27, 35] are factors that affect the depressive patients, which was in line with the systematic review study in Africa [23]. The reason might be due to the fact that those who did not share their problems with other people had stress, which means that when the problems were shared with others, stress reduced by half. Poor medication adherence and last time missed any of medication were risk factors for depression in PLWHIV in Ethiopia [26, 35]. The possible reason might be due to worsening of the symptoms. Clinical stage, stage III of HIV [28, 35], and stage IV of HIV/AIDS [28] were risk factors for depression. The reason might be due to the fact that psychiatric complications of HIV/AIDS signify a significant additional burden for mental health services [6]. Patients who had low income [26, 28, 36] and

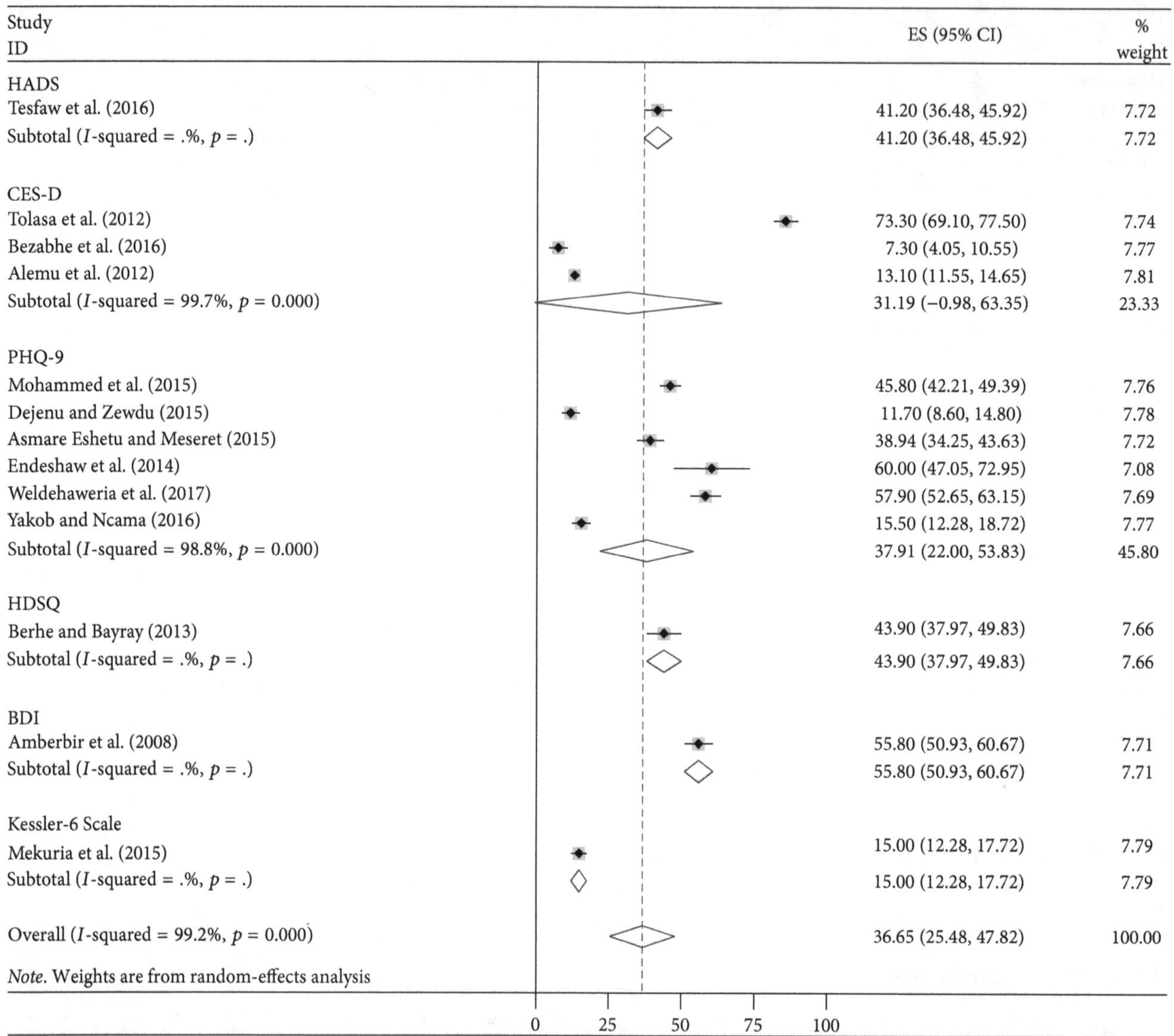


Figure 3: Forest plot presenting subgroup analysis of pooled estimated prevalence of depression according to the tool used among PLWHIV in Ethiopia, 2017.

experience of quitting work were significantly affected [27]. The reason might be that unfulfillment of human needs leads to depression. Being hospitalized in the past one month [28] was also another factor. The reason might be due to the fact that readmission indicates the complication of the problems. Being female was not statistically significant, 1.45 (0.91, 2.31), for depression, which contradicts with the finding of Uganda [14] and sub-Saharan Africa systematic review [23]. The possible justification was that in this finding we considered the pooled random-effect size of the four studies but in Uganda, which had a single study, and in Sub-Saharan Africa it was described qualitatively. Therefore, this finding has implication for clinicians as baseline data to link cases to psychiatry side, to reduce risks like suicide, to increase antiretroviral drug adherence, to reduce treatment delay, and to develop depression screening tool. For policymakers, it is used as baseline data to plan integrating HIV clinic with mental health and to prepare the guideline for HIV and mentally ill patients care.

## 6. Conclusion and Recommendation

The pooled estimate prevalence of depression among PLWHIV was higher than that in the general population. It is better to offer special attention to these populations.

## Ethical Approval

Since the review was concerned with the research articles, there was no need for ethical approval and/or additional consent from participants.

Table 2: Associated factors for depression among PLWHIV in Ethiopia, 2017.

| Variables | Factors that affect depression in PLWHIV | First author |
|---|---|---|
| Sex | Being male (AOR = 1.633; 95% CI: 1.138, 2.342) | Mohammed [26] |
| | Being female (AOR = 2.071; 95% CI: 1.077, 3.985) | Asmare Eshetu [28] |
| Age | 30–39 years (AOR = 2.761; 95% CI: 1.165, 6.540),<br>40–49 years (AOR = 3.847; 95% CI: 1.489, 9.942),<br>60–69 years (AOR = 19.645; 95% CI: 4.020, 95.991) compared to age 20–29<br>As the age increases, depression also increases | Asmare Eshetu [28] |
| Marital status | Being widowed (AOR = 3.128; 95% CI: 1.700, 5.757) | Mohammed [26] |
| Living arrangement | Living alone (AOR = 2.465; 95% CI: 1.196, 5.078) | Dejenu [27] |
| | Urban dwellers (AOR = 3.19; 95% CI: 1.5, 6.65) compared to rural dwellers | Berhe [36] |
| Social support | Poor social support (AOR = 2.02; 95% CI: 1.25, 3.27) compared to strong social support | Tesfaw [35] |
| Monthly income | Earning 500–1000 (AOR = 1.924; 95% CI: 1.159, 3.195) compared to >1500 birrs | Mohammed [26] |
| | Lower socioeconomic class (AOR = 4.43; 95% CI: 1.35, 14.58) | Berhe [36] |
| | Income < 200 birrs (AOR = 3.917; 95% CI: 1.559, 9.845), 201–400 birrs (AOR = 2.796; 95% CI: 1.139, 6.865), 401–700 birrs (AOR = 2.590; 95% CI: 1.058, 6.340) compared to >700 birrs | Asmare Eshetu [28] |
| Occupation | Unemployed (AOR = 2.74; 95% CI: 1.34, 5.57) and government employees (AOR = 3.56; 95% CI: 1.73, 7.30) compared to privately employed | Berhe [36] |
| | Quitting work (AOR = 2.73; 95% CI: 1.778, 6.329) compared to those in work | Dejenu [27] |
| Stigma and discrimination | Perceived HIV stigma (AOR = 3.60; 95% CI: 2.23, 5.80) compared to not having perceived HIV stigma | Tesfaw [35] |
| | Being teased, insulted, or sworn at (AOR = 2.286; 95% CI: 1.216, 4.297)<br>Gossiped about (AOR = 2.990; 95% CI: 1.682, 5.313) | Mohammed [26] |
| | Stigma and discrimination from the community were 3 times more likely to have depression than their counterparts (AOR = 3.42; 95% CI: 1.628, 7.188) | Dejenu [27] |
| | Felt stigmatized were about 4 times (AOR = 3.597; 95% CI: 1.861, 6.954) more likely to feel stigma than the counterparts | Asmare Eshetu [28] |
| Medication adherence | Poor medication adherence around 2 times (AOR = 1.61; 95% CI: 1.02, 2.55) had depression compared to good medication adherence | Tesfaw [35] |
| | Last time missed any of medication (AOR = 5.274; 95% CI: 2.583, 10.768) compared to those who take medication regularly | Mohammed [26] |
| Clinical stage of HIV/AIDS | Stage III HIV/AIDS (AOR = 2.317; 95% CI: 1.108, 4.848)<br>Stage IV HIV/AIDS (AOR = 8.769; 95% CI: 1.928, 39.872) | Asmare Eshetu [28] |
| | HIV stage III (AOR = 2.80; 95% CI: 1.50, 5.21) when compared to clinical stage I of HIV/AIDS | Tesfaw [35] |
| Hospitalization | In the past one month was (AOR = 15.262; 95% CI: 1.463, 159.219) | Asmare Eshetu [28] |

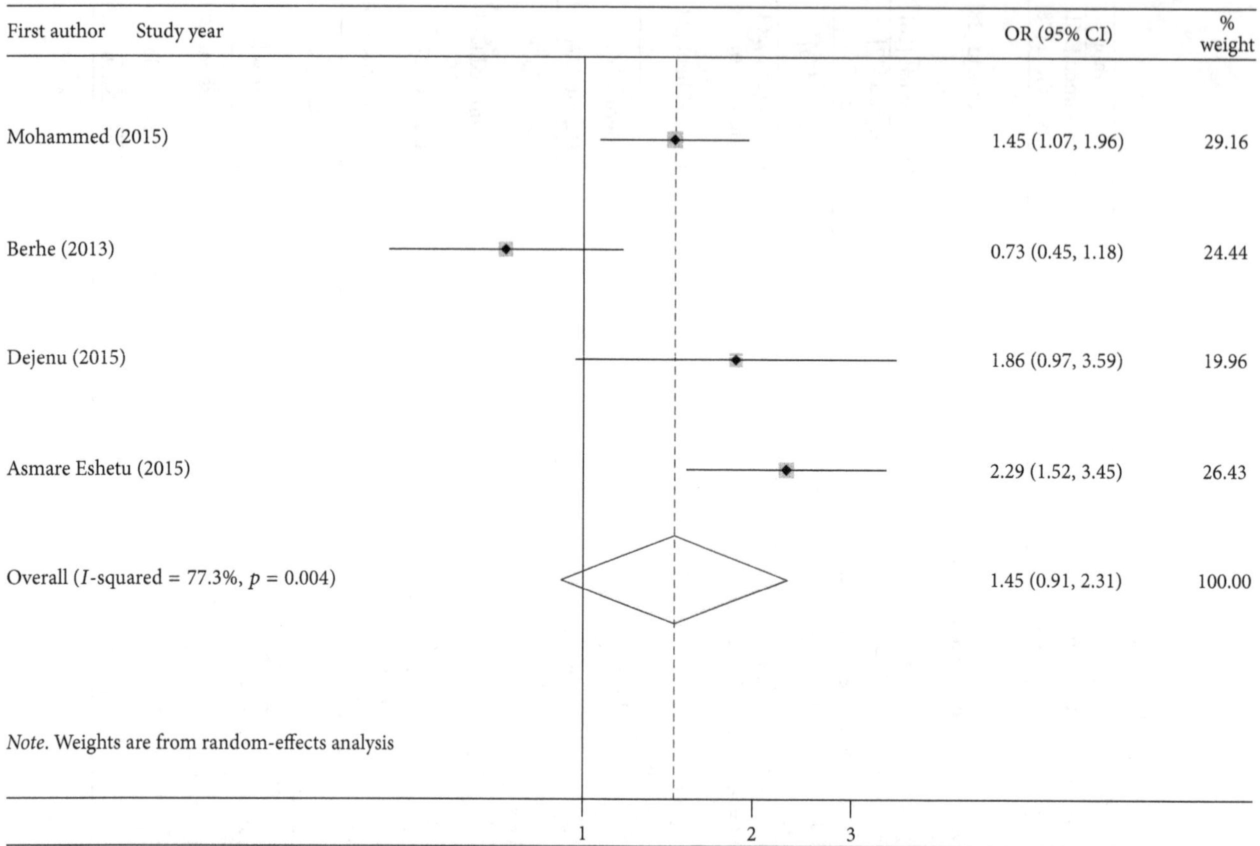


FIGURE 4: Forest plot presenting pooled random-effect size (OR) of females related to males in depressive PLWHIV patients in Ethiopia, 2017.

## Conflicts of Interest

The authors declare that there are no conflicts of interest.

## Authors' Contributions

Tadele Amare had a primary role in conceptualization, data review, data extraction, data analysis, and writing and editing of this manuscript. Wondale Getinet, Shegaye Shumet, and Biksegn Asrat had a role in data review, data extraction, and writing and editing of this manuscript.

## References


[1] J. A. Ciesla and J. E. Roberts, "Meta-analysis of the relationship between HIV infection and risk for depressive disorders," *The American Journal of Psychiatry*, vol. 158, no. 5, pp. 725–730, 2001.

[2] Disorders WGoSU, H. Kleber, R. Weiss, R. Anton, B. Rounsaville, and T. George, *American Psychiatric Association Steering Committee on Practice Guidelines*, J. McIntyre, S. Charles, D. Anzia, and et al., Eds., 2006.

[3] J. Leserman, "Role of depression, stress, and trauma in HIV disease progression," *Psychosomatic Medicine*, vol. 70, no. 5, pp. 539–545, 2008.

[4] M. Marcus, M. T. Yasamy, M. van Ommeren, D. Chisholm, and S. Saxena, *Depression: A global public health concern*, WHO Department of Mental Health and Substance Abuse, 2012.

[5] K. Miller and M. J. Massie, "Depression and anxiety," *Cancer Journal*, vol. 12, no. 5, pp. 388–397, 2006.

[6] J. K. Burns, "Mental health challenges rela th challenges rela th challenges related to hiv ted to hiv ted to hiv-aids in developing countries oping countries," *Journal Publishing Practices and Standards*, vol. 9, no. 1, pp. 3-4, 2012.

[7] OWH, "Suicide Prevention Across the Globe: Strengthening Protective Factors and Instilling Hope," in *International Association for Suicide Prevention*, 2012.

[8] OWH, "HIV/AIDS and Mental Health," Report by the Secretariat, WHO Google Scholar, Geneva, Switzerland, 2008.

[9] C. J. Berg, S. E. Michelson, and S. A. Safren, "Behavioral Aspects of HIV Care: Adherence, Depression, Substance Use, and HIV-Transmission Behaviors," *Infectious Disease Clinics of North America*, vol. 21, no. 1, pp. 181–200, 2007.

[10] M. Funk, *Global burden of mental disorders and the need for a comprehensive, coordinated response from health and social sectors at the country level*, 2016, Global burden of mental disorders and the need for a comprehensive, coordinated response from health and social sectors at the country level.

[11] P. S. Chandra, V. Ravi, A. Desai, and D. K. Subbakrishna, "Anxiety and depression among HIV-infected heterosexuals - A report from India," *Journal of Psychosomatic Research*, vol. 45, no. 5, pp. 401–409, 1998.

[12] C. Bernard, F. Dabis, and N. De Rekeneire, "Prevalence and factors associated with depression in people living with HIV in sub-Saharan Africa: A systematic review and meta-analysis," *PLoS ONE*, vol. 12, no. 8, Article ID e0181960, 2017.

[13] R. O. Shittu, M. K. Alabi, L. O. Odeigah et al., "Suicidal ideation among depressed people living with HIV/AIDS in Nigeria, West Africa," *Open Journal of Medical Psychology*, vol. 3, no. 3, pp. 262–270, 2014.

[14] F. M. Kaharuza, R. Bunnell, S. Moss et al., "Depression and CD4 cell count among persons with HIV infection in Uganda," *AIDS and Behavior*, vol. 10, no. 7, pp. S105–S111, 2006.

[15] A. Kagee and L. Martin, "Symptoms of depression and anxiety among a sample of South African patients living with HIV," *AIDS Care Psychological and Socio-medical Aspects of AIDS/HIV*, vol. 22, no. 2, pp. 159–165, 2010.

[16] N. Nakasujja, R. L Skolasky, S. Musisi et al., "Depression symptoms and cognitive function among individuals with advanced HIV infection initiating HAART in Uganda," *BMC Psychiatry*, vol. 10, article no. 44, 2010.

[17] O. A. Uthman, J. F. Magidson, S. A. Safren, and J. B. Nachega, "Depression and adherence to antiretroviral therapy in low-, middle- and high-income countries: a systematic review and meta-analysis," *Current HIV/AIDS Reports*, vol. 11, no. 3, pp. 291–307, 2014.

[18] P. Feuillet, F. Lert, L. Tron, C. Aubriere, B. Spire, and R. Dray-Spira, "Prevalence of and factors associated with depression among people living with HIV in France," *HIV Medicine*, vol. 18, no. 6, pp. 383–394, 2017.

[19] P. Seth, D. Kidder, S. Pals et al., "Psychosocial Functioning and Depressive Symptoms Among HIV-Positive Persons Receiving Care and Treatment in Kenya, Namibia, and Tanzania," *Prevention Science*, vol. 15, no. 3, pp. 318–328, 2014.

[20] D. E. Lyon and C. Munro, "Disease severity and symptoms of depression in Black Americans infected with HIV," *Applied Nursing Research*, vol. 14, no. 1, pp. 3–10, 2001.

[21] Worlad Health Organization, *HIV/AIDS Progress in Update/ Ethiopia 2014. Department of Health and Human service USA*, 2015.

[22] Program World Bank Global HIV/AIDS, "HIV/AIDS in Ethiopia an Epidemiological Synthesis," Washington, DC, USA, 2008, http://www.worldbank.org/AIDS.

[23] R. Brandt, "The mental health of people living with HIV/AIDS in Africa: A systematic review," *African Journal of AIDS Research*, vol. 8, no. 2, pp. 123–133, 2009.

[24] D. Moher, A. Liberati, J. Tetzlaff, and D. G. Altman, "Preferred reporting items for systematic reviews and meta-analyses: the PRISMA statement," *PLoS Medicine*, vol. 6, no. 7, Article ID e1000097, 2009.

[25] J. B. Institute, "The Joanna Briggs Institute Critical Appraisal Tools for Use in JBI Systematic Reviews Checklist for Analytical Cross Sectional Studies," 2016.

[26] M. Mohammed, B. Mengistie, Y. Dessie, and W. Godana, "Prevalence of depression and associated factors among HIV patients seeking treatments in ART clinics at Harar Town, Eastern Ethiopia," *Journal of AIDS and Clinical Research*, vol. 6, no. 474, p. 2, 2015.

[27] G. Dejenu and S. Zewdu, "Prevalence and Associated Factors of Depression among HIV Infected Patients in Debre Markos Town Northwest Ethiopia," *International Journal of Emergency Mental Health and Human Resilience*, vol. 17, no. 1522-4821, pp. 714–716, 2015.

[28] D. Asmare Eshetu and S. Meseret, "Prevalence of Depression and Associated Factors among HIV/ AIDS Patients Attending ART Clinic at Debrebirhan Referral Hospital, North Showa, Amhara Region, Ethiopia," *Journal of Clinical Psychiatry*, vol. 1, no. 1, 2015.

[29] M. Endeshaw, J. Walson, S. Rawlins et al., "Stigma in Ethiopia: Association with depressive symptoms in people with HIV," *AIDS Care Psychological and Socio-medical Aspects of AIDS/ HIV*, vol. 26, no. 8, pp. 935–939, 2014.

[30] N. B. Weldehaweria, E. H. Abreha, M. G. Weldu, and K. H. Misgina, "Psychosocial correlates of nutritional status among people living with HIV on antiretroviral therapy: A matched case-control study in Central zone of Tigray, Northern Ethiopia," *PLoS ONE*, vol. 12, no. 3, Article ID e0174082, 2017.

[31] B. Yakob and B. P. Ncama, "Client satisfaction: Correlates and implications for improving HIV/AIDS treatment and care services in southern Ethiopia," *International Health*, vol. 8, no. 4, pp. 292–298, 2016.

[32] B. Tolasa, D. B. Demissie, T. Tesfaye, and T. Belachew, *Food Insecurity and Associated Factors among People Living with HIV Attending ART Clinic in Fitche Zonal Hospital*, Ethiopia, 2016.

[33] W. M. Bezabhe, L. Chalmers, L. R. Bereznicki, P. Gee, and G. M. Peterson, "Antiretroviral adherence and treatment outcomes among adult Ethiopian patients," *AIDS Care Psychological and Socio-medical Aspects of AIDS/HIV*, vol. 28, no. 8, pp. 1018–1022, 2016.

[34] H. Alemu, D. Haile Mariam, A. Tsui, S. Ahmed, and A. Shewamare, "Effect of depressive symptoms and social support on weight and CD4 count increase at HIV clinic in Ethiopia," *AIDS Care Psychological and Socio-medical Aspects of AIDS/HIV*, vol. 24, no. 7, pp. 866–876, 2012.

[35] G. Tesfaw, G. Ayano, T. Awoke et al., "Prevalence and correlates of depression and anxiety among patients with HIV on-follow up at Alert Hospital, Addis Ababa, Ethiopia," *BMC Psychiatry*, vol. 16, no. 1, article no. 368, 2016.

[36] H. Berhe and A. Bayray, "Prevalence of depression and associated factors among people living with HIV/AIDS in Tigray, north ethiopia: a cross sectional hospital based study," *International Journal of Pharmaceutical Sciences and Research*, vol. 4, no. 2, p. 765, 2013.

[37] A. Amberbir, K. Woldemichael, S. Getachew, B. Girma, and K. Deribe, "Predictors of adherence to antiretroviral therapy among HIV-infected persons: a prospective study in Southwest Ethiopia," *BMC Public Health*, vol. 8, article 265, 2008.

[38] L. A. Mekuria, M. A. G. Sprangers, J. M. Prins, A. W. Yalew, and P. T. Nieuwkerk, "Health-related quality of life of HIV-infected adults receiving combination antiretroviral therapy in Addis Ababa," *AIDS Care Psychological and Socio-medical Aspects of AIDS/HIV*, vol. 27, no. 8, pp. 934–945, 2015.

# 9

# Male Partners Involvement in Prevention of Mother-to-Child Transmission of HIV Services in Southern Central Ethiopia: In Case of Lemo District, Hadiya Zone

**Degefa Tadele Belato,[1] Abera Beyamo Mekiso,[2] and Bayu Begashaw[3,4]**

[1] *Hadiya Zone Health Department, Hadiya Zone, Ethiopia*
[2] *Public Health Department, College of Health Sciences, Wolayta Sodo University, Wolayta Sodo, Ethiopia*
[3] *Public Health Department, College of Health Sciences, Mizan-Tepi University, Mizan-Aman, Ethiopia*
[4] *College of Medicine and Health Sciences, Institute of Public Health, University of Gondar, Gondar, Ethiopia*

Correspondence should be addressed to Degefa Tadele Belato; degefa04@gmail.com

Academic Editor: Robert R. Redfield

Male partners' involvement is a vital issue to prevent human immunodeficiency virus (HIV) transmission from mother to child; because it is much expectable that women were more vulnerable and high risk group of population portion. Therefore, to save lives of mothers and their newborn from acquiring HIV, male partners should do their maximum endeavor regardless of any determinant factors as our results revealed its status in our study context and elsewhere at past time too.

## 1. Background

Mother-to-child transmission is the most common mode of human immunodeficiency virus (HIV) transmission in children which can be vertically transmitted from HIV positive pregnant women to their unborn babies during pregnancy, labour, and delivery or through breastfeeding after delivery [1–3]. HIV remains a major challenge globally regardless of decades of advocacy and investment in programs to control the spread of the virus [4, 5]. Globally, an estimated 35.3 million people were living with HIV in 2012 [6, 7]. The number of newly infected children in 2012 was 260,000 in low- and middle-income countries [7]. Nearly all of these children acquired HIV through mother-to-child transmission and ninety percent of them live in Sub-Saharan Africa [8, 9]. Beyond this HIV/AIDS mainly affects people of reproductive age and increasingly affects women whose newborn babies will be victims of the disease [9]. Consequently, maximum efforts to improve programs for prevention of mother-to-child transmission (PMTCT) of HIV have been focused primarily at the health facility level on defining an effective set of community interventions to increase demand and uptake of services and retention [10]. Among communities male partners have greater roles but their participation is low in PMTCT [11].

Uptake of PMTCT services by the pregnant mothers is affected both by factors related to the health system such as accessibility of voluntary counselling and testing (VCT) services and by individual factors such as fear of disclosure of HIV results, lack of male partner support, fear of domestic violence, rejection, and negligence [1, 5, 11–14]. In Ethiopia, mother-to-child transmission (MTCT) accounts for 95% of childhood HIV infections. It poses a significant threat to child health and survival [11, 13, 15]. In 2013, there were an estimated 793,700 people living with HIV including 200,300 children and the paediatric HIV population. In the country there were mostly older children who were vertically infected in earlier years when the coverage and effectiveness of PMTCT in the country were low [11]. To halt the problem their male partners and mostly husbands should play a vital role besides mothers [16].

In Ethiopia, lack of male partner involvement in PMTCT undermined the potential benefits of antenatal HIV preventive efforts [16], thus representing a missed opportunity to effectively prevent vertical HIV transmission [17]. However, the factors associated with poor male participation are not well known in Ethiopia and need to be investigated to help the country develop reasonable strategies to address these bottlenecks. Male involvement is said to be very low in many health facilities in Ethiopia and it is one of the potential program gaps unfavourably affecting PMTCT services uptake in the country [18]. For this reason, previously in a country it was highlighted as involving male partners in ANC/PMTCT can often be utilized as an entry point for the provision of additional PMTCT services notably partner testing, condom use, and infant feeding recommendations for both male and female participants [6, 14].

There is global consensus that the world must strive towards elimination of new HIV infections among children by 2015 to keep mothers and children living with HIV alive. Many low- and middle-income countries have already moved significantly towards achieving these goals [19]. In spite of this in Southern Ethiopia, only 45% mothers brought their partner to HIV counselling and testing. Among these only 25% were tested and the HIV prevalence was 6.5%. This can also increase the likelihood of HIV infection among the newborns [17, 20].

As a result, in Lemo district, there is no clear evidence that could show level of male partners involvement in the PMTCT service. Thus, this study was conducted to determine the level of male involvement in PMTCT and factors which affect male involvement in PMTCT of HIV among males whose wives were attending ANC in previous six months before the study was conducted in Lemo district, Hadiya Zone, southern central Ethiopia.

## 2. Materials and Methods

*2.1. Study Design, Setting, and Participants.* Community based cross-sectional study was conducted in Lemo district from March 15/2015 to April 15/2015. Lemo district is located about 213 km from Addis Ababa, the capital city of Ethiopia. Based on 2007 national census, projection for 2014/15 the total population of the District is 148,339. From this 73,390 were males and 74,950 were females. There were 34,563 women in reproductive age group from which 5133 is expected pregnancy and 4732 were under one-year children [21].

*2.2. Sampling.* The sample size was calculated using a single population proportion formula, considering 50% proportion of male partner involvement in PMTCT of HIV service, 5% margin of error, design effect 2, correction formula, and 10% estimated nonresponse rate.

Multistage stratified sampling technique was used to select the study units. First, all the *kebeles* (the smallest administrative unit in Ethiopian government system below a district) in the district was stratified into urban and rural kebeles. Then 1 out of 2 urban kebeles and 10 out of 33 rural kebeles were selected randomly. The number of male partners was proportionally allocated based on the average number of male partners whose pregnant mothers were attending ANC services in previous six months before the study was conducted. Family folder in the health posts was used to identify households with eligible male partners. Households with eligible male partners were identified and sampling frame was created based on house numbers. Finally computer generated simple random sampling method was employed to select and approach each male partner.

*2.3. Variables in the Study and Its Measurement.* Data was collected by using interviewer administered structured questionnaire that was initially adapted from previous studies in English (questionnaire, in Supplementary Material available online at https://doi.org/10.1155/2017/8617540) and then was translated to both Hadiyigna and Amharic by language experts in Hadiyigna and Amharic and translated back to English by another language expert to ensure consistency. The tool includes five sections; sociodemographic and socioeconomic factors of the respondents, sociocultural norms of the respondents, service related factors of PMTCT, knowledge of respondents in PMTCT of HIV, and level of male involvement in PMTCT services. Those who responded to five and above male involvement items were recorded as "yes = 1" and those who responded to less than five items were recorded as "no = 0"; respondents' [11] total score on male involvement was calculated by summing up the scores of ten items designed to assess level of male involvement. All items had an equal weight of score 1. For all items, a score of 1 was given for "yes" responses for positive connotation and 0 (zero) for "no" or "uncertain" responses for negative connotation.

*2.4. Data Collection and Processing.* Eight diploma nurses for data collection and two health officers for supervision were recruited. One day training on how to fill the questionnaire, request the consent, and assure confidentiality of information of the study participants was given to data collectors and supervisors to ensure the quality of the field operation by principal investigator. During data collection, the supervisors had supervised the data collection process in daily base and performed quality checks. The instrument was pretested on 5% of the sample in Misha District which is 18 km far from the study area to check reliability of the tool. The pretest data was not included in the main data analysis.

All collected data from questionnaire was checked manually before entry to software. Then, the data was entered into a computer using EpiData version 3.1 software. The software was created based on data type and size, categories, validating permitted values and ranges, and codes to missing value. Corrections were made according to the original data.

*2.5. Data Analysis.* The data was analyzed by using SPSS version 16 software. Descriptive analysis was carried out for each of the variables to check frequency, distribution, and missing value. Bivariate analysis was employed to check crude association between level of male partner involvement in PMTCT of HIV services and independent variables. Chi-square test was conducted to see variables fulfilling assumption. Variable with $p$ value $< 0.25$ on bivariate analysis was entered to multivariable logistic regression to identify the factors that affect male involvement in PMTCT. Binary logistic regression test was used to assess association between independent variables and male involvement in PMTCT. Odds ratio and corresponding 95% confidence intervals were used to quantify the degrees of association between independent variable and level of male partner involvement in PMTCT of HIV services. Results with $p$ value $\leq 0.05$ were considered as being statistically significant and the rest was refuted. Multicollinearity among independently associated variables was checked by multicollinearity diagnostic test VIF in linear regression and none was collinear.

*2.6. Ethical Statement.* Ethical clearance and formal letters were obtained from Hadiya Zonal Health Department; then letter of permission was produced from administrative bodies of the zone to the district administration hierarchically. Verbal consent was preferred rather than written consent for the following reasons. Firstly, this was cross-sectional study that found out descriptive data. Secondly, their responses had no personal, cultural, social, or political impacts. Thirdly, there would not be significant risk/s to the participants. Finally, a significant number of people living in the study area have no educational status. The IRB approved the proposed verbal consent procedure. The confidentiality of the data was ensured by not asking their names.

## 3. Results

*3.1. Study Participant Characteristics.* Total of 401 male partners of pregnant mothers had participated in thestudy making the response rate of 95%. The remaining 5% were not taking part during interview due to lack of consent, withdraw, and fear of social neglect. The majority, 173 (43.1%), of respondents belong to the age group below 34 years with median age of 35 years. Regarding the ethnic background the predominant ethnic group, 341 (85%), was Hadiya followed by Kambata, 30 (7.5), while the dominant religion, 242 (60.2%), was protestant followed by orthodox 85 (21.2%). The majority, 378 (94.4%), of male partners were from the rural areas; the remaining 23 (5.7%) of respondents were from the urban areas. With regard to occupation, 176 (68.8%) of the participants were farmers followed by merchants 75 (18.7%) and the largest number of the respondents, 297 (74.1%), had earned family monthly income above 1170 ETB (Table 1).

Table 1: Showing sociodemographic and economic characteristic of male partners' involvement in PMTCT of HIV services in Lemo District, Hadiya Zone, southern central Ethiopia, 2015.

| Sociodemographic variables | Frequency ($n$ = 401) | Percent (%) |
|---|---|---|
| Residence | | |
| Urban | 23 | 5.7 |
| Rural | 378 | 94.3 |
| Age | | |
| ≤34 years | 173 | 43.1 |
| 35–44 years | 157 | 39.2 |
| ≥45 years | 71 | 17.7 |
| Marital status | | |
| Traditional married | 371 | 92.5 |
| Registered married | 30 | 7.5 |
| Duration of living relationship | | |
| <5 years | 143 | 35.7 |
| 5–10 years | 132 | 32.9 |
| >10 years | 126 | 31.4 |
| Religion | | |
| Protestant | 242 | 60.3 |
| Orthodox | 85 | 21.2 |
| Muslim | 54 | 13.5 |
| Others[a] | 20 | 5.0 |
| Ethnicity | | |
| Hadiya | 341 | 85.0 |
| Kambata | 30 | 7.5 |
| Silte | 16 | 4.0 |
| Others[b] | 14 | 3.5 |
| Educational | | |
| Illiterate | 18 | 4.5 |
| Able to read and write | 26 | 6.5 |
| Grades 1–4 | 58 | 14.5 |
| Grades 5–8 | 134 | 33.4 |
| Grades 9-10 | 84 | 20.9 |
| Grade 11 and higher | 81 | 20.2 |
| Occupation | | |
| Farmers | 276 | 68.8 |
| Governmental employees | 36 | 9.0 |
| Merchants | 75 | 18.7 |
| Daily labourers | 14 | 3.5 |
| Monthly income | | |
| ≤1170 ETB | 104 | 25.9 |
| >1170 ETB | 297 | 74.1 |

[a]Catholic and Adventist [b]Wolayta and Halaba.

*3.2. Sociocultural Factors Influence on Male Involvement in PMTCT of HIV Services.* Only 123/401 (30.9%) were accompanied by their male partner at the ANC/PMTCT. Among male partners who accompany their pregnant wives, 117/123 (95.2%) of husbands who accompany their pregnant wives have tested and counselled for HIV in the current pregnancy of their wives at ANC. Three-fourth of the respondents (64.1%) agreed that it was taboo for men to discuss with women HIV testing during pregnancy, delivery, and breastfeeding. Nearly half of the respondents, 183 (45.6%), agreed that it is better to postpone HIV testing to postdelivery due to fear of stress during pregnancy and 252 (62.8%) of respondent approved that it is enough that a pregnant woman come to ANC clinic by less busy relatives or friends. Nearly half of respondents, 196 (48.8%), agreed that the maternal and child health clinics should focus only on the health care service of women and children excluding male partners and 174 (43.4%) of the respondents decided that if the pregnant woman was found to be HIV positive she should be divorced.

*3.3. Male Partners Knowledge in PMTCT of HIV Services.* Three hundred forty-seven (86.5%) of male partners knew that HIV could be transmitted by an unprotected sexual intercourse. Almost half, (50.4%) and (50.6%), of male partners knew that MTCT of HIV could be during pregnancy and labour, respectively, and 169 (42.1%) of respondents approved that HIV could be transmitted during breastfeeding. Nearly half, 182 (45%), of male partners knew that HIV counselling and testing of pregnant women could reduce MTCT of HIV and almost one-fourth (27.4%) of male partners knew that HIV counselling and testing of pregnant women could reduce MTCT of HIV and nearly three-fourth (72.6%) of the male partners knew that provision of ARV could reduce MTCT of HIV. About half (49.6%) of male partners knew and heard about PMTCT services and almost half (51.9%) of male partners knew that HIV counselling and testing service was provided for pregnant women in ANC clinics.

*3.4. Service Related Factors to Male Partner Involvement in PMTCT of HIV.* Two hundred nineteen (54.6%) of male partners disproved that antenatal clinics should be opened on weekends and evening for men to attend ANC clinics with their partner and 72 (17.9%) of respondents agreed that distance from health facility was major obstacle to have attend ANC/PMTCT clinic with their partners and also 214 (53.4%) of male partners disagreed that couple HIV counselling and testing for PMTCT should be conducted at villages.

Majority, 249 (62.0%), of the respondents agreed that there should be separate waiting areas for men and women visiting maternal and child health clinics and 214 (53.4%) of male partners approved that there should be a different exit for male and female partners after HIV testing to avoid being identified by the crowded waiting for service. Nearly two-thirds of the respondents (66.0%) agreed that service providers did not request men to enter into ANC room together with their partner and nearly one-fifth and 79 (19.7%) of male partners agreed that health facilities did give men medical certificate of ANC attendance and invited verbally or in written form for their attendance at ANC clinic by the antenatal clinic, respectively.

*3.5. Level of Male Partner's Involvement in PMTCT of HIV Services.* Nearly two-thirds, 124 (30.9), of male partners supported ANC follow-up of their partners by arranging transport cost, 122 (30.4%) of male partners were self-initiated to discuss HIV testing with their partner during pregnancy, 125 (31.2%) of male partners participated by remembering the follow-up schedule, and 117 (29.2%) of male partners were accompanying the partner to ANC clinics at least once; out of those who came to ANC clinic with their partners only 61 (15.2%) of male partners entered into ANC room together with their partner. Only one hundred eleven (28.0%) male partners were counselled and tested for HIV during their partners' pregnancy; out of those counselled and tested only 45 (38.9%) of male partners were counselled and tested together with their female partner.

Almost three-fourth of the respondents (76.8%) agreed to support the medical follow-up of newborn until their HIV status was known while nearly two-thirds of the respondents, 259 (64.6%), were confident of using a condom consistently in case of discordant HIV status but nearly one-fourth of the male partners (24.4%) decided to discontinue conjugal or love relationship if their partners' HIV status was positive.

*3.6. Factors Affecting Male Partners Involvement in PMTCT of HIV Service.* The bivariate analysis revealed that residence, level of education, occupation and family monthly income, sociocultural factors influence, level of knowledge, and service related factors influences were candidates for further analysis in multivariable logistic regression. Variables such as level of education, occupation, family monthly income, sociocultural factors influence, level of knowledge, and service related factors influences were significantly associated with male partners involvement in PMTCT of HIV service.

*3.7. Factors Independently Affecting Male Partners Involvement in PMTCT Services.* Variables which significantly predict the level of male partners' involvement in PMTCT of HIV services were family monthly income, level of education, sociocultural factor influence, level of knowledge, and service related factors influence. See Table 2.

Those male partners educated from grades 1 to 4 were (AOR, 0.27, 95% CI: 0.08–0.90) less likely involved in PMTCT of HIV services when compared with grade 11 and higher. Male partners who had family income ≤ 1170 ETB monthly were 84% (AOR, 0.16, 95% CI: 0.1–0.4) less likely involved in PMTCT service when compared to those who had earned 1170 ETB. Male partners who had low sociocultural factor influence to involve in PMTCT services were almost four (AOR = 4.09, 95% CI: 2.28–7.34) times more likely involved in PMTCT services when compared with their counterparts. Moreover, the participants who had high knowledge in PMTCT of HIV service were nearly seven (AOR = 6.65, 95%: 3.67–12.08) times more likely involved in PMTCT service when compared with their counterparts and the respondents who had better service related factors influence to involve in PMTCT service were almost three (AOR, 3.2, 95% CI: 1.78–5.63) times more likely involved in PMTCT services when compared with those who had high service related factor influence to be involved in PMTCT of HIV services.

## 4. Discussion

In this study the level of male partner involvement in prevention of mother-to-child transmission of human immune deficiency virus service among participated male partners was 30.9%. The findings of this study were higher than the studies result which were conducted in Gondar and Mekelle which revealed that 20.9% and 20.1% of male partners come to ANC/PMTCT clinic with their female partners, respectively [11, 20]. The discrepancy of these findings might be attributed to difference in method used and study settings, sociodemographic characteristics of the study participants, and availability and accessibility of the infrastructures.

In this study, 15.2% of male partners who had come to ANC/PMTCT clinic with their partners were entered into ANC room together with their partners. This finding is lower than that of the study conducted in Deremarkos town which revealed that out of respondents who had come with their

Table 2: Showing bivariate and multivariable logistic regression of factors associated with male partners' involvement in PMTCT of HIV among males in Lemo district, Hadiya Zone, southern central Ethiopia, 2015.

| Variables | Male partner involvement in PMTCT of HIV services | | | | |
|---|---|---|---|---|---|
| | High Number (%) | Low Number (%) | COR (95% C.I) | AOR (95% C.I) | $p$ value |
| Residence | | | | | |
| Urban | 10 (43.5) | 13 (56.5) | 1.81 (0.77, 4.24) | 3.08 (0.91, 10.42) | 0.071 |
| Rural | 113 (29.9) | 265 (70.1) | | 1 | |
| Educational status | | | | | |
| Illiterate | 5 (27.8) | 13 (72.2) | 1.28 (0.42, 3.86) | 0.72 (0.19, 2.64) | 0.619 |
| Able to read and write | 6 (23.1) | 20 (76.9) | 0.99 (0.37, 2.70) | 0.49 (0.14, 1.74) | 0.276 |
| Grades 1–4 | 5 (8.6) | 53 (91.4) | 0.31 (0.12, 0.85) | 0.27 (0.08, 0.90) | 0. 033* |
| Grades 5–8 | 31 (23.1) | 103 (76.9) | 1.41 (0.76, 2.61) | 0.76 (0.35, 1.64) | 0.22 |
| Grades 9-10 | 25 (29.8) | 59 (70.2) | 5.61 (3.09, 10.33) | 3.19 (0.54, 6.64) | 0.488 |
| Grade 11 and higher | 51 (63) | 30 (30.0) | | 1 | |
| Occupation | | | | | |
| Farmer | 62 (22.5) | 214 (77.5) | | 1 | |
| Governmental employee | 30 (83.3) | 6 (16.7) | 17.26 (6.87, 43.35) | 1.75 (0.47, 6.47) | 0.403 |
| Merchant | 28 (37.3) | 47 (62.7) | 2.06 (1.19, 3.55) | 0.67 (0.31, 1.46) | 0.413 |
| Daily laborer | 3 (21.7) | 11 (78.9) | 0.94 (0.26, 3.48) | 1.11 (0.17, 7.39) | 0.915 |
| Monthly income | | | | | |
| ≤1170 ETB | 11 (10.6) | 93 (89.4) | 0.19 (0.1, 0.38) | 0.16 (0.1, 0.4) | 0.000* |
| >1170 ETB | 112 (37.7) | 185 (62.3) | | 1 | |
| Sociocultural factors | | | | | |
| High cultural | 42 (10.6) | 176 (44.2) | | 1 | |
| Low cultural | 80 (20.1) | 100 (25.1) | 3.35 (2.14, 5.24) | 4.09 (2.28, 7.34) | 0.000* |
| Level of knowledge | | | | | |
| High knowledge | 96 (30.7) | 89 (69.3) | 7.55 (4.60, 12.40) | 6.65 (3.67, 12.08) | 0.000* |
| Low knowledge | 27 (6.7) | 189 (47.1) | | 1 | |
| Service related factors | | | | | |
| Poor service | 44 (11.0) | 176 (44.1) | | 1 | |
| Better service | 78 (19.5) | 101 (25.3) | 3.09 (1.98, 4.81) | 3.17 (1.78, 5.63) | 0.000* |

*Note.* * = statistically significant at ($p \leq 0.05$); 1 = reference group.

partners to ANC clinic, 69.3% of male partners were entered into ANC room together with their female partners [22].

One hundred twenty-three (30.7%) of male partners were highly involved in the PMTCT of HIV services in this study. This finding is nearly similar with the study conducted in four districts in Addis Ababa which found that 28.1% of male partners were highly involved in PMTCT of HIV services and the study in Eastern Uganda found that 99 (26%) of the male partners were highly involved in PMTCT services. However, the finding of this study is lower than the study conducted in Debre Markos town and three public hospitals in Addis Ababa which revealed that male partner involvement in the PMTCT services was 72.26% and 88, respectively. This difference might be due to the fact that those studies were conducted in urban area, with probable higher access to information on PMTCT of HIV services. This implies that efforts should be made to disseminate information through different mechanisms to community about PMTCT of HIV services in the study area.

Male partners educated from grades 1 to 4 were 73% less likely involved in PMTCT services when compared with grades 5 to 8, whereas, male partners educated till grade 11 and higher were almost three times more likely involved in PMTC services when compared with grades 5 to 8 in this study. The findings of this study are supported by the study findings conducted in Eastern Uganda which found that male partners who had attended secondary education or higher education were twice more likely involved in PMTCT of HIV services. The findings of this study imply that formal education has impact on male partners involvement in PMTCT services; therefore, more efforte should be made to increase awareness to low educated individuals about PMTCT services to increase PMTCT uptake in the study area.

This study found that male partners who had earned average family monthly income less than or equal 1170 ETB were 84% less likely involved in PMTCT of HIV service when compared to those who earned monthly income above 1170 ETB. The findings of this study supported the study conducted in South Africa which revealed that the male partners who had high monthly income were more involved in PMTCT of HIV services than respondents who had low monthly income [1]. This low involvement might be due to lack of awareness about PMTCT service which are given free of fee in all governmental health facilities and sociodemographic characteristics of the respondents. This implies that more efforts should be made to create awareness to community as PMTCT service is given free of fee for both pregnant mothers and their partners found in any economical status to increase level of male partners involvement in PMTCT services in the study area.

This study found that 180 (45.2%) of male partners had low sociocultural factors influence to be involved in PMTCT services. The findings of this study are inconsistence with the study finding in Debre Markos town which revealed 99.3% of male partners were within the range of low sociocultural factors influence [22]. This discrepancy might be attributed to different sociodemographic characteristics of respondents; in the later study more than two-thirds of the respondents were farmers whereas in previous study more than half of the respondents were government employees and study context also has its own impact for the observed discrepancy.

In the current study male partners who had low sociocultural factors influence on being involved in PMTCT services were almost four times more likely to be involved in PMTCT of HIV service when compared to male partners who had high sociocultural factors influence on being involved in PMTCT services. The finding of this study was comparable with the findings of studies conducted in Addis Ababa which revealed that as the sociocultural influence decreases the males involvement in PMTCT increases [23]. The findings of this study are also supported by the study findings in South Africa, which state that the barriers to male partner testing during pregnancy, delivery, and breast feeding were fear, guilt, and subsequent denial associated with a positive test result and lack of social expectation for a man to get tested during his partner's pregnancy [24].

This study found that 46.1% of male partners had high knowledge in PMTCT of HIV services. The findings of this study are lower than the study finding from four districts of Addis Ababa which revealed that 77% of male partners had high knowledge in PMTCT of HIV services [23]. The discrepancy might be attributed to difference in sociodemographic characteristics of the study participants and lack of access and availability of infrastructures like mass media and others.

Moreover, this study revealed that male partners who had high knowledge in PMTCT of HIV service were nearly seven times more likely involved in PMTCT of HIV services when compared to those who had low knowledge in PMTCT services. The findings of this study are comparable to the study findings from four districts of Addis Ababa which revealed that participants who had high knowledge were 14% more likely to have high involvement in PMTCT services when compared to those who had low knowledge [23]. Furthermore, the findings of this study are supported by the study findings in Debre Markos town which revealed that male partners who had moderate and good knowledge about PMTCT services were 4.4 and 3.2 times more likely involved in PMTCT services than male partners with low knowledge about PMTCT services, respectively [22].

Male partners having better service related factor influence to be involved in PMTCT services were 44.9%. This finding is lower than study conducted in Nigeria which revealed that 82.4% of male partners had low service related factor influence to involve in PMTCT services [5].

Moreover, respondents who had better service related factors influence on PMTCT service were almost three times more likely involved in PMTCT services when compared to their counterparts. The findings of the study are consistent with the study findings from Debre Markos town which showed that the respondents who had low service related factor influence to involve in PMTCT service were 14 times more likely involved in PMTCT of HIV services [24]. Lastly, our study revealed that, among male partners who accompany their pregnant wives, 117 (95.2%) of husbands who accompany their pregnant wives have tested and counselled for HIV in the current pregnancy of their wives at ANC. This is higher than findings from Mekele and Tanzania [11, 25]. This inconsistency might be due to current improvement in maternal and child health activities when compared to those studies period.

## 5. Conclusions

In this study majority of male partners had low involvement in PMTCT services. Male partners who are highly educated and have high family monthly income, high knowledge, low sociocultural influence toward male partners' involvement in PMTCT services, and low service related factor influence toward male partner involvement in PMTCT services were more likely involved in PMTCT of HIV services than their counterparts. But lack of awareness and knowledge about PMTCT services, cultural influence, and service related factors influence were some of the reasons that hinder higher male partner involvement in PMTCT of HIV services. Low male involvement in PMTCT service affects successful implementation of the PMTCT program. Additional consideration should also be given for the risk factors which may increase maternal and child mortality due to high expansion of HIV from mother-to-child. Availability of PMTCT service should be disseminated to community in different media with local language to increase the knowledge of male partners and to decrease sociocultural factors influence in PMTCT service. We also recommend further countrywide research on the issue.

## Abbreviations

ANC: Antenatal care
ETB: Ethiopian birr
HIV: Human immune deficiency syndrome
MTCT: Mother-to-child transmission
PMTCT: Prevention of mother-to-child transmission
SNNPR: Southern nation nationalities and peoples region.

## Data Access

All relevant data are within the paper and its supporting information files but any additional data required by the journal can be available anytime.

## Conflicts of Interest

The authors declare that they have no conflicts of interest.

## Authors' Contributions

Degefa Tadele Belato, Bayu Begashaw, and Abera Beyamo Mekiso conceived and designed the experiments. Degefa Tadele Belato conducted formal analysis. Degefa Tadele Belato was responsible for funding acquisition. Degefa Tadele Belato analyzed the data. Degefa Tadele Belato, Bayu Begashaw, and Abera Beyamo Mekiso contributed materials/analysis tools. Degefa Tadele Belato wrote original draft. Degefa Tadele Belato, Bayu Begashaw, and Abera Beyamo Mekiso were responsible for writing, reviewing, and editing.

## Acknowledgments

The authors thank every and each participant who took part in this study. Study participants, data collectors, and supervisors are acknowledged for their cooperation during data collection.

## References

[1] W. Van Den Berg, K. Brittain, G. Mercer, and D. Peacock, "Improving men's participation in preventing mother-to-child transmission of HIV as a maternal, neonatal, and child health priority in South Africa," *PLoS Medicine*, vol. 12, no. 4, pp. 1–8, 2015.

[2] E. Morden, K.-G. Technau, J. Giddy, N. Maxwell, O. Keiser, and M.-A. Davies, "Growth of HIV-exposed uninfected infants in the first 6 months of life in South Africa: the IeDEA-SA collaboration," *PLoS ONE*, vol. 11, no. 4, Article ID e0151762, 2016.

[3] G. B. Woelk, M. P. Kieffer, D. Walker, D. Mpofu, and R. Machekano, "Evaluating the effectiveness of selected community-level interventions on key maternal, child health, and prevention of mother-to-child transmission of HIV outcomes in three countries (the ACCLAIM Project): a study protocol for a randomized controlled trial," *Trials*, vol. 17, no. 1, article 88, 2016.

[4] L. Sherr and N. Croome, "Review article Involving fathers in prevention of mother to child transmission initiatives Á what the evidence suggests," *Journal of the International AIDS Society*, vol. 15, supplement 2, pp. 1–9, 2012.

[5] E. Ademola, "Barriers to uptake of prevention of mother-to-child transmission of HIV services among mothers of vertically infected HIV-seropositive infants in," *Patient Preference and Adherence*, vol. 10, pp. 57–72, 2016.

[6] Z. Namukwaya, L. Barlow-Mosha, P. Mudiope et al., "Use of peers, community lay persons and Village Health Team (VHT) members improves six-week postnatal clinic (PNC) follow-up and Early Infant HIV Diagnosis (EID) in urban and rural health units in Uganda: a one-year implementation study," *BMC Health Services Research*, pp. 1–11, 2015.

[7] T. Kendall and I. Danel, "Research and evaluation agenda for HIV and maternal health in sub-Saharan Africa," Women and Health Initiative Working Paper 1, Women and Health Initiative, Harvard School of Public Health, Boston, Mass, USA, 2014.

[8] K. Peltzer, D. Jones, S. M. Weiss, and E. Shikwane, "Promoting male involvement to improve PMTCT uptake and reduce antenatal HIV infection: a cluster randomized controlled trial protocol," *BMC Public Health*, vol. 11, article 778, 2011.

[9] E. Nicol, L. Dudley, and D. Bradshaw, "Assessing the quality of routine data for the prevention of mother-to-child transmission of HIV: An analytical observational study in two health districts with high HIV prevalence in South Africa," *International Journal of Medical Informatics*, vol. 95, pp. 60–70, 2016.

[10] G. B. Woelk, D. Ndatimana, S. Behan et al., "Retention of mothers and infants in the prevention of mother-Tochild transmission of HIV programme is associated with individual and facility-level factors in Rwanda," *Journal of the International AIDS Society*, vol. 19, no. 4, 2016.

[11] A. Amano and A. Musa, "Male involvement in PMTCT and associated factors among men whom their wives had ANC visit 12 months prior to the study in Gondar town, North west Ethiopia, December, 2014," *Pan African Medical Journal*, vol. 24, no. 239, pp. 1–8, 2016.

[12] A. Gourlay, A. Wringe, I. Birdthistle, G. Mshana, D. Michael, and M. Urassa, "'It is like that, we didn't understand each other': exploring the influence of patient-provider interactions on prevention of mother-to-child transmission of HIV service use in rural tanzania," *PLoS ONE*, vol. 9, no. 9, 2014.

[13] H. Balisanga, M. Mutagoma, E. Remera et al., "HIV surveillance in Rwanda: readiness assessment to transition from antenatal care-based to prevention of mother-to-child transmission program-based HIV surveillance," *International Journal of Infectious Diseases*, vol. 52, pp. 62–67, 2016.

[14] F. Mohammed and N. Assefa, "Determinants of desire for children among HIV-Positive women in the afar region, Ethiopia: case control study," *PLOS ONE*, vol. 11, no. 3, pp. 1–9, 2016.

[15] Y. A. D. Melaku, E. G. E. Zeleke, J. Kinsman, and A. K. E. Abraha, "Fertility desire among HIV-positive women in Tigray region, Ethiopia: implications for the provision of reproductive health and prevention of mother-to-child HIV transmission services," *BMC women's health*, vol. 14, p. 137, 2014.

[16] M. Al-Mujtaba, L. J. Cornelius, H. Galadanci et al., "Evaluating religious influences on the utilization of maternal health services among muslim and christian women in North-Central Nigeria," *BioMed Research International*, vol. 2016, Article ID 3645415, 8 pages, 2016.

[17] M. Coulibaly, E. Thio, C. Yonaba et al., "Prevention and care of paediatric HIV infection in Ouagadougou, Burkina Faso: knowledge, attitudes and practices of the caregivers," *BMC Pediatrics*, vol. 16, no. 1, article 33, 2016.

[18] A. L. Nyondo, A. F. Chimwaza, and A. S. Muula, "Stakeholders' perceptions on factors influencing male involvement in prevention of mother to child transmission of HIV services in Blantyre, Malawi," *BMC Public Health*, vol. 14, no. 1, article 691, 2014.

[19] UNAIDS, *Global Plan Towards the Elimination of New HIV Infections*, 2015.

[20] E. F. Falnes, K. M. Moland, T. Tylleskär, M. M. De Paoli, S. E. Msuya, and I. M. S. Engebretsen, "'It is her responsibility': partner involvement in prevention of mother to child transmission of HIV programmes, northern Tanzania," *Journal of the International AIDS Society*, vol. 14, no. 1, article 21, 2011.

[21] Hadya Zone Vitals Statistics Bureau, "Haydya zone annual population data," 2015.

[22] E. Amsalu, G. Tiruneh, and A. A. Abajobir, "Level of male partner involvement and associated factors in prevention of mother to child transmission of HIV/AIDS services in Debremarkos town, Northwest Ethiopia," *BMC Pediatrics*, vol. 10, pp. 16–25, 2013.

[23] Y. Abuhay, L. Abebe, and N. Fentahun, "Male involvement in prevention of mother to child transmission of HIV and associated factors among males in Addis Ababa, Ethiopia," *American Journal of Health Research*, vol. 2, no. 6, pp. 338–343, 2014.

[24] K. Koo, J. D. Makin, and B. W. C. Forsyth, "Barriers to male-partner participation in programs to prevent mother-to-child HIV transmission in south Africa," *AIDS Education and Prevention*, vol. 25, no. 1, 2013.

[25] F. Haile and Y. Brhan, "Male partner involvements in PMTCT: a cross sectional study, Mekelle, Northern Ethiopia," *BMC Pregnancy and Childbirth*, vol. 14, no. 1, article 65, 2014.

# 10

# Factors Affecting Utilization of Voluntary HIV Counseling and Testing Services among Teachers in Awi Zone, Northwest Ethiopia

**Woudneh Gereme Desta,[1] Mulusew Alemneh Sinishaw,[2] and Kelemu Dessie Bizuneh[3]**

[1]*Health Promotion and Disease Prevention Core Process, Amhara National Regional State Health Bureau, Bahir Dar, Ethiopia*
[2]*Clinical Chemistry, Amhara Public Health Institute, Bahir Dar, Ethiopia*
[3]*Public Health Emergency Management, Awi Zone Health Department, Injibara, Ethiopia*

Correspondence should be addressed to Mulusew Alemneh Sinishaw; mulusewalemneh@yahoo.com

Academic Editor: Soraya Seedat

HIV/AIDS affects the basic educational sector which is the most productive segment of the population and vital to the creation of human capital. The loss of skilled and experienced teachers due to the problem is increasingly compromising the provision of quality education in most African countries. The study was proposed to determine the magnitude of VCT utilization and assess contributing factors that affect VCT service utilization among secondary school teachers in Awi Zone. A cross-sectional study design was conducted among 588 participants in 2014. Self-administered questionnaire was used to collect data. Data was analyzed using SPSS version 16, presented as frequencies and summary statistics, and tested for presence of significant association with odds ratio at 95% CI. More than half (53.6%) of study participants were tested for HIV. Those who had sexual intercourse, had good knowledge about VCT, were divorced/widowed, were in the age group of 20–29 years, and were married utilized VCT services two, three, four, three, and two times better than their counterparts, respectively. Actions targeting unmarried status, increase of educational level, and teachers with age groups above 30 years are necessary to follow their counterparts to utilize VCT service in order to save loss of teachers.

## 1. Introduction

Assumption of Human Immunodeficiency Virus/Acquired Immune Deficiency Syndrome (HIV/AIDS) as a serious health crisis in the past few decades shifted to its impact on social and economic structures especially of developing countries as it affects adult populations in the productive and reproductive age groups [1].

HIV/AIDS epidemic stage was reached globally at different times according to different risk factors that undermine general productivity and production of the household as well as community, scrotal, and national economic securities is being affected [2].

According to UNAIDS report on the global AIDS epidemic in 2010, globally in 2009 about 33.3 million people (2.5 million children) were living with HIV/AIDS; among these 2.5 million people are newly infected with the virus; in the same year 1.8 million people (260,000 children less than 15 years) died due to HIV/AIDS [3].

Sub-Saharan Africa remains hardest hit and has just over 10% of the world population but is the home of 24.7 million people (1.5 million new infections) living with HIV/AIDS. Sub-Saharan Africa constituted 71% of people living with HIV/AIDS in the world; among these women are more affected than men; at the same time 1.1 million people lost their life as a result of HIV/AIDS [3, 4].

Ethiopia is one of the highly affected countries with HIV/AIDS pandemic in the world. Since the first two reported AIDS cases in 1986, the disease has spread at alarming rate throughout the country [5].

Eastern African country Ethiopia was a home of 1,116,216 people (336,160 were eligible for antiretroviral treatment (ART)) living with HIV/AIDS out of which 72,945 (20,522 needed ART) were children less than 15 years. Due to the combined effect of poverty and HIV/AIDS, more than 5.4 million children under the age of 18 years were orphaned, out of which 855,720 (16%) lost at least one parent due to HIV/AIDS [6].

Different professionals are victims for HIV/AIDS disease in all sectors; particularly the basic education sector which is vital to the creation of human capital is also equally affected. The loss of skilled and experienced teachers due to HIV/AIDS related deaths and long term HIV/AIDS related illnesses are affecting the provision of quality education in most African countries [7].

The impact of HIV/AIDS in education sector causes multifaceted effect. Evidence obtained in 1998–2003 among teachers in Addis Ababa showed that HIV/AIDS related illnesses were the leading cause of death accounting for half of all mortalities [8].

Since the issue not only is a health concern, but also has social, economic, and political implications, the Federal Ministry of Health has undertaken various appropriate reversing measures [9]. One strategy for prevention and control of HIV/AIDS is provision of extensive voluntary HIV counseling and testing services.

Voluntary HIV counseling and testing is the process by which an individual undergoes counseling enabling him or her to make an informed choice about being tested for HIV [1]. Voluntary HIV counseling and testing allows teachers to know their HIV serostatus and, if the result is positive, prepare for treatment as well as care and support services [10].

Many people in Ethiopia living with HIV/AIDS do not know their serostatus including teachers. Various studies undertaken in Ethiopia have shown different factors that contributed to nonacceptance of voluntary counseling and testing (VCT) services; among these factors are lack of perception of being at risk, no consideration given for VCT services, fear of HIV positive results, and fear of stigma and discrimination. Another study in Bethzatha project indicated that individuals having educational status of secondary school and above, being female, and Christian religion were associated with willingness to take VCT [11–13].

The 2013 Awi Zone Health Department annual report showed that the coverage of VCT utilization was 70% [14]. However, teachers were very few in the utilization of VCT services as compared to other professionals. There was scarcity of such studies conducted in Awi Zone especially in higher professional population groups. Hence, this study was initiated to fill the knowledge gap in identifying the factors that affect the acceptability of VCT services among teachers for exerting multidirectional HIV/AIDS prevention and controlling efforts, responsible professionals for creating human capital for next generation, involving shaping of school adolescents. Furthermore, the findings of this study were intended to help policy makers and planners as an input for their future program planning by identifying factors associated with VCT utilization among secondary school teachers.

This study was intended to determine magnitude of VCT service utilization and assess the associated factors among secondary school teachers in terms of sociodemographic, cognitive, and service delivery factors (Figure 1).

*Note.* Respondents were considered to have comprehensive knowledge about HIV/AIDS if they knew about the three HIV prevention methods (abstinence, being faithful to one HIV uninfected partner, and condom use).

## 2. Methods and Materials

*2.1. Study Period and Setting.* A cross-sectional study was conducted in secondary school teachers from September to October 2014 in Awi Zone. Awi Zone, one of the eleven zones in Amhara National Regional State, located 447 km away from Addis Ababa at north west direction along Bahir Dar highway. There were 13 secondary schools (7 high schools and 6 preparatory schools) and 1004 teachers in the zone in all its 11 district administrations. The potential health service coverage by public health facilities of the zone was 98%. VCT, PMTCT, and ART services were also given in 28, 15, and 9 health centers, respectively.

*2.2. Study Population.* All secondary school teachers, who worked at the time of the study, were included in the study whereas unconsciously sick ones at the specified period were excluded.

*2.3. Sample Size Determination and Sampling Technique.* The number of study participants required for the study was determined using single population proportion formula in consideration of 95% confidence level, 5% precision, design effect of 2, 10% nonresponse rate, and 46.3% practice rate of VCT among teachers obtained from pervious study in Ethiopia [7] from a source population of 1004. The calculated final sample size was 609.

A two-stage sampling procedure was employed in order to get representative sample size from the source population. In the first stage, seven out of 13 secondary schools (6 preparatory and 7 high schools) were selected using lottery method simple random sampling technique. The determined sample size was allocated to each school proportional to the size of study population. Secondly, to pick individual participant from each selected school, lists of teachers were taken from the school Administration Office and codes were given. Then the required sample sizes were selected using systematic random sampling. To determine the $K$th value for systematic random sampling a total number of teachers were divided into each cluster sample size. The first participant was selected using lottery method simple random sampling technique.

*2.4. Data Collection Instruments and Procedure.* The data were collected using face-to-face structured questionnaire adopted from HIV/AIDS behavioral surveillance survey (BSS) [15] and demographic health survey (DHS) [16]. The questionnaire was initially prepared in English, translated to Amharic version and back to English to ensure its consistency and comparability. Pretest was conducted on 30 secondary

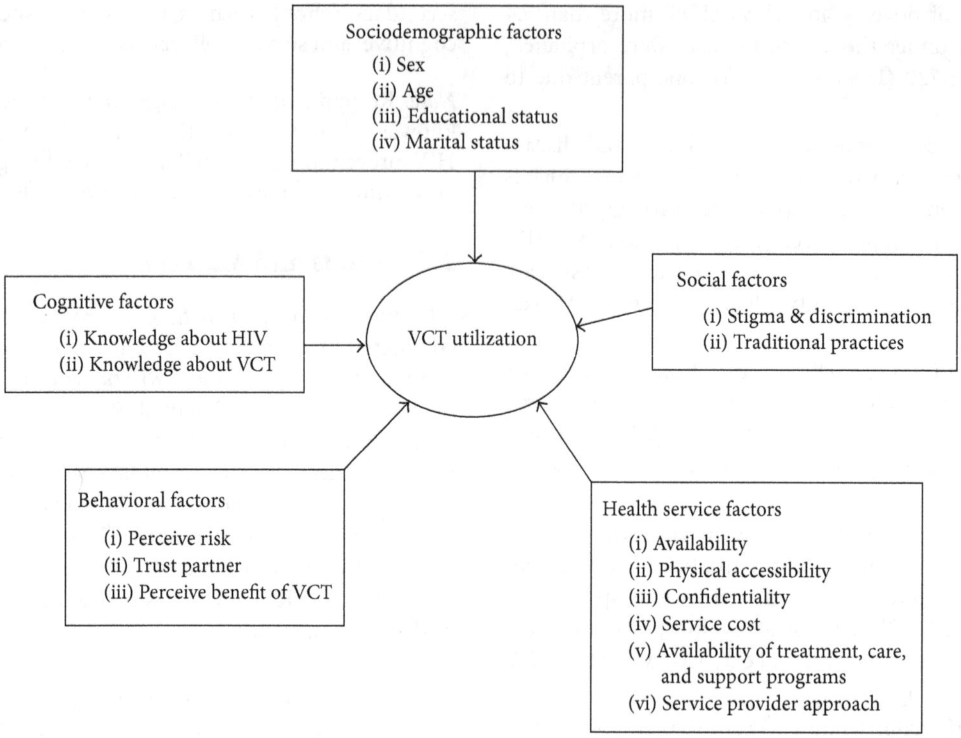


FIGURE 1: Conceptual framework for factors influencing VCT service utilization among secondary school teachers in Awi Zone, Amhara Region, 2014.

school teachers out of the study area to prevent information contamination. After the necessary modifications were made for ambiguous questions the actual data collection had taken place among study subjects.

Two supervisors and five data collectors, who have Bachelor of Science and diploma level nurses, respectively, were recruited and trained about the process of data collection for two days and collected the data.

*2.5. Data Management and Analysis.* Precoded data were entered and cleaned using Epi-info version 3.5.1 software. The entered data were exported to SPSS version 16 software and analysis was done. The data were presented using description, tables and graphs. Presence and strength of associations between dependent and independent variables were determined using odds ratio with 95% CI. Multivariable model logistic regression was employed to control possible confounding effects among variables that had $p$ value < 0.2 at bivariate regression.

*2.6. Ethical Consideration.* Ethical clearance was obtained from ethical clearance committee, Addis Continental Institute of Public Health, and University of Gondar joint MPH program. Permission letters were obtained from Amhara National Regional State Education Bureau and other substructures of education sector wrote a permission letter to study institutions accordingly. Verbal informed consent of the study participants was secured after explaining the purpose of the study. All the communications with study subjects were made with strict privacy and confidentiality. To keep confidentiality no individual identifiers were used and the collected data were put in lockable cupboard and password protected computer.

## 3. Results

*3.1. Sociodemographic Characteristics.* A total of 588 individuals with a response rate of 96.5% participated in this study. The mean age of study subjects was 29.8 ranging from 20 to 55 years with standard deviation of 6.3. Most of the respondents were males (85.2%) and 55% were single in marital status. The majority (94%) was first degree and most (86.7%) were Christian by religion. More than half of (52.4%) respondents were Agew by ethnicity (Table 1).

*3.2. Sexual History of Study Subjects.* Four hundred eighty-nine (83.1%) reported that they ever had sex at the time of the survey. From those who had sexual experience, 248 (50.7%) reported that they had more than one sexual partner. Among them, 230 (92.7%) reported that they had used condom (Table 2).

*3.3. Knowledge, Attitude, and Practice on VCT.* Regarding HIV counseling and testing services all have heard about confidential VCT services. The common sources of information about HIV counseling and testing services reported by secondary school teachers were mass media 525 (89.3%)

TABLE 1: Sociodemographic characteristics of secondary school teachers in Awi Zone, Amhara Region, Ethiopia, 2014.

| Characteristics | Category | Frequency | Percent |
|---|---|---|---|
| Sex | Male | 501 | 85.2 |
| | Female | 87 | 14.8 |
| Age group | 20–29 | 346 | 58.8 |
| | 30–39 | 191 | 32.5 |
| | 40–55 | 51 | 8.7 |
| Marital status | Single | 329 | 55.9 |
| | Married | 249 | 42.4 |
| | Widowed/divorced | 10 | 1.7 |
| Educational level | First degree and above | 553 | 94.0 |
| | Diploma and certificate | 35 | 6.0 |
| Religion | Orthodox Christian | 510 | 86.7 |
| | Muslim | 58 | 9.9 |
| | Others | 20 | 3.4 |
| Ethnicity | Agew | 308 | 52.4 |
| | Amhara | 252 | 42.8 |
| | Others | 28 | 4.8 |
| Monthly income | <1000 birr | 12 | 2.0 |
| | 1000–2000 birr | 352 | 59.9 |
| | >2000 birr | 224 | 38.1 |

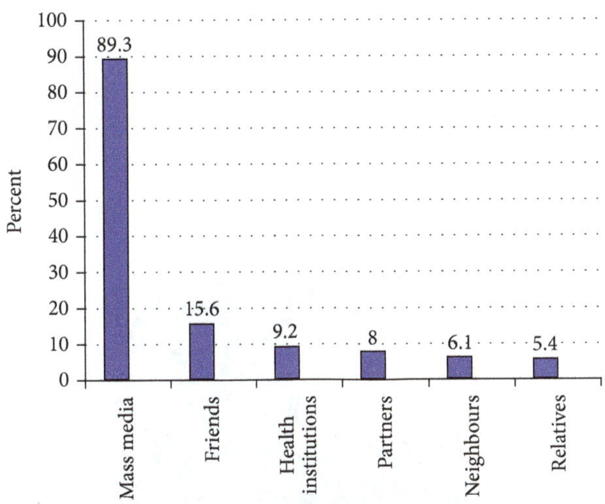


FIGURE 2: Sources of information about VCT among secondary school teachers in Awi Zone, Amhara Region, 2014.

and the other 63 (10.7%) were from health institutions, friends/peers, relatives, spouse, and neighbors (Figure 2).

Of the participants who had awareness about VCT services, 575 (100%) knew that voluntary counseling and testing service is available in their localities. Of them, 425 (72%) reported that the service process could take more than 30 minutes including walking time to reach the service site while others, 163 (28%) teachers, reported that they could have got the service within less than 30 minutes (Table 3). The main sites stated by teachers to get VCT service other than their localities were the said hospital, 438 (74.5%), private clinics, 307 (52.2%), health centers, 233 (39.9%), family guidance clinics, 208 (35.4%), and mobile sites, 8 (1.4%) and those who did not know other sites to get VCT services were 40 (6.8%).

Seventy-two percent, 472 (72.4%), of the respondents had good knowledge about VCT. Almost all, 569 (96.7%), of respondents agreed that HIV counseling and testing service is important and the reasons given for the importance of services were as follows: to know one's own health status, 460 (78.2%), to protect oneself from being infected, 267 (45.5%), if positive not to transmit to others, 225 (38.3%), if positive mothers to protect the child from HIV transmission, 202 (34.4%), to choose partner, 173 (29.4%), to plan future life, 235 (40%), and if positive to get treatment, care, and support services, 7 (1.2%).

Regarding targets for HIV counseling and testing services, 147 (25%) said any sexually active person, 144 (24.5%) anyone expected to be at risk, 135 (22.9%) those who are to be married, 128 (21.8%) those people who have more than one partner, 107 (18.8%) partners of commercial sex worker, 68 (11.5%) people who are sick, and 17 (2.9%) all people.

Three hundred fifteen (53.6%; 95% CI: 49.4%, 57.7%) of study subjects ever had HIV test. From those study participants who had HIV test 83 (26.3%) underwent HIV test before three months, 60 (19.1%) before six months, 138 (43.8%) before one year, 13 (4.1%) before two years, 8 (2.5%) before three years, and 13 (4.1%) before four years. Of the HIV tested study subjects, 298 (93.9%) utilized counseling service. Among these participants 166 (56.3%), 106 (35.9%), and 29 (9.8%) had received both pre- and posttest, pretest, and posttest counseling services in that order.

About the service delivery, 281 (89.2%) study subjects who were tested stated that they were satisfied with the service; 33 (10.5%) claimed that they were not satisfied by the given service. The reasons reported for being satisfied are as follows: 180 (57.1%) quick service, 180 (34.3%) confidentiality, 111 (35%) privacy, 89 (28.3%) warm reception, 84 (26.7%) health workers competency, 118 (37.5%) brief counseling, 80 (25.4%) free service, and 31 (9.8%) referral linkage for treatment, care, and support services.

On the other hand, the reason mentioned for dissatisfaction of VCT services were, 18 (90%), no warm reception, 13 (65%), lack of confidentiality, 13 (65%), health workers competency, 7 (35%), no clear counseling service, 6 (30%), long waiting time, 5 (25%), no referral linkage for treatment and other care and support services, and, 4 (20%), lack of privacy.

*3.4. Reasons for HIV Counseling and Testing.* Among respondents who utilized HIV counseling and testing services the reasons given for being tested were for knowing self-status, 161 (51.1%), for planning future life, 129 (40.9%), for premarital cases, 80 (25.4%), for blood donation, 9 (2.8%), and for starting antiretroviral treatment, 7 (2.2%) (Figure 3). On the other hand, respondents' reasons reported for not being tested were fear of result, 80.6%, fear of stigma, 17.2%, and other reasons, 17.2% (Figure 4).

TABLE 2: Sexual history of secondary school teachers in Awi Zone, Amhara Region, Ethiopia, 2014.

| Characteristics | Category | Frequency | Percent |
|---|---|---|---|
| Ever had sex ($n = 588$) | Yes | 490 | 83.3 |
| | No | 98 | 16.7 |
| Ever had sex with multiple sexual partners in the last five years ($n = 489$) | Yes | 248 | 50.7 |
| | No | 241 | 49.3 |
| Ever used condom with multiple sexual partners in the last five years ($n = 248$) | Yes | 230 | 92.7 |
| | No | 18 | 7.3 |
| How often they used condom with multiple sexual partners ($n = 230$) | Always | 136 | 58.7 |
| | Sometimes | 95 | 41.3 |

TABLE 3: Knowledge, attitude, and practice of secondary school teachers on VCT, Awi Zone, Amhara Region, Ethiopia, 2014.

| Characteristics | Category | Frequency | Percent |
|---|---|---|---|
| VCT available in your locality | Yes | 575 | 97.8 |
| | No | 13 | 2.2 |
| Time to take the service | Less than 30 minutes | 163 | 27.7 |
| | More than 30 minutes | 425 | 72.3 |
| Comprehensive knowledge about VCT | Good knowledge | 426 | 72.4 |
| | Poor knowledge | 162 | 27.6 |
| VCT mentioned as important ($n = 588$) | Yes | 569 | 96.7 |
| | No | 10 | 1.7 |
| | Neutral | 9 | 1.7 |
| Ever had VCT test ($n = 569$) | Yes | 315 | 53.6 |
| | No | 273 | 46.4 |
| Place where HIV test was performed ($n = 315$) | Government health center | 263 | 83.5 |
| | Other health institutions | 52 | 16.5 |

VCT: voluntary counseling and testing; HIV: Human Immunodeficiency Virus.

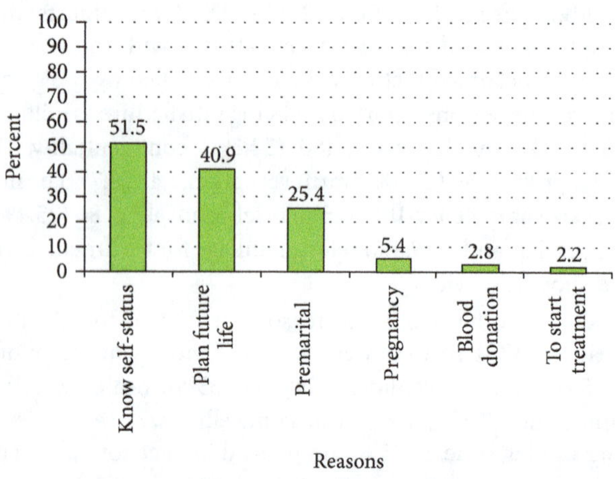


FIGURE 3: Reason mentioned to get tested for HIV among secondary school teachers in Awi Zone, Amhara Region, 2014.

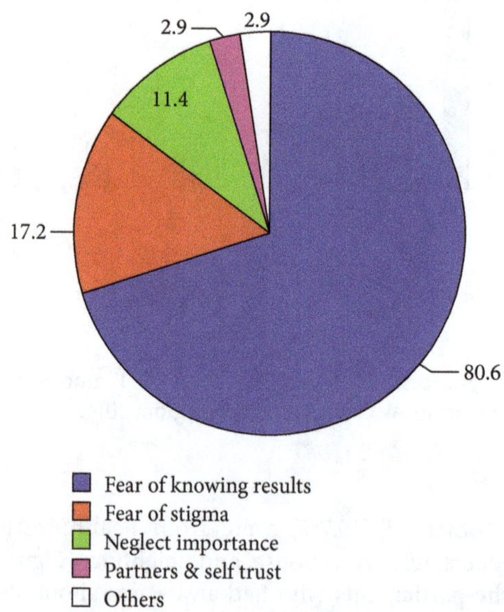


FIGURE 4: Reasons mentioned not to get tested for HIV among secondary school teachers in Awi Zone, Amhara Region, 2014.

*3.5. Factors Associated with VCT Service Utilization.* Respondents of age group 20–29 utilized VCT services 3 times better than 40 years and above (AOR: 3.03; 95% CI: 1.4, 6.13).

Divorced/widowed and married study participants were more than four and two times extra utilizing VCT services than unmarried counterparts (AOR: 4.38; 95% CI: 1.0, 18.32 and AOR: 2.29; 95% CI: 1.51, 3.49), respectively. In terms of education level of respondents who had first degree and above they used VCT services less as compared to the respondents of diploma and certificate holders (AOR: 0.29; 95% CI: 0.11,

TABLE 4: Associations of selected sociodemographic variables with VCT service utilization among secondary school teachers in Awi Zone, Amhara Region, Ethiopia, 2014.

| Characteristics | Category | Had VCT | | COR (95% CI) | AOR (95% CI) |
|---|---|---|---|---|---|
| | | Yes | No | | |
| Sex | Male | 266 | 235 | 0.88 (0.56, 1.39) | 1.07 (0.66, 1.74) |
| | Female | 49 | 38 | 1 | 1 |
| Age group | 20–29 | 201 | 145 | 1.69 (0.90, 3.18) | 3.03 (1.40, 6.13)* |
| | 30–39 | 91 | 100 | 1.11 (0.57, 2.16) | 1.44 (0.76, 2.75) |
| | 40–60 | 23 | 28 | 1 | 1 |
| Marital status | Single | 162 | 167 | 1 | 1 |
| | Married | 146 | 103 | 1.46 (1.03, 2.07) | 2.29 (1.50, 3.49)* |
| | Divorced/widowed | 7 | 3 | 2.41 (0.55, 11.95) | 4.38 (1.05, 18.32)* |
| Educational level | Above first degree | 286 | 267 | 0.22 (0.08, 0.57)* | 0.29 (0.11, 0.75)* |
| | Diploma and certificate | 29 | 6 | 1 | 1 |
| Religion | Orthodox | 278 | 232 | 1 | 1 |
| | Muslim | 30 | 28 | 0.89 (0.50, 1.59) | 1.01 (0.58, 1.78) |
| | Others | 7 | 13 | 0.45 (0.16, 1.23) | 0.48 (0.18, 1.25) |
| Monthly income | <1000 birr | 10 | 2 | 1 | 1 |
| | 1000–2000 birr | 196 | 160 | 0.24 (0.04, 1.21)* | 0.47 (0.077, 2.15) |
| | >2000 birr | 109 | 111 | 0.20 (0.03, 0.99)* | 0.37 (0.07, 2.05) |

*Significantly associated; VCT: voluntary counseling and testing.

0.75). However, VCT service vitalization was not significantly associated ($p > 0.05$) with sex, religion, and income of respondents (Table 4).

Respondents who had practiced sexual intercourse utilized VCT services two times greater than those who had not (AOR: 2.25; 95% CI: 1.09, 4.61). Similarly, the participants who had multiple sexual partners utilized VCT services about 2 times more than those who do not (AOR: 1.96; 95% CI: 1.37, 2.81) (Table 5). However, significant association was not observed among partners who used condom during intercourse with multiple sexual partners compared to their counterparts.

Knowledge about VCT was significantly associated with VCT service utilization. Respondents who had good knowledge utilized VCT services 3 times higher than those who had poor knowledge about VCT services (AOR: 3.05; 95% CI: 1.72, 7.21).

Respondents perceived to be discriminated by family and unwilling to disclose themselves utilized VCT services about 22% and 62% less than their counterparts (AOR: 0.22; 95% CI: 0.055, 1.01 and AOR: 0.62; 95% CI: 0.44, 0.88), respectively (Table 6).

## 4. Discussion

VCT is one of those approaches that are adopted at the national level for HIV/AIDS prevention and control strategies. This study tried to look into some of the important factors that affect the utilization of VCT among secondary school teachers in Awi Zone.

In this study we found that the proportion of VCT service utilization was 53.6%, which is still low as compared to VCT service utilized by the general community (70%) in Awi Zone [14]. This figure is considerably higher when compared to the study conducted in Harari Administrative region and the 2005 BSS-Ethiopia findings which were 46.3% and 41.3%, respectively [7, 15]. Similar study conducted among teachers in Tanzania also showed about 20% of the participants had utilized voluntary testing for HIV [17]. The increased uptake could be due to the intensive advocacy, health education, and expansion of VCT site and other related activities which have been conducted on HIV/AIDS prevention and control interventions assisted by health extension programs.

In this study, teachers aged between 20 and 29 years utilized VCT services 3 times better than 40 years and above. A study conducted among teachers in Tanzania also indicated that teachers who were aged between 21 and 30 years were significantly associated with an increased rate of having been tested for HIV [17]. Another study conducted in Kagera Region, Tanzania, also revealed an increasing tendency for young people to be tested for HIV especially before marriage [18]. Along with our findings, several population based studies conducted in Ethiopia revealed an association between testing for HIV and age; as age increases, the rate of testing for HIV decreases. The significant positive association of the younger age group may be due to the fact that they perceive themselves at risk of HIV infection.

In this study, respondents with education levels of first degree and above used VCT services less than diploma and certificate holders. This finding supported a study conducted in Gonder among different professional and community groups that showed high school teachers were found to have less acceptance of VCT compared with the other community groups [10]. This could be due to the fact that as people's

TABLE 5: Association of sexual behaviors with VCT service utilization among secondary school teachers in Awi Zone, Amhara Region, Ethiopia, 2014.

| Characteristics | Category | Had VCT | | COR (95% CI) | AOR (95% CI) |
|---|---|---|---|---|---|
| | | Yes | No | | |
| Ever had sexual intercourse | Yes | 271 | 219 | 1.52 (0.96, 2.40)* | 2.25 (1.09, 4.61)* |
| | No | 44 | 54 | 1 | 1 |
| Had sex with multiple sexual partners | Yes | 181 | 112 | 1.51 (1.05, 2.03)* | 1.96 (1.37, 2.81)* |
| | No | 112 | 136 | 1 | 1 |
| | No response | 22 | 25 | 0.54 (0.28, 1.08) | 1.38 (0.53, 3.67) |
| Frequency of condom use during sexual intercourse with multiple partners | Yes | 117 | 133 | 0.54 (0.38, 0.77)* | 0.69 (0.24, 2.05) |
| | No | 176 | 108 | 1 | 1 |
| | No response | 22 | 32 | 0.42 (0.22, 0.79)* | 0.48 (0.27, 1.12) |
| Frequency of condom use with the multiple sexual partners | Always | 69 | 66 | 1 | 1 |
| | Sometimes | 50 | 65 | 0.69 (0.41, 0.41) | 0.5 (0.31, 0.8) |
| | No response | 143 | 64 | 1.45 (0.49, 4.3) | 0.5 (0.31, 0.8) |

*Significantly associated; VCT: voluntary counseling and testing.

TABLE 6: Association of knowledge, attitude, and practices towards VCT service utilization, among secondary school teachers in Awi Zone, Amhara Region, Ethiopia, 2014.

| Characteristics | Category | Had VCT | | Crude OR (95% CI) | Adjusted AOR (95% CI) |
|---|---|---|---|---|---|
| | | Yes | No | | |
| Educational level | Above first degree | 286 | 267 | 0.22 (0.08, 0.57)* | 0.16 (0.17, 2.42) |
| | Diploma and certificate | 29 | 6 | 1 | 1 |
| Knowledge of VCT | Poor knowledge | 51 | 111 | 1 | 1 |
| | Good knowledge | 246 | 180 | 2.97 (1.99, 4.45)* | 3.05 (1.72, 7.21)* |
| Unwillingness to disclose HIV test results for anyone | Yes | 20 | 82 | 0.16 (0.09, 0.27)* | 0.22 (0.055, 1.01) |
| | No | 295 | 191 | 1 | 1 |
| Attitude of discriminating by family | Yes | 127 | 142 | 0.62 (0.44, 0.88)* | 1.26 (0.54, 2.79) |
| | No | 188 | 131 | 1 | 1 |

VCT: voluntary counseling and testing; HIV: Human Immunodeficiency Virus; *significantly associated.

knowledge increases about the serious health consequences to the extent of death and the society's reaction to the disease, people could decline to accept VCT despite good knowledge. On the other hand, the study conducted in Tanzania has showed teachers who had a college or university education have been tested for HIV greater than those who had secondary or primary education [17]. The increased uptake of VCT utilization among Tanzanian teachers might be due to the fact that in urban areas those with higher levels of education anticipated reactions of HIV/AIDS related stigma and discrimination less.

Married individuals showed utilizing VCT services 2 times more than unmarried counterparts. Moreover, those who were divorced/widowed utilized VCT services 4 times more than unmarried counterparts. Similar findings were reported from the study conducted in North Wollo Zone, Amhara Region, and in Rakai, Uganda [19, 20]. Individuals who had practiced sex ever and had multiple sexual partners were also depicted to utilize VCT services 2 times more than those who had not. Parallel finding was also reported from a study conducted among 15–49-year age group in Mersa Town of North Wollo Zone, Ambo and Bahir Dar University Students [19, 21, 22]. This might be due to the fact that those who had practiced sex with multiple sexual partners perceived that HIV is transmitted through high-risk sexual practices.

The present study indicated that individuals who had good knowledge about VCT were three times more likely to utilize VCT service than those who had not. Similar finding was reported from a study among Debre Markos University students [23]. In contrast to this, a study in Harari among teachers indicated that knowing about VCT was not significantly associated with utilization of VCT [7]. This might be because knowledgeable individuals might perceive the benefits gained from being tested for HIV at this time.

In this study individuals with discriminating attitude and fear of stigma were less likely to utilize VCT service than those who had not such perceptions. This finding is inconsistent with other study findings [19, 24, 25]. This could be due to the fact that many years of social mobilization, extensive education, and counseling bring behavioral change on stigma and discrimination attitude.

The limitation of this study was confined to one zone which may not represent other zones in the region as well as in Ethiopia.

## 5. Conclusions and Recommendation

VCT utilization rate among teachers was still low. Therefore, strengthening coordinated efforts for convincing teachers to perceive their risk behavior and to utilize VCT service is recommended with a special attention to educational level holders of first degree and above who utilized VCT less.

Focused group appropriate activities are necessary using local resources like school community conversation and HIV/AIDS clubs that will bring behavioral change regarding utilization of VCT service to sustain more utilization of VCT among age groups 20–29, those being married and windowed/divorced, those having good knowledge about VCT, and those who had ever sexual intercourse.

## Conflicts of Interest

The authors declare that there are no conflicts of interest regarding the publication of this paper.

## Authors' Contributions

Woudneh Gereme Desta and Kelemu Dessie Bizuneh designed the study and collected data. Woudneh Gereme Desta, Mulusew Alemneh Sinishaw, and Kelemu Dessie Bizuneh performed analysis and wrote the manuscript. All authors read and agreed on the final manuscript submitted.

## Acknowledgments

First and foremost the authors would like to acknowledge Amhara National Regional State Health Bureau, Awi Zone Health Department, Awi Zone Education Department, and all Awi Zone secondary schools for their unreserved support and Amhara National Regional State HAPCO for the financial support of this study. Their heartfelt thanks go to Professor Meaza Demissie, Ato saketa Borru, Dr. Abebe Eshetu, and Miss Banchayehu Atakilt for their technical support. They would also like to extend their thanks to the study participants, without whom the study would not have been a reality. Finally they are interested in acknowledging data collectors and supervisors who provided their devotion to the successful completion of the field activities.

## References

[1] Ministry of Health, *National Guide Lines for Voluntary HIV Counseling and Testing in Ethiopia*, Ministry of Health, Addis Ababa, Ethiopia, 2007, http://www.ilo.org/wcmsp5/groups/public/—ed_protect/—protrav/—ilo_aids/documents/legaldocument/wcms_125384.pdf.

[2] E. O. Ogunbodede, "HIV/AIDS situation in Africa," *International Dental Journal*, vol. 54, no. 6, supplement 1, pp. 352–360, 2004.

[3] UNAIDS, "UNAIDS report on the Global AIDS epidemic 2010," http://www.unaids.org/globalreport/Global_report.htm.

[4] "Global information and advice on HIV & AIDS: HIV and AIDS in Sub-Saharan Africa Regional Overview," 2013, http://www.avert.org/professionals/hiv-around-world/sub-saharan-africa/overview.

[5] Federal Democratic Republic of Ethiopia, *Report on Progress Towards Implementation of the Declaration of Commitment on HIV/AIDS*, HAPCO, Addis Ababa, Ethiopia, 2005, http://data.unaids.org/pub/Report/2006/2006_country_progress_report_ethiopia_en.pdf.

[6] Federal Democratic Republic of Ethiopia/Federal HIV/AIDS Prevention and Control Office, *Report on Progress Towards Implementation of the Declaration of Commitment on HIV/AIDS*, Federal HIV/AIDS Prevention and Control Office, Addis Ababa, Ethiopia, 2010, http://data.unaids.org/pub/Report/2010/ethiopia_2010_country_progress_report_en.pdf.

[7] S. Omer and J. Haidar, "VCT uptake and associated factors among teachers from Harari Administrative Region," *Ethiopian Journal of Health Development*, vol. 23, no. 3, 2010.

[8] A. Asmelash, *Assessment of HIV/AIDS related mortality among primary and secondary school teachers in Addis Ababa, using verbal Autopsy [MPH thesis]*, Addis Ababa University, Addis A baba, Ethiopia, 2004, http://etd.aau.edu.et/bitstream/123456789/8482/1/Abebe%20Asmelash.PDF.

[9] Federal Ministry of Health/Federal HIV/AIDS Prevention and Control Office, *AIDS in Ethiopia: Sixth Report*, Federal Ministry of Health/Federal HIV/AIDS Prevention and Control Office, Addis Ababa, Ethiopia, 2006, http://www.etharc.org/aidsineth/publications/AIDSinEth6th_en.pdf.

[10] M. Admassu and Y. Fitaw, "Factors affecting acceptance of VCT among different professional and community groups in North and South Gondar Administrative zones, north west Ethiopia," *Ethiopian Journal of Health Development*, vol. 20, no. 1, pp. 24–31, 2006.

[11] UNAIDS, "Voluntary counseling and testing (VCT): technical update," 2000, http://data.unaids.org/Publications/IRC-pub01/jc379-vct_en.pdf.

[12] E. Mulugeta, "Socio demographic characteristics, sexual behavior, and reasons for attending VCT service at Bethzatha VCT project," EPHA Abstract 5, 2003.

[13] D. Zerihun, "Trends of HIV infection and profiles of voluntary HIV counseling and testing (VCT) acceptance in seven branch clinics of the Family Guidance Association of Ethiopia," in *Proceedings of the 14th EPHA Annual Public Health Conference*, Addis Ababa, Ethiopia, October 2003.

[14] Awi Zone Health Department, "Zonal Health Department Annual Report," 2013.

[15] G. Mitike, T. Mekonnen, R. Ayele et al., *HIV/AIDS Behavioral Surveillance Survey (BSS), Round Two*, Federal Ministry of Health, Addis Ababa, Ethiopia, 2005, http://www.etharc.org/resources/download/view.download/33/50.

[16] CSA and ICF International, *Ethiopia Demographic and Health Survey 2011*, Central Statistical Agency and ICF International, Addis Ababa, Ethiopia, 2012, http://www.unicef.org/ethiopia/ET_2011_EDHS.pdf.

[17] D. C. Kakoko, W. L. Lugoe, and G. T. Lie, "Voluntary testing for HIV among a sample of Tanzanian teachers: a search for socio-demographic and socio-psychological correlates," *AIDS Care*, vol. 18, no. 6, pp. 554–560, 2006.

[18] J. Lugalla, M. Emmelin, A. Mutembei et al., "Social, cultural and sexual behavioral determinants of observed decline in HIV

infection trends: lessons from the Kagera Region, Tanzania," *Social Science and Medicine*, vol. 59, no. 1, pp. 185–198, 2004.

[19] S. Bekele, *Assessment of Voluntary HIV Counseling and Testing (VCT) Service Utilization Among 15–49 Years Age Group*, AAU, Amhara Region, Ethiopia, 2007, http://etd.aau.edu.et/handle/123456789/3015.

[20] J. K. B. Matovu, R. H. Gray, F. Makumbi et al., "Voluntary HIV counseling and testing acceptance, sexual risk behavior and HIV incidence in Rakai, Uganda," *AIDS*, vol. 19, no. 5, pp. 503–511, 2005.

[21] G. Endazenaw Bekele, K. Kensa, M. Abebe, and K. T/Mariam, "Assessment of Knowledge, Attitude, Practice and Determinants of VCT utilization for HIV/AIDS among ambo university students, West Shoa Zone, Oromia Region, Ethiopia: Cross Sectional Study," *Science Journal of Public Health*, vol. 3, no. 2, pp. 259–264, 2015.

[22] G. Fikadie, M. Bedimo, and Z. Alamrew, "Prevalence of voluntary counseling and testing utilization and its associated factors among bahirdar university students," *Advances in Preventive Medicine*, vol. 2014, Article ID 906107, 9 pages, 2014.

[23] G. Tsegay, M. Edris, and S. Meseret, "Assessment of voluntary counseling and testing service utilization and associated factors among Debre Markos University Students, North West Ethiopia: a cross-sectional survey in 2011," *BMC Public Health*, vol. 13, no. 1, article 243, 2013.

[24] S. D. Weiser, M. Heisler, K. Leiter et al., "Routine HIV testing in Botswana: a population-based study on attitudes, practices, and human rights concerns," *PLOS Medicine*, vol. 3, no. 7, article e261, 2016.

[25] S. C. Kalichman and L. C. Simbayi, "HIV testing attitudes, AIDS stigma, and voluntary HIV counselling and testing in a black township in Cape Town, South Africa," *Sexually Transmitted Infections*, vol. 79, no. 6, pp. 442–447, 2003.

11

# HIV among Female Sex Workers in Five Cities in Burkina Faso: A Cross-Sectional Baseline Survey to Inform HIV/AIDS Programs

**Henri Gautier Ouedraogo,[1,2,3] Odette Ky-Zerbo,[4] Adama Baguiya,[1] Ashley Grosso,[5] Sara Goodman,[5] Benoît Cesaire Samadoulougou,[4] Marcel Lougue,[4] Nongoba Sawadogo,[6] Yves Traore,[2] Nicolas Barro,[2] Stefan Baral,[5] and Seni Kouanda[1,3]**

[1]*Institut de Recherche en Sciences de la Santé (IRSS), Ouagadougou, West Africa, Burkina Faso*
[2]*University Ouaga 1 Joseph Ki-Zerbo, Ouagadougou, West Africa, Burkina Faso*
[3]*Institut Africain de Santé Publique, Ouagadougou, West Africa, Burkina Faso*
[4]*Programme d'Appui au Monde Associatif et Communautaire, Ouagadougou, West Africa, Burkina Faso*
[5]*Department of Epidemiology, Johns Hopkins Bloomberg School of Public Health, Baltimore, MD, USA*
[6]*Centre Hospitalier Regional de Kaya, West Africa, Burkina Faso*

Correspondence should be addressed to Henri Gautier Ouedraogo; gouedraogo@irss.bf

Academic Editor: Glenda Gray

*Background.* Female sex workers (FSWs) are considered a vulnerable population for HIV infection and a priority for HIV/AIDS response programs. This study aimed to determine HIV prevalence among FSWs in five cities in Burkina Faso. *Methods.* FSWs aged 18 and older were recruited using respondent driven sampling (RDS) in five cities (Ouagadougou, Bobo-Dioulasso, Koudougou, Ouahigouya, and Tenkodogo) in Burkina Faso from 2013 to 2014. HIV testing was performed using the HIV testing national algorithm. We conducted bivariate and multivariate logistic regression analysis to assess correlates of HIV in all cities combined (not RDS-adjusted). *Results.* Among Ouagadougou, Koudougou, and Ouahigouya FSWs, RDS-adjusted HIV prevalence was 13.5% (95% Confidence Interval [CI]: 9.6–18.7), 13.3% (95% CI: 7.6–22.4), and 13.0% (95% CI: 7.6–21.3), respectively, compared to 30.1% (95% CI: 25.5–35.1) among Bobo-Dioulasso FSWs. Factors associated with HIV infection were age (adjusted odds ratio [aOR] = 7.84 95% CI: 3.78–16.20), being married or cohabitating (aOR = 2.43, 95% CI: 1.31–4.49), and history of pregnancy (aOR = 5.24, 95% CI: 1.44–18.97). *Conclusion.* These results highlight the need to strengthen HIV prevention among FSWs, through behavior change strategies, and improve access to sexual and reproductive health services.

## 1. Introduction

The HIV epidemic is still a major concern in low- and middle-income countries, specifically in sub-Saharan Africa [1]. The World Health Organization (WHO) African Region is the most affected globally, with 25.6 million people living with HIV out of the 36.7 million people living with HIV worldwide at the end of 2016 [2]. Although the global burden of HIV has significantly decreased, in West Africa, the epidemic is concentrated mainly in specific groups and vulnerable populations including female sex workers (FSWs) [3, 4]. Female sex workers are defined as women aged 18 and older who sell consensual sexual services in return for cash or payment in kind and who may sell sex formally or informally, regularly or occasionally [5]. Compared to women not practicing sex work, FSWs are at increased vulnerability to contract HIV and sexually transmitted infections (STIs) [5–12].

A review of FSW studies in low- to middle-income countries indicated that FSWs in sub-Saharan Africa had more than 12 times the risk of contracting HIV compared with all women of reproductive age [13]. Studies conducted in

Swaziland (70.4%) and Uganda (37%) among FSWs showed higher HIV prevalence [14, 15]. Papworth et al. reported, in a systematic review on HIV among FSWs, their clients, men who have sex with men, and people who inject drugs in 24 countries of Central and Western Africa, an overall HIV prevalence of 34.9% among FSWs with differences across countries [8]. HIV prevalence among FSWs varies within and across African settings [8, 16]. In West and Central Africa, epidemiological data on vulnerable populations remain either outdated or partial and are mostly from the largest cities with no data from smaller cities. Several studies largely conducted in urban areas in West and Central Africa have reported HIV prevalence among FSWs to be 15.9% in Gambia, 20.0% in Nigeria, 45.4% in Togo, 68.6% in Ghana and Benin, and 58.2% in Burkina Faso [14–18].

In Burkina Faso, the Joint United Nations Programme on HIV/AIDS (UNAIDS) consecutive reports on the HIV epidemic show a decline in HIV prevalence in the overall population of Burkina Faso over time, from 2.7% in 2003 to 1.0% in 2010 and then to 0.9% in late 2014 [19]. Although the HIV prevalence in Burkina Faso among people of reproductive age (ages 15 to 49) is low, the epidemic is concentrated in vulnerable groups such as FSWs [20]. One study reported that HIV prevalence was 6.5% among part-time sex workers in Burkina Faso and 10.3% among full-time sex workers, much higher than the national rates for people of reproductive age [20]. However, this study was limited to FSWs aged 18 to 25 in Ouagadougou alone. National and international programs addressing HIV in regard to FSWs lack basic information regarding this population which impedes evidence-based program planning, implementation, monitoring, and evaluation. This study aimed to determine HIV prevalence and correlates of HIV infection among FSWs in two large and three small cities in Burkina Faso.

## 2. Materials and Methods

*2.1. Study Design.* We conducted a cross-sectional biological and behavioral study among FSWs in Burkina Faso, using respondent driven sampling (RDS) [21, 22]. Eligibility criteria included the following: (1) being at least 18 years old, (2) assigned female sex at birth, (3) having at least 50% of annual income from sex work in the past 12 months, (4) having stayed in the city at least for the past three months, (5) having a valid study coupon, and (6) being able to provide informed consent for participation in study activities.

*2.2. Setting.* We selected the two largest cities: the capital, Ouagadougou in the Central region, and Bobo-Dioulasso in the Hauts-Bassins region (western Burkina Faso), and three smaller cities: Koudougou in the West Central region, Ouahigouya in the North region, and Tenkodogo in the East Central region. These cities were selected for their level of urbanization, HIV prevalence, and geographic location. Formative research with FSWs, local FSW organizations, and government officials took place using a formal meeting in each site to inform the study procedures. Data were collected from February 2013 to May 2014.

*2.3. Study Size.* The sample size was calculated to recruit 345 FSWs in the two largest cities (Ouagadougou and Bobo-Dioulasso) and 126 FSWs in the smaller ones (Koudougou, Ouahigouya, and Tenkodogo). Sample size calculations were based on the assumption that populations that always use condoms have a 75% lower HIV prevalence than populations who do not, and the effectiveness of condoms is roughly 80%, with 73% as a conservative estimate [23]. Overall, across all cities, HIV prevalence was estimated at 15%, with a 19% prevalence among those who did not consistently use condoms [24, 25]. A design effect of 1.5 associated with RDS and significance level of 0.05 and a power of 80% were employed.

*2.4. Study Participants.* Respondent driven sampling, a peer-driven sampling method designed to reach hidden populations such as FSWs [21, 26], was selected in order to collect rigorous, representative data. Respondent driven sampling starts with eligible "seeds" to start recruitment chains [21, 26]. For each site, three to ten seeds were selected based on diverse sociodemographic selection criteria, including popularity, sociability, age, location, type of sex work, and nationality, with the assumption that each individual represented a different social network within the FSW population as a whole in each study site. After completing study procedures, these seeds were each provided with three coded coupons, valid for four weeks, to recruit peer FSWs from their social network. This process continued until the desired sample size was reached.

All participants received male condoms, condom-compatible lubricants, HIV education materials, and information regarding existing services. They also received 2000 West African CFA franc (XOF) (United States [US] $4) for their time and transportation costs for each study visit and 1500 XOF (US$3) per successfully recruited eligible peer (for up to three peers). To avoid individuals participating multiple times, a single study office was used in each study site in addition to the use of a unique identification code. Trained staff at each site included a site manager, a coupon manager, two data collectors, an HIV test counsellor, and a lab technician. Full details of the study methodology have been previously described [27].

*2.5. Data Collection.* Data were collected from February 2013 to May 2014. After informed consent, each participant completed a private interviewer-administered questionnaire in French or the local language. Topics included demographic and socioeconomic characteristics, sexual partnerships and behaviors (including condom use during the last 12 months and condom use at last sex with a new client), and knowledge, attitudes, and practices related to STIs and HIV based on the modified social ecological model [28]. After the questionnaire, pre- and posttest HIV counselling, based on the standard national counselling protocol, was conducted. A venous blood specimen (~5 milliliters) was collected from each consenting participant for HIV testing.

*2.6. HIV Testing.* HIV testing was performed using the national Burkina Faso HIV testing algorithm (Presidency of Burkina Faso/CNLS: HIV testing and diagnosis algorithm in Burkina Faso. Oct. 2004.). The first step was to perform a rapid test using Alere Determine™ HIV-1/2 kit (Alere, Inc., Waltham, Massachusetts). This was followed by ImmunoComb® II HIV 1&2 BiSpot kit (Alere, Inc.) as a second test for differential detection of antibodies to HIV types 1 and 2, only if the first test was positive. Four discordant results were further tested and confirmed negative through use of the ImmunoComb II HIV 1&2 CombFirm kit (Alere, Inc.).

*2.7. Data Processing and Analysis.* Data were entered using double data entry into EpiData 3.1 (The EpiData Association, Odense, Denmark) and exported into Stata 14 (StataCorp, College Station, TX) for analysis. Descriptive statistics were used to describe participants' characteristics, sexual behaviors, condom use, and HIV prevalence. We adjusted all proportions separately for each city to account for the RDS method. This adjustment takes into consideration the probability of each participant to be included in the study. This probability was measured through weighting based on the size of each participant's network. Network size was determined using the survey question: "how many different people do you know personally who are female sex workers or sell sex? i.e., you know them and they know you, and you could contact them if you needed to?" The mean network size was 39: the network size by city was 69 in Ouagadougou, 21 in Bobo-Dioulasso, 39 in Koudougou, 13 in Ouahigouya, and 27 in Tenkodogo. Network size ranged from 1 to 1000. We presented population estimates and 95% confidence intervals (CI) adjusted for RDS design using the RDS Analysis Tools (RDSAT) version 6.0.1 (RDS, Inc., Ithaca, NY). Bivariate and multivariate logistic regression analyses were performed using Stata to identify factors associated with HIV infection at the $p < 0.05$ level of significance along with their 95% confidence interval (CI). These pooled bivariate and multivariate analyses were not RDS-adjusted because data from all cities were combined. Multivariate analyses were not conducted separately for each city due to smaller sample sizes in Koudougou, Ouahigouya, and Tenkodogo. Age categories were generated according to existing HIV planning goals with adolescent FSWs categorized as age 24 and younger.

Our outcome variable was HIV status (positive or negative) as determined by blood tests. Predictor variables included sociodemographic variables including age, education level, marital status, employment, and migration to Burkina Faso. Other predictor variables included those related to sex work including experience, number of clients, and condom use. First, sociodemographic and behavioral variables associated with HIV infection at the significance level of $p < 0.2$ in bivariate analyses were included in a backward elimination model selection procedure, and variables independently associated with HIV infection were retained in the multivariate model to produce the final results.

## 3. Results

*3.1. Descriptive Statistics.* As shown in Table 1, overall, 1073 FSWs (349 in Ouagadougou, 350 in Bobo-Dioulasso, 117 in Koudougou, 121 in Ouahigouya and 136 in Tenkodogo) were included in this study. The mean age of participants varied across cities, from 23.9 (±5.1) years in Tenkodogo to 30.7 (±8.6) years in Bobo-Dioulasso.

*3.1.1. RDS-Adjusted Descriptive Statistics*

*Sociodemographic Characteristics of FSWs.* Participants' education level was low in general with many who never attended school. Almost one-third of those of Ouagadougou (31.6%, 95% CI: 26.5–37.2) and in Koudougou (32.3%, 95% CI: 24.0–41.9) as well as half (49.2%, 95% CI: 43.8–54.5) of those of Bobo-Dioulasso had never been to school. The majority of FSWs in each city had no other job besides sex work. In terms of marital status, more than half of FSWs were single ranging from the lowest frequency of 52% (95% CI: 46.6–57.1) in Bobo-Dioulasso to 74% (95% CI: 65.2–81.2) in Tenkodogo. More than a third of them were divorced, separated, or widowed in Ouagadougou and Bobo-Dioulasso, whereas, in Koudougou, Ouahigouya, and Tenkodogo, this group represented less than a quarter of participants.

More than half of FSWs in Tenkodogo (59.8%, 95% CI: 44.7–55.4) and Ouagadougou (50.0%, 95% CI: 44.7–55.4) FSWs reported that both of their biological parents were alive compared to a third (31.8%, 95% CI: 27.0–36.9) in Bobo-Dioulasso. Almost half of FSWs were foreigners, except in Bobo-Dioulasso where non-Burkina Faso nationals were 19.6% of participants (95% CI: 15.7–24.2).

*Socioprofessional Characteristics.* As shown in Table 2, earlier age of initiation to sex work was observed in Ouagadougou and Tenkodogo. The time spent in sex work varied across cities. In Ouagadougou, 40.9% (95% CI: 35.8–46.3) of FSWs had been doing this work for two years whereas, in Bobo-Dioulasso, 27.7% (95% CI: 23.1–32.9) had worked for two years. Those who had done sex work for two to five years were estimated to be 38.2% (95% CI: 34.2–44.6) in Ouagadougou and 33.0% (95% CI: 28.1–38.3) in Bobo-Dioulasso. Conversely, the majority of FSWs had been in sex work for less than two years in smaller cities as seen in Koudougou (61.0%, 95% CI: 51.7–69.6), Ouahigouya (73.3%, 95% CI: 65.1–80.2), and Tenkodogo (60.4%, 95% CI: 51.2–68.9).

*HIV Prevalence.* As shown in Table 3, among Ouagadougou, Koudougou, and Ouahigouya FSWs, RDS-weighted HIV prevalence was 13.5% (95% CI: 9.6–18.7), 13.3% (95% CI: 7.6–22.4), and 13.0% (95% CI: 7.6–21.3), respectively, as compared to 30.1% (95% CI: 25.5–35.1) in Bobo-Dioulasso. The lowest prevalence was observed in Tenkodogo with 4.4% (95% CI: 2.2–8.8).

*3.2. Bivariate.* As also shown in Table 3, in unweighted bivariate logistic regression analyses, the HIV prevalence was statistically significantly different across the cities ($p = 0.001$)

and age groups within the same city. Among FSWs who were less than 25 years old, 9.3% (95% CI: 5.3–15.9) tested positive for HIV as compared to 31.8% (95% CI: 20.2–46.3) among those 30 years old and above in Ouagadougou ($p = 0.001$). Likewise, in all the other cities, FSWs aged 30 years and above were the most likely to test positive for HIV.

As shown in Table 4, in the bivariate analysis, FSWs who had symptoms of STIs in the past 12 months were 64% more likely to test positive for HIV compared to those who did not have symptoms (odds ratio [OR] = 1.64, 95% CI: 1.18–2.30).

*3.3. Multivariate.* As also shown in Table 4, the association between STI symptoms and HIV was not significant in the multivariate analysis (adjusted odds ratio [aOR] = 1.44, 95% CI: 0.98–2.13, $p = 0.063$). Our multivariate analysis showed that FSWs aged 30 years old and above were more likely to test positive for HIV (aOR = 7.84, 95% CI: 3.78–16.20) compared to those aged 18 to 24 years. Those married or cohabitating were also more likely to test positive for HIV than single FSWs (aOR = 2.43, 95% CI: 1.31–4.49). There was an association between divorced or widow status and HIV infection; however, it was not statistically significant in the multivariate analysis (aOR = 1.58, 95% CI: 0.99–2.51, $p = 0.052$).

Compared to FSWs who had between one and 14 clients per week, those who had more than 30 clients per week were less likely to test positive for HIV (aOR = 0.49, 95% CI: 0.27–0.87). The likelihood of testing positive for HIV was higher among those who had previously been pregnant (aOR = 5.24, 95% CI: 1.44–18.97), as well as those who reported a condom broke during sexual intercourse in the last 12 months (aOR = 1.78, 95% CI: 1.16–2.73).

## 4. Discussion

FSWs who lived in larger cities, were older, and engaged in condomless intercourse or became pregnant were more likely to be HIV positive in this sample. This data shows that, despite the continuous decline of HIV prevalence among the general population of reproductive age, dropping from 2.7% in 2003 to 0.9% in 2014, the prevalence among FSWs is still very high in the country.

In this study, the HIV prevalence was higher in the larger cities compared to the smaller cities which is concurrent with other West African settings. In a study conducted in Côte d'Ivoire in the following cities, Abidjan, Yamoussoukro, Gagnoa, and San Pedro, HIV prevalence was 17.5%. But in Abidjan, the largest city, it was 31.1% [29].

In this study, older FSW, aged 25 and older, had a higher prevalence of HIV, with those over 30 having the highest prevalence at 31.8% compared to younger FSW aged 24 and younger. HIV prevalence among FSWs remains five times higher than the prevalence in the same age group in the general population of reproductive age in Burkina Faso [19]. Some previous studies have shown that HIV is less prevalent among younger FSWs compared to older ones. Older FSWs may have greater accumulated vulnerability because they have engaged in sex work longer, potentially with more clients over time making them more likely to acquire HIV [30].

FSWs in Burkina Faso engaged in behavior increasing the likelihood of HIV transmission, including condomless sex with some clients [27]. In the study sample, condom breakage during sexual intercourse and history of previous pregnancies were associated with HIV infection among FSWs. Pregnancy increases vulnerability to HIV among FSWs. A pregnancy in the context of sex work assumes that the FSW engaged in condomless vaginal intercourse with clients or nonpaying partners, which can lead to HIV infection. In fact, FSWs who intend to conceive are more likely to have condomless sex and therefore more likely to contract HIV [31]. Although the design of this study could not establish whether HIV or condomless sexual intercourse occurred first, systematic and regular use of condoms remains a reliable method to prevent both HIV infection and unintended pregnancies during sex work [32, 33].

These results illustrate a need to strengthen HIV and STI prevention programs among FSWs in general. In particular, interventions focusing on older FSWs who have been working longer are needed to create a safe working environment. HIV response programs should reinforce HIV awareness and communication for behavior change strategies and access to preexposure prophylaxis among FSWs and their clients. These strategies should include access to condoms and education on correct utilization in order to prevent condom breakage which can lead to HIV transmission [27, 34, 35]. Previous studies indicate the importance of peer-based education. As seen in the Yerelon cohort in Bobo-Dioulasso, peer-based education intervention can result in positive changes in sexual behavior and low HIV incidence among FSWs [36]. This data helps us better understand the needs of FSW that are opportunities for improved future interventions.

## 5. Limitations

Our study has some limitations pertaining to the RDS method [31–34] specifically that the data across cities cannot be pooled because the networks, chains, and seeds are unique to each city. In addition, self-reported data are subject to inaccurate recall and social desirability bias. Despite these limitations, this study shows that the RDS method is feasible among FSWs in both large and small cities in Burkina Faso as it has been in other countries and settings.

## 6. Conclusions

In Burkina Faso, HIV prevention programs for vulnerable populations, namely, FSWs, are crucial, as HIV prevalence in West Africa is concentrated in these groups. With current interventions, we are still seeing high prevalence among this vulnerable population and we should take these results as an opportunity to change HIV prevention efforts towards FSWs. The results of this study suggest innovative, evidence-based HIV prevention interventions are needed especially

Table 1: Sociodemographic characteristics of female sex workers by city.

| Variables | | Ouagadougou ($n$ = 349) $n$ (% unadjusted) | Ouagadougou ($n$ = 349) RDS-adjusted% (95% CI) | Bobo-Dioulasso ($n$ = 350) $n$ (% unadjusted) | Bobo-Dioulasso ($n$ = 350) RDS-adjusted% (95% CI) | Koudougou ($n$ = 117) $n$ (% unadjusted) | Koudougou ($n$ = 117) RDS-adjusted% (95% CI) | Ouahigouya ($n$ = 121) $n$ (% unadjusted) | Ouahigouya ($n$ = 121) RDS-adjusted% (95% CI) | Tenkodogo ($n$ = 136) $n$ (% unadjusted) | Tenkodogo ($n$ = 136) RDS-adjusted% (95% CI) |
|---|---|---|---|---|---|---|---|---|---|---|---|
| Age (years) | 18–24 | 203 (58.2) | 63.6 (58.1–68.1) | 101 (28.9) | 32.1 (27.2–37.3) | 47 (40.2) | 32.2 (24.6–40.9) | 59 (48.8) | 44.9 (36.2–53.9) | 86 (63.2) | 65.5 (57.1–73.1) |
| | 25–29 | 83 (23.8) | 18.9 (15.4–23.0) | 67 (19.1) | 21.5 (17.3–26.4) | 37 (31.6) | 40.9 (31.8–50.7) | 31 (25.6) | 25.5 (18.5–34.2) | 33 (24.3) | 25.5 (18.7–33.7) |
| | 30–55 | 63 (18.1) | 17.5 (13.9–21.8) | 182 (52.0) | 46.5 (41.3–51.7) | 33 (28.2) | 26.8 (19.5–35.6) | 31 (25.6) | 29.6 (21.7–38.8) | 17 (12.5) | 9.0 (5.6–14.2) |
| Education | None | 82 (23.8) | 31.6 (26.5–37.2) | 145 (41.5) | 49.2 (43.8–54.5) | 32 (27.4) | 32.3 (24.0–41.9) | 40 (33.1) | 41.5 (32.6–51.0) | 37 (27.2) | 23.4 (17.2–30.9) |
| | Primary | 131 (38.0) | 35.7 (30.9–41.0) | 130 (37.1) | 34.9 (30.1–40.0) | 47 (40.2) | 40.7 (32.0–50.0) | 28 (23.1) | 21.3 (15.0–29.4) | 48 (35.3) | 33.0 (25.6–41.3) |
| | Secondary and above | 132 (38.3) | 32.7 (28.0–37.7) | 75 (21.4) | 15.9 (12.8–19.7) | 38 (32.5) | 27.1 (20.0–35.5) | 53 (43.8) | 37.2 (29.1–46.0) | 51 (37.5) | 43.6 (35.2–52.3) |
| Marital status | Single | 220 (63.0) | 55.7 (50.2–61.0) | 156 (44.6) | 51.9 (46.6–57.1) | 81 (69.2) | 72.0 (63.1–79.4) | 83 (68.6) | 66.8 (57.7–74.9) | 103 (75.7) | 74.0 (65.2–81.2) |
| | Married/cohabitating | 33 (9.5) | 8.7 (6.3–12.1) | 43 (12.3) | 12.5 (9.4–16.4) | 11 (9.4) | 5.4 (3.0–9.7) | 13 (10.7) | 10.3 (6.0–17.1) | 6 (4.4) | 8.4 (3.8–17.4) |
| | Divorced/separated/widowed | 96 (27.5) | 35.6 (30.4–41.2) | 151 (43.1) | 35.7 (30.9–40.7) | 25 (21.4) | 22.6 (15.7–31.4) | 25 (20.7) | 22.8 (15.9–31.6) | 27 (19.9) | 17.6 (12.2–24.7) |
| Occupation | Student/pupil | 20 (5.8) | 5.6 (3.6–8.6) | 8 (2.3) | 1.5 (0.7–3.0) | 6 (5.1) | 5.1 (2.3–11.1) | 4 (3.3) | 4.7 (1.8–11.9) | 13 (9.6) | 14.1 (8.4–22.7) |
| | Employed (public or private) | 151 (43.5) | 44.3 (39.1–49.6) | 100 (28.6) | 24.0 (20.0–28.5) | 58 (49.6) | 49.6 (40.5–58.7) | 46 (38.0) | 36.3 (28.2–45.3) | 44 (32.4) | 21.5 (16.0–28.3) |
| | Unemployed | 176 (50.7) | 50.1 (44.8–55.3) | 242 (69.1) | 74.5 (70.0–78.6) | 53.0 (45.3) | 45.3 (36.4–54.5) | 71 (58.7) | 59.0 (49.0–67.5) | 79 (58.1) | 64.4 (55.7–72.1) |
| Number of children | 0 | 107 (30.7) | 30.4 (25.8–35.4) | 58 (16.6) | 16.2 (12.7–20.4) | 29 (25.2) | 25.0 (18.0–34.0) | 30 (29.1) | 28.8 (20.9–38.3) | 55 (40.7) | 40.3 (32.4–48.8) |
| | 1 | 157 (45.0) | 44.9 (39.7–50.2) | 103 (29.4) | 29.1 (24.5–34.0) | 48 (41.7) | 41.3 (32.7–50.5) | 42 (40.8) | 40.5 (31.5–50.3) | 48 (35.6) | 36.1 (28.4–44.6) |
| | ≥2 | 85 (24.4) | 24.7 (20.4–29.5) | 189 (54.0) | 54.8 (49.5–59.9) | 38 (33.0) | 33.6 (25.5–42.8) | 48 (35.6) | 30.7 (22.5–40.3) | 32 (23.7) | 23.6 (17.2–31.5) |
| Parents alive | Both alive | 174 (50.6) | 50.0 (44.7–55.4) | 105 (30.0) | 31.8 (27–36.9) | 47 (40.9) | 39.1 (30.6–48.4) | 59 (49.6) | 47.1 (38.2–56.3) | 71 (52.2) | 59.8 (51.4–67.6) |
| | Only one alive | 129 (37.5) | 32.5 (27.9–37.5) | 158 (45.1) | 43.8 (38.6–49.0) | 51 (44.3) | 44.9 (35.9–54.2) | 43 (36.1) | 33.0 (25.1–41.9) | 46 (33.8) | 29.4 (22.5–37.4) |
| | None alive | 41 (11.9) | 17.4 (13.2–22.7) | 87 (24.9) | 24.5 (20.3–29.3) | 17 (14.8) | 16.0 (10.1–24.3) | 17 (14.3) | 19.9 (12.9–29.5) | 19 (14.0) | 10.8 (6.9–16.5) |
| Migrated into Burkina Faso | No | 232 (67.1) | 66.9 (61.7–71.7) | 284 (81.1) | 81.0 (76.5–84.8) | 54 (47.4) | 47.1 (38.1–56.3) | 44 (43.1) | 43.4 (34.1–53.2) | 68 (54.0) | 52.0 (41.8–58.6) |
| | Yes | 114 (32.9) | 42.7 (37.3–48.3) | 66 (18.9) | 19.6 (15.7–24.2) | 62 (53.4) | 51.3 (42.1–64.0) | 61 (58.0) | 53.7 (44.6–62.5) | 67 (49.3) | 47.9 (39.5–56.4) |

TABLE 2: Socioprofessional and behavioral characteristics of female sex workers by city.

| Variables | | Ouagadougou ($n$ = 349) $n$ (% unadjusted) | Ouagadougou RDS-adjusted% (95% CI) | Bobo-Dioulasso ($n$ = 350) $n$ (% unadjusted) | Bobo-Dioulasso RDS-adjusted% (95% CI) | Koudougou ($n$ = 117) $n$ (% unadjusted) | Koudougou RDS-adjusted% (95% CI) | Ouahigouya ($n$ = 121) $n$ (% unadjusted) | Ouahigouya RDS-adjusted% (95% CI) | Tenkodogo ($n$ = 136) $n$ (% unadjusted) | Tenkodogo RDS-adjusted% (95% CI) |
|---|---|---|---|---|---|---|---|---|---|---|---|
| Age at start of selling sex (years) | <20 | 226 (64.9) | 64.8 (59.6–69.6) | 173 (49.4) | 48.5 (43.2–53.7) | 44 (39.6) | 39.7 (31.1–49.1) | 38 (38.0) | 37.7 (28.8–47.6) | 81 (60.4) | 60.3 (51.8–68.3) |
| | 20–24 | 81.0 (23.3) | 23.4 (19.2–28.1) | 67 (19.1) | 19.1 (15.3–23.6) | 41 (36.9) | 36.9 (28.5–46.3) | 34 (34.0) | 34.0 (25.4–43.8) | 36 (26.9) | 27.0 (20.1–35.2) |
| | ≥25 | 41.0 (11.8) | 11.9 (8.9–15.7) | 110 (31.4) | 32.4 (27.7–37.6) | 26 (23.4) | 23.3 (16.4–32.1) | 28 (28.0) | 28.3 (20.3–38.0) | 17 (12.7) | 12.7 (8.0–19.5) |
| Experience in sex work (years) | <1 | 59 (17.1) | 17.0 (13.4–21.3) | 35 (10.0) | 09.7 (07.0–13.2) | 35 (37.0) | 30.1 (22.5–39.1) | 52 (54.2) | 53.9 (43.8–63.6) | 62 (47.7) | 47.6 (39.2–56.2) |
| | 1–5 | 204 (59.0) | 59.0 (53.7–64.1) | 154 (44.0) | 43.3 (38.2–48.5) | 63 (55.3) | 55.3 (46.0–64.1) | 37 (38.5) | 39.0 (29.7–49.1) | 49 (37.7) | 37.7 (29.8–46.4) |
| | ≥6 | 83 (24.0) | 24.0 (19.8–28.8) | 161 (46.0) | 47.0 (41.8–52.3) | 16 (14.0) | 14.6 (09.1–22.5) | 7 (7.3) | 07.1 (03.4–14.2) | 19 (14.6) | 14.6 (09.5–21.8) |
| Number of clients per week | 1–14 | 214 (61.5) | 61.8 (56.6–66.8) | 146 (41.7) | 42.2 (37.1–47.4) | 73 (63.5) | 63.5 (54.3–71.8) | 50 (48.5) | 48.5 (39.0–58.1) | 82 (1.2) | 61.2 (52.7–69.1) |
| | 15–29 | 92 (26.4) | 26.3 (21.9–31.2) | 132 (37.7) | 37.8 (32.9–43.0) | 25 (21.7) | 21.8 (15.2–30.4) | 9 (8.7) | 08.7 (04.6–15.9) | 18 (13.4) | 13.3 (08.5–20.1) |
| | ≥30 | 42 (12.1) | 11.9 (08.9–15.7) | 72 (26.0) | 20.0 (16.2–24.5) | 17 (14.8) | 14.7 (09.3–22.4) | 44 (42.7) | 42.8 (33.6–52.5) | 34 (25.4) | 25.5 (18.8–33.6) |
| Mean income per week (XOF, $US 1~500 XOF) | <15000 | 29 (8.3) | 20.0 (14.6–26.8) | 59 (16.9) | 23.7 (19.0–29.1) | 21 (17.9) | 27 (18.6–37.4) | 41 (35.3) | 35.3 (27.1–44.6) | 36 (27.1) | 27.1 (20.1–35.4) |
| | 15000–35000 | 147 (42.1) | 35.3 (30.4–40.6) | 178 (50.9) | 47.9 (42.6–53.2) | 35 (29.9) | 29.5 (21.7–38.6) | 43 (37.1) | 37.1 (28.7–46.3) | 76 (57.1) | 57.1 (48.5–65.4) |
| | 35001–99999 | 127 (36.4) | 34.8 (29.7–40.1) | 103 (29.4) | 27.1 (22.7–31.9) | 43 (36.8) | 24.5 (18.1–32.3) | 27 (23.3) | 23.3 (16.4–32.0) | 20 (15.0) | 15.0 (9.9–22.3) |
| | ≥100000 | 46 (13.2) | 9.9 (7.4–13.1) | 10 (2.8) | 1.4 (0.7–2.5) | 18 (15.4) | 19.0 (12.3–28.2) | 5 (4.3) | 4.3 (1.8–10.1) | 1 (0.8) | 0.8 (0.1–5.3) |
| STI symptoms over the last 12 months | No | 175 (50.3) | 52 (45.0–55.5) | 166 (47.8) | 47.8 (42.5–53.0) | 69 (60) | 59.6 (50.3–68.2) | 67 (65.0) | 64.2 (54.5–73.0) | 101 (75.9) | 75.8 (67.7–82.3) |
| | Yes | 172 (49.4) | 49.5 (44.2–54.7) | 181 (52.2) | 52.2 (47.0–57.5) | 46 (40) | 40.4 (31.8–49.7) | 34 (33.0) | 33.9 (25.3–43.6) | 32 (24.1) | 24.2 (17.7–32.3) |
| | Don't know | 01 (0.3) | 0.3 (00–02.0) | — | | — | | 02 (02.0) | 00.9 (00.1–06.4) | — | |
| Ever got pregnant | No | 74 (21.3) | 21.0 (17.0–25.6) | 29 (8.3) | 07.9 (05.6–11.2) | 22 (19.1) | 18.8 (12.7–26.9) | 20 (19.4) | 19.1 (12.7–27.9) | 44 (32.6) | 32.2 (24.9–40.5) |
| | Yes | 274 (78.7) | 79.0 (74.4–83.0) | 321 (91.7) | 92.1 (88.8–94.4) | 93 (89.0) | 81.2 (73.1–87.3) | 83 (86.0) | 80.9 (72.1–87.3) | 91 (67.4) | 67.8 (59.5–75.1) |
| Ease of requesting client to wear a condom | Easy | 238 (68.4) | 68.4 (63.4–73.1) | 246 (71.1) | 71.0 (65.9–75.5) | 83 (75.5) | 75.2 (66.3–82.4) | 96 (93.2) | 93.4 (86.7–96.8) | 124 (92.5) | 92.6 (86.8–96.0) |
| | Not easy | 110 (31.6) | 31.6 (26.9–36.6) | 100 (28.9) | 29.0 (24.5–34.1) | 27 (24.5) | 24.8 (17.6–33.7) | 7 (6.8) | 06.6 (03.2–13.3) | 10 (7.5) | 07.4 (04.0–13.2) |
| Consistent condom use during the last 12 months | No | 129 (37.7) | 37.6 (32.6–42.8) | 150 (43.1) | 43.2 (38.0–48.5) | 20 (17.9) | 17.7 (11.7–25.9) | 54 (56.8) | 56.9 (46.7–66.5) | 53 (48.0) | 40.9 (32.7–49.5) |
| | Yes | 213 (62.3) | 62.4 (57.2–67.4) | 198 (56.9) | 56.8 (51.5–62.0) | 92 (82.1) | 82.3 (74.1–88.3) | 41 (43.2) | 43.1 (33.5–53.3) | 77 (59.2) | 59.1 (50.5–67.3) |
| Condom use during the last intercourse with new client | No | 36 (17) | 15 (07.7–14.3) | 29 (8.6) | 08.8 (06.2–12.4) | 9 (7.9) | 07.9 (04.2–14.5) | 16 (15.8) | 15.6 (09.8–24.1) | 4 (3.0) | 02.9 (01.1–07.6) |
| | Yes | 301 (89.3) | 89.5 (85.7–92.3) | 309 (91.4) | 91.2 (87.6–93.8) | 105 (92.1) | 92.1 (85.5–95.8) | 85 (84.2) | 84.4 (75.9–90.2) | 131 (97.0) | 97.1 (92.4–98.9) |
| Condom breakage over the last 12 months | No | 128 (36.7) | 36.6 (31.7–41.7) | 134 (38.3) | 37.8 (32.9–43.0) | 47 (49) | 32.8 (24.4–42.4) | 34 (33.0) | 40.5 (31.9–49.7) | 70 (51.9) | 51.4 (43.0–59.7) |
| | Yes | 221 (63.3) | 63.4 (58.3–68.3) | 216 (61.7) | 62.2 (57.0–67.1) | 68 (59.1) | 59.5 (50.3–68.1) | 69 (67.0) | 67.2 (57.6–75.6) | 65 (48.1) | 48.6 (40.3–57.0) |

TABLE 3: HIV prevalence among female sex workers by city.

| Variables | | Ouagadougou | | | Bobo-Dioulasso | | | Koudougou | | | Ouahigouya | | | Tenkodogo | | |
|---|---|---|---|---|---|---|---|---|---|---|---|---|---|---|---|---|
| | Age (years) | *n* | % unadjusted | RDS-adjusted% (95% CI) | *n* | % unadjusted | RDS-adjusted% (95% CI) | *n* | % unadjusted | RDS-adjusted% (95% CI) | *n* | % unadjusted | RDS-adjusted% (95% CI) | *n* | % unadjusted | RDS-adjusted% (95% CI) |
| HIV prevalence | 18–24 | 203 | 5.4 | 9.3 (5.3–15.9) | 101 | 4.0 | 3.8 (1.4–9.7) | 46 | 6.5 | 9.2 (3.0–25.0) | 51 | 5.9 | 6.1 (1.9–17.0) | 85 | 3.5 | 2.6 (0.8–8.0) |
| | 25–29 | 83 | 4.8 | 8.3 (3.2–20.0) | 37 | 6.4 | 15.8 (8.9–26.4) | 36 | 8.3 | 11.7 (3.8–30.5) | 27 | 22.2 | 22.8 (10.5–42.7) | 33 | 9.1 | 6.9 (2.2–19.8) |
| | 30–55 | 63 | 20.6 | 31.8 (20.2–46.3) | 182 | 51.6 | 50.4 (43.2–57.7) | 33 | 15.2 | 20.6 (9.0–40.6) | 25 | 16.0 | 16.5 (6.2–36.9) | 17 | 11.8 | 9,0 (2.2–30.9) |
| | Total | 349 | 8.0 | 13.5 (9.6–18.7) | 350 | 31.1 | 30.1 (25.5–35.1) | 115 | 9.6 | 13.3 (7.6–22.4) | 103 | 12.6 | 13 (7.6–21.3) | 135 | 5.9 | 4.4 (2.2–8.8) |

TABLE 4: Factors associated with HIV positive status among female sex workers in five cities in Burkina Faso ($n$ = 1052).

| | Variables | $n$ (% HIV positive) | Bivariate analysis OR | Bivariate analysis 95% CI | Bivariate analysis $p$ | Multivariate analysis aOR | Multivariate analysis 95% CI | Multivariate analysis $p$ |
|---|---|---|---|---|---|---|---|---|
| Sociodemographic characteristics | *Total* | 1052 (16.1) | — | — | — | — | — | — |
| | *Age (years)* | | | | | | | |
| | 18–24 | 486 (4.9) | 1 | | | 1 | | |
| | 25–29 | 246 (27.0) | 2.37 | 1.33–4.21 | *0.003* | 1.76 | 0.90–3.45 | *0.095* |
| | 30–55 | 320 (36.9) | 11.24 | 7.02–18.00 | *0.001* | 7.84 | 3.78–16.20 | *0.001* |
| | *Education* | | | | | | | |
| | None | 243 (7.0) | 1 | | | 1 | | |
| | Primary | 507 (13.2) | 0.79 | 0.55–1.16 | *0.242* | 0.88 | 0.57–1.36 | *0.585* |
| | Secondary and above | 286 (29.0) | 0.39 | 0.25–0.62 | *0.001* | 0.71 | 0.42–1.19 | *0.199* |
| | *Marital status* | | | | | | | |
| | Single | 630 (8.9) | 1 | | | 1 | | |
| | Married/cohabitating | 102 (27.5) | 3.87 | 2.32–6.48 | *0.001* | 2.43 | 1.31–4.49 | *0.005* |
| | Divorced/separated/widowed | 320 (26.6) | 3.71 | 2.56–3.37 | *0.001* | 1.58 | 0.99–2.51 | *0.052* |
| | *Occupation* | | | | | | | |
| | Student/pupil | 49 (0.0) | — | | | — | — | — |
| | Employed (public or private) | 391 (15.9) | 0.88 | 0.63–1.25 | *0.488* | — | — | — |
| | Unemployed | 610 (17.5) | 1 | | | — | — | — |
| | *Number of children* | | | | | | | |
| | 0 | 279 (6.5) | 1 | | | 1 | | |
| | 1 | 398 (12.3) | 2.03 | 1.16–3.58 | *0.013* | 0.82 | 0.40–1.65 | *0.583* |
| | ≥2 | 375 (27.2) | 2.41 | 3.19–9.19 | *0.001* | 0.74 | 0.35–1.56 | *0.440* |
| | *Parents alive* | | | | | | | |
| | One died | 596 (19.3) | 1 | | | 1 | | |
| | Both alive | 447 (11.6) | 0.55 | 0.38–0.78 | *0.001* | 1.25 | 0.81–1.94 | *0.307* |

Table 4: Continued.

| | Variables | *n* (% HIV positive) | Bivariate analysis OR | Bivariate analysis 95% CI | Bivariate analysis *p* | Multivariate analysis aOR | Multivariate analysis 95% CI | Multivariate analysis *p* |
|---|---|---|---|---|---|---|---|---|
| Sex work-related characteristics | *Migrated into Burkina Faso* | | | | | | | |
| | No | 682 (16.7) | 1 | | | | | |
| | Yes | 365 (14.8) | 0.86 | 0.61–1.23 | *0.420* | — | — | — |
| | *Age at start of selling sex (years)* | | | | | | | |
| | <20 | 562 (11.0) | 1 | | | 1 | | |
| | 20–24 | 259 (15.1) | 1.42 | 0.92–2.19 | *0.104* | 1.27 | 0.74–2.17 | *0.376* |
| | ≥25 | 222 (30.2) | 3.48 | 2.36–5.14 | *0.001* | 1.06 | 0.59–1.90 | *0.844* |
| | *Experience in sex work (years)* | | | | | | | |
| | Less than one year | 243 (7.0) | 1 | | | 1 | | |
| | 1–5 years | 507 (13.2) | 2.02 | 1.16–3.52 | *0.013* | 1.33 | 0.70–2.53 | *0.375* |
| | 6 years and more | 286 (29.0) | 5.43 | 3.11–9.46 | *0.001* | 1.57 | 0.76–3.22 | *0.223* |
| | *Number of clients per week* | | | | | | | |
| | 1–14 | 565 (16.8) | 1 | | | 1 | | |
| | 15–29 | 276 (18.8) | 1.14 | 0.79–1.66 | *0.468* | 0.91 | 0.59–1.41 | *0.691* |
| | 30 and more | 209 (10.5) | 0.58 | 0.35–0.95 | *0.032* | 0.49 | 0.27–0.87 | *0.015* |
| | *STI symptoms over the last 12 months* | | | | | | | |
| | No | 578 (13.0) | 1 | | | 1 | | |
| | Yes | 465 (19.8) | 1.64 | 1.18–2.30 | *0.003* | 1.44 | 0.98–2.13 | *0.063* |
| | *Ever got pregnant* | | | | | | | |
| | No | 189 (2.1) | 1 | | | 1 | | |
| | Yes | 862 (19.1) | 10.94 | 4.00–29.9 | *0.001* | 5.24 | 1.44–18.97 | *0.012* |
| | *Ease of requesting client to wear a condom* | | | | | | | |
| | Easy | 787 (15.5) | 1 | | | | | |
| | Difficult | 254 (18.1) | 1.20 | 0.83–1.75 | *0.326* | — | — | — |
| | *Consistent condom use during the last 12 months* | | | | | | | |
| | No | 406 (16,5) | 1 | | | | | |
| | Yes | 621 (15.7) | 0.95 | 0.67–1.33 | *0.758* | — | — | — |
| | *Condom use during the last intercourse with new client* | | | | | | | |
| | No | 94 (16.0) | 1 | | | | | |
| | Yes | 931 (15.9) | 0.99 | 0.57–1.77 | *0.988* | — | — | — |
| | *Condom breakage over the last 12 months* | | | | | | | |
| | No | 413 (11.4) | 1 | | | 1 | | |
| | Yes | 639 (19.1) | 1.84 | 1.27–2.64 | *0.001* | 1.78 | 1.16–2.73 | *0.007* |

in larger cities particularly among older FSWs because the prevalence is high. These interventions should benefit FSWs of all ages, especially older FSWs aged 25 and older in different locations throughout the country. Programs supporting FSWs could offer increased services to this population including increasing availability of STI testing, self-testing for HIV, mental health counselling and support, condom and lubricant distribution, and evaluation of FSWs as candidates for preexposure prophylaxis as it becomes available in Burkina Faso. Preexposure prophylaxis would provide FSWs an additional way to protect themselves from HIV and create a safer environment for them to work in. There has been previous success with peer-based education which could potentially be scaled up to a larger level and to more cities. The cost effectiveness of comprehensive HIV prevention programs for FSWs needs further evaluation to inform potential scale-up of these interventions in Burkina Faso.

## Ethical Approval

Ethical approval for this study was received from the Johns Hopkins University Bloomberg School of Public Health Institutional Review Board and the Health Research Ethics Committee (Comité d'Éthique pour la Recherche en Santé) of Burkina Faso.

## Consent

The survey was presented and explained to FSWs in each of the cities before the start of the study. Participating in this study was voluntary. Signed, informed, consent was sought from all participants. Participants were counseled before and after the HIV test. All those who tested positive for HIV got a referral to an appropriate treatment clinic.

## Conflicts of Interest

The authors declare that there are no conflicts of interest regarding the publication of this article.

## Authors' Contributions

S. Baral, S. Kouanda, H. G. Ouedraogo, O. Ky-Zerbo, A. Grosso, and M. Lougue contributed to study design, implementation, and manuscript writing; S. Goodman assisted in manuscript writing; B. C. Samadoulougou helped in study implementation, data cleaning, and manuscript review; A. Baguiya, N. Sawadogo, Y. Traore, and Nicolas Barro conducted the manuscript review.

## Funding

The USAID and Project SEARCH, Task Order No. 2, is funded by the US Agency for International Development under Contract No. GHH-I-00-0700,032-00, beginning September 30, 2008, and supported by the President's Emergency Plan for AIDS Relief. The Research to Prevention Project is led by the Johns Hopkins Center for Global Health and managed by the Johns Hopkins Bloomberg School of Public Health Center for Communication Programs. Additional funding was from Global Fund to Fight AIDS, Tuberculosis and Malaria, and the Permanent Secretary of the National Council against AIDS (SP/CNLS), Burkina Faso.

## Acknowledgments

The authors acknowledge the USAID-Project SEARCH, the Global Fund to Fight AIDS, Tuberculosis and Malaria, the Permanent Secretary of the National Council against AIDS (SP/CNLS), Burkina Faso, the Yerelon Association in Bobo-Dioulasso, and all other associations that were involved in this study. They are grateful to all the study participants. The USAID and Project SEARCH, Task Order no. 2, is funded by the US Agency for International Development under Contract no. GHH-I-00-0700,032-00, beginning September 30, 2008, and supported by the President's Emergency Plan for AIDS Relief. The Research to Prevention Project is led by the Johns Hopkins Center for Global Health and managed by the Johns Hopkins Bloomberg School of Public Health Center for Communication Programs.

## References

[1] "WHO — HIV/AIDS prevalence in sub-Saharan Africa [Internet]. WHO," http://www.who.int/gho/urban_health/outcomes/hiv_prevalence/en/.

[2] "WHO — HIV/AIDS [Internet]. WHO," http://www.who.int/mediacentre/factsheets/fs360/en/.

[3] E. Gouws and P. Cuchi, "Focusing the HIV response through estimating the major modes of HIV transmission: a multi-country analysis," *Sexually Transmitted Infections*, vol. 88, no. Suppl 2, pp. i76–i85, 2012.

[4] S. Baral and N. Phaswana-Mafuya, "Rewriting the narrative of the epidemiology of HIV in sub-Saharan Africa," *Sahara J*, vol. 9, no. 3, pp. 127–130, 2012.

[5] "Sex work and HIV/AIDS: UNAIDS technical update - jc705-sexwork-tu_en.pdf," http://data.unaids.org/publications/irc-pub02/jc705-sexwork-tu_en.pdf.

[6] D. Kang, M. Liao, Z. Jiang et al., "Commercial sex venues, syphilis and methamphetamine use among female sex workers," *AIDS Care—Psychological and Socio-Medical Aspects of AIDS/HIV*, vol. 23, no. 1, pp. 26–36, 2011.

[7] L. Zohrabyan, L. G. Johnston, O. Scutelniciuc et al., "Determinants of HIV infection among female sex workers in two cities in the republic of Moldova: The role of injection drug use and sexual risk," *AIDS and Behavior*, vol. 17, no. 8, pp. 2588–2596, 2013.

[8] E. Papworth, N. Ceesay, L. An et al., "Epidemiology of HIV among female sex workers, their clients, men who have sex with men and people who inject drugs in West and Central Africa," *Journal of the International AIDS Society*, vol. 16, no. 4(Suppl 3), 2013.

[9] "HIV & AIDS Information: Female sex workers have 14 times the risk of having HIV as other women," http://www.aidsmap.com/Female-sex-workers-have-14-times-the-risk-of-having-HIV-as-other-women/page/2457223/.

[10] A. Prüss-Ustün, J. Wolf, T. Driscoll, L. Degenhardt, M. Neira, and J. M. G. Calleja, "HIV Due to Female Sex Work: Regional and Global Estimates," *PLoS ONE*, vol. 8, no. 5, Article ID e63476, 2013.

[11] A. Scheibe, F. M. Drame, and K. Shannon, "HIV prevention among female sex workers in Africa," *SAHARA-J: Journal of Social Aspects of HIV/AIDS*, vol. 9, no. 3, pp. 167–172, 2012.

[12] Y. Li, R. Detels, P. Lin et al., "Prevalence of HIV and STIs and associated risk factors among female sex workers in guangdong Province, China," *Journal of Acquired Immune Deficiency Syndromes*, vol. 53, no. 1, pp. S48–S53, 2010.

[13] S. Baral, C. Beyrer, K. Muessig et al., "Burden of HIV among female sex workers in low-income and middle-income countries: a systematic review and meta-analysis," *The Lancet Infectious Diseases*, vol. 12, no. 7, pp. 538–549, 2012.

[14] J. Vandepitte, J. Bukenya, H. A. Weiss et al., "HIV and other sexually transmitted infections in a cohort of women involved in high-risk sexual behavior in Kampala, Uganda," *Sexually Transmitted Diseases*, vol. 38, no. 4, pp. 316–323, 2011.

[15] V. A. Fonner, D. Kerrigan, Z. Mnisi, S. Ketende, C. E. Kennedy, and S. Baral, "Social cohesion, social participation, and HIV related risk among female sex workers in Swaziland," *PLoS ONE*, vol. 9, no. 1, Article ID e87527, 2014.

[16] South African Health Monitoring Study (SAHMS), *Final Report: The Integrated Biological and Behavioural Survey among Female Sex Workers, South Africa 2013-2014*, UCSF, San Francisco, 2015.

[17] S. Peitzmeier, K. Mason, N. Ceesay et al., "A cross-sectional evaluation of the prevalence and associations of HIV among female sex workers in the Gambia," *International Journal of STD & AIDS*, vol. 25, no. 4, pp. 244–252, 2014.

[18] F. Sobéla, J. Pépin, S. Gbéléou et al., "A tale of two countries: HIV among core groups in Togo," *Journal of Acquired Immune Deficiency Syndromes*, vol. 51, no. 2, pp. 216–223, 2009.

[19] "Burkina Faso Enquête Démographique et de Santé et à Indicateurs Multiples (EDSBF-MICS IV) 2010 [FR256] - FR256.pdf," http://www.dhsprogram.com/pubs/pdf/FR256/FR256.pdf.

[20] I. T. Traore, N. M. Hema, A. Sanon et al., "HIV risk and behaviour among part-time versus professional FSW: Baseline report of an interventional cohort in Burkina Faso," *Sexually Transmitted Infections*, vol. 92, no. 7, pp. 550–553, 2016.

[21] D. D. Heckathorn, "Respondent-driven sampling: a new approach to the study of hidden populations," *Social Problems*, vol. 44, no. 2, pp. 174–199, 1997.

[22] N. McCreesh, A. Copas, J. Seeley et al., "Respondent driven sampling: determinants of recruitment and a method to improve point estimation," *PLoS ONE*, vol. 8, no. 10, p. e78402, 2013.

[23] S. C. Weller and K. Davis-Beaty, "Condom effectiveness in reducing het erosexual HIV transmission," *Cochrane Database Systematic Reviews*, vol. 1, 2002.

[24] S. Lankoandé, N. Meda, L. Sangaré et al., "Prevalence and risk of HIV infection among female sex workers in Burkina Faso," *International Journal of STD & AIDS*, vol. 9, no. 3, pp. 146–150, 1998.

[25] N. Nagot, A. Ouangré, A. Ouedraogo et al., "Spectrum of Commercial Sex Activity in Burkina Faso: Classification Model and Risk of Exposure to HIV," *Journal of Acquired Immune Deficiency Syndromes*, vol. 29, no. 5, pp. 517–521, 2002.

[26] D. D. Heckathorn, "Respondent-driven sampling II: deriving valid population estimates from chain-referral samples of hidden populations," *Social Problems*, vol. 49, no. 1, pp. 11–34, 2002.

[27] A. L. Wirtz, S. Schwartz, S. Ketende et al., "Sexual violence, condom negotiation, and condom use in the context of sex work: Results from two West African countries," *Journal of Acquired Immune Deficiency Syndromes*, vol. 68, pp. S171–S179, 2015.

[28] S. Baral, C. H. Logie, A. Grosso, A. L. Wirtz, and C. Beyrer, "Modified social ecological model: A tool to guide the assessment of the risks and risk contexts of HIV epidemics," *BMC Public Health*, vol. 13, no. 1, article no. 482, 2013.

[29] B. Vuylsteke, G. Semdé, L. Sika et al., "HIV and STI prevalence among female sex workers in côte d'ivoire: Why targeted prevention programs should be continued and strengthened," *PLoS ONE*, vol. 7, no. 3, Article ID e32627, 2012.

[30] C. Inguane, R. Z. Horth, A. E. Miranda et al., "Sociodemographic, Behavioral and Health Characteristics of Underage Female Sex Workers in Mozambique: The Need to Protect a Generation from HIV Risk," *AIDS and Behavior*, vol. 19, no. 12, pp. 2184–2193, 2015.

[31] S. R. Schwartz, E. Papworth, O. Ky-Zerbo et al., "Safer conception needs for HIV prevention among female sex workers in Burkina Faso and Togo," *Infectious Diseases in Obstetrics and Gynecology*, vol. 2014, Article ID 296245, 2014.

[32] J. R. Williams, M. Alary, C. M. Lowndes et al., "Positive impact of increases in condom use among female sex workers and clients in a medium HIV prevalence epidemic: Modelling results from project SIDA1/2/3 in Cotonou, Benin," *PLoS ONE*, vol. 9, no. 7, Article ID e102643, 2014.

[33] M. F. Chersich, S. Luchters, I. Ntaganira et al., "Priority interventions to reduce HIV transmission in sex work settings in sub-Saharan Africa and delivery of these services," *Journal of the International AIDS Society*, vol. 16, Article ID 17980, 2013.

[34] J. Bradley, S. Rajaram, M. Alary et al., "Determinants of condom breakage among female sex workers in Karnataka, India," *BMC Public Health*, vol. 11, no. 6, article no. S14, 2011.

[35] F. K. Tounkara, S. Diabaté, F. A. Guédou et al., "Violence, condom breakage, and HIV infection among female sex workers in Benin, West Africa," *Sexually Transmitted Diseases*, vol. 41, no. 5, pp. 312–318, 2014.

[36] I. Konate, L. Traore, A. Ouedraogo et al., "Linking HIV prevention and care for community interventions among high-risk women in Burkina Faso-the ARNS 1222 yerelon cohort," *Journal of Acquired Immune Deficiency Syndromes*, vol. 57, no. 1, pp. S50–S54, 2011.

# 12

# Trauma and Growth: Impact of AIDS Activism

**Judith G. Rabkin,[1,2] Martin C. McElhiney,[1,2] Mark Harrington,[3] and Tim Horn[3]**

[1]*New York State Psychiatric Institute, New York, NY, USA*
[2]*Department of Psychiatry, Columbia University, New York, NY, USA*
[3]*Treatment Action Group, New York, NY, USA*

Correspondence should be addressed to Martin C. McElhiney; mcelhin@nyspi.columbia.edu

Academic Editor: Glenda Gray

*Introduction.* Our goal was to assess the long-term impact of AIDS activism of ACT UP/New York on the current adjustment of those who were members during its peak years (1987–1992), including assessment of trauma sequelae as well as posttraumatic growth. *Methods.* A 90-minute semistructured interview and 6 validated self-report scales were administered. We relied on purposive and snowball sampling to recruit potential participants. Areas covered include demographics, ACT UP participation, and psychiatric problems. Self-report scales provided approximate diagnoses of PTSD and depression, as well as coping, optimism, and related concepts. *Results.* Participants included 102 men (40% HIV-positive) and 23 women. Seventeen percent reported current symptoms suggesting PTSD, slightly above the range in general population studies. Symptoms consistent with depression were reported by 8% overall, with higher rates for HIV+ men. Enhanced sense of self, belief in change, and empowerment were reported by 93% of respondents, independent of concurrent PTSD or depression. *Conclusions.* Twenty-eight years later, ACT UP study participants recall their activist days during the AIDS epidemic as the peak experience of their lives. While some continue to have symptoms of stress and depression, most found that their activism has enriched their subsequent lives.

## 1. Introduction

In the early years of the HIV/AIDS epidemic in the United States, activists played a unique and unprecedented role. Confronting a new, lethal, and highly stigmatized disease, they became caregivers, advocates, "citizen scientists," and the voice of an outraged community [1]. While the history of organizations such as ACT UP (the AIDS Coalition to Unleash Power) continues to be documented [2], the long-term psychosocial effects of AIDS activism on activists themselves have yet to be well studied. What happens when members of a marginalized community, threatened both by a rapidly fatal disease and by an unresponsive government, organize to fight for survival and survive? We examined the prevalence of posttraumatic stress disorder (PTSD), depression, and posttraumatic growth among men and women who participated in ACT UP between 1987 and 1992.

ACT UP was founded in 1987 in New York City as a radical protest organization; peak membership and activity occurred between 1987 and 1992. Its members were exposed to extensive loss and trauma because of the intensity of their work, the high mortality within their extended networks of HIV-exposed fellow activists and friends, their own risk of illness and death, and their confrontational demonstrations. At the same time, they had the opportunity to connect with a network, find emotional support, and act on behalf of their own and their community's lives. ACT UP survivors thus constitute a distinctive sample with which to address key questions of long-term trauma and growth.

ACT UP members were predominantly young, gay, and often but not always HIV-infected, although women (often but not always lesbian) also played leading roles. ACT UP members conducted major, very visible demonstrations, starting within a month of its formation by Larry Kramer in March 1987. In September of that year, a demonstration took place inside the New York Stock Exchange, protesting the high cost of AZT, the only medication at that time approved to treat AIDS. Few people with AIDS had health insurance or access to medical care and were sometimes evicted, fired, and rejected by their families. ACT UP had committees whose members pioneered innovative housing for people with AIDS, piloted syringe exchanges and other harm reduction projects for drug users, and worked with the FDA and NIH-funded AIDS trial networks, to plan drug trials and facilitate medication access at a time when no effective treatments were available. ACT UP was loud; it was confrontational; it was effective.

The long-term effects of ACT UP participation are unclear. Those who were engaged in the years 1987–1992 today are all "long-term" survivors of the epidemic years and, for some, survivors with HIV/AIDS. Some have proposed that community activism has a protective effect, often leading to posttraumatic growth [3], while others such as Spencer Cox ("Living on the Edge: Gay men in mid-life, and the impact of HIV/AIDS," unpublished) emphasized negative outcomes including posttraumatic stress disorder, clinical depression, and substance use.

Following the Cox initiative, we included measures of posttraumatic stress disorder, major depression, and substance use to assess long-term negative sequelae of ACT UP participation, acknowledging that neither we nor respondents would be able to rule out the concurrent effects of living in the midst of the AIDS epidemic itself. Major depressive disorder has been recognized as a significant psychiatric problem since the development of formal diagnostic criteria. PTSD has been an official psychiatric disorder since 1980 [4], although the concept of shell shock in combat veterans has a much longer history. The formal definition of PTSD requires exposure to "actual or threatened death, serious injury, or sexual violence, either by direct experience, witnessing, learning that such an event occurred to someone close, or experiencing repeated exposure to aversive details of the traumatic event" [5], along with associated symptoms such as numbness, intrusive recollections, and hyperarousal. Symptom duration varies. Among American soldiers deployed in Iraq assessed 7 years later and Romanian political prisoners 40 years later, 25–30% still had PTSD symptoms [6, 7]. For both PTSD and depression, diagnosis requires clinically significant distress or impairment in major areas of functioning.

In addition to formal psychiatric diagnoses such as depressive disorder and PTSD, the lay term "AIDS Survivor Syndrome" (ASS) is defined by its proponents as a "spectrum of sustained trauma of survivorship, the psychological state resulting from living through the HIV/AIDS pandemic" [8]. It is intended to represent a different phenomenon than PTSD and is conceptualized as a normal response to an exceptional experience [9].

Some survivors of the earliest days of the AIDS epidemic continue to report ongoing distress and "long-term survivor" support groups continue to exist. Overall, however, the limited evidence, largely published in the early 1990s, reflects the prominence of resiliency over pathology [10–13]. In the general population, an estimated 60% to 80% of those who endure traumatic or highly stressful events do not develop psychiatric disorders [14, 15].

Protective conditions, relations, or circumstances have been examined in various contexts. A major factor is "unit cohesion." Junger [16] observed that membership in tribes and communities provides a powerful protective effect during wartime, noting that admissions to psychiatric hospitals actually declined during the London Blitz of 1940-41 and the Dutch famine of 1944-45. The same has been observed in wartime among elite frontline troops most directly exposed to danger, who have lower rates of psychiatric breakdown compared to rear-base troops. "Unit cohesion," strong emotional bonds of friendship, and mutual trust within a community, company, or platoon are considered to protect against otherwise virtually intolerable experiences [17].

Although the negative effects of trauma have been studied for years, the concept of "posttraumatic growth" [18, 19] and the study of "positive psychology" have evolved more recently [20]. Folkman [21] added the concept of positive reappraisal to her model of stress and coping, in which the significance of a stressful event is reinterpreted in a positive way. Reappraisal is similar to cognitive reframing, a standard component of cognitive behavioral therapy [22]. PTSD and posttraumatic growth can be conceptualized, not as poles of one continuum, but as two independent constructs that can coexist.

Building on these observations, we assessed the current rates of PTSD, depression, and substance abuse, as well as posttraumatic growth, among ACT UP survivors. We explored their association with exposure to losses and other experiences associated with AIDS activism. We attempted to determine the extent to which the alternative model of AIDS Survivor Syndrome overlaps with measures of depression and PTSD. We also evaluated the protective effects of "unit cohesion" and posttraumatic growth with respect to sense of self, relationships, and life outlook.

## 2. Methods

*2.1. Sampling and Recruitment.* ACT UP New York drew several hundred members to its weekly meetings in its peak years [31], but there was no official membership list and no way to obtain a random sample of survivors. Instead, we used purposive sampling followed by snowball sampling to identify study participants. We relied on Community Advisory Board members to contact their social networks and to post notices about the study on the ACT UP Alumni Facebook page to recruit volunteers. Controls (defined as those present in NYC between 1987 and 1992 who identified with the lesbian/gay community but who chose not to join ACT UP) were identified by ACT UP study participants.

*2.2. Measures.* Study tools were selected and a semistructured interview was developed following preliminary discussions with seven key informants (six were prominent in HIV research or treatment including two psychiatrists, and one was a former HIV+ activist). We asked about experiences during ACT UP participation as well as past and current medical and psychological problems. Participants completed six validated self-report scales [23–30] assessing current coping, optimism, loneliness, depression and PTSD symptoms and DSM-IV diagnoses, and alcohol use (Table 1). Algorithms for the measures of PTSD (PCL using Ruggiero's [26, p. 500] preferred method of deriving DSM-IV diagnosis) and depression (PHQ) were used to determine approximate DSM-IV diagnoses; formal psychiatric interviews were not conducted. Continuous scores on the PCL and PHQ also were used.

TABLE 1: Study measures: items, content, score range, and cut-offs (if applicable)*.

| Scale | Number of items | Content | Score range* | Cut-offs |
|---|---|---|---|---|
| Patient Health Questionnaire (PHQ-9) (depression) [23] | 9 | Consists of the 9 criteria for diagnosis of major depression and minor depression (DSM-IV and 5); provides a provisional diagnosis and also a symptom severity score. Diagnosis of major depression requires ratings of "most days" (3) or "almost every day" (4) on 5+ items including either depressed mood or loss of interest. Minor depression requires only 3 items. Time frame: past 2 weeks. | 0–27 | <10 = absent/mild<br>10–14 = moderate<br>15–19 = moderately severe<br>≥20 = severe<br>Diagnosis: algorithm |
| PTSD Checklist (PCL) [24–26] | 17 | Consists of DSM-IV symptoms of PTSD. It generates an approximate diagnosis, using an algorithm that requires 1+ symptoms scored 3+ on individual items from each of 3 symptom clusters. Time frame: past month. | 17–85 | >50 = "case"<br>Diagnosis: algorithm |
| Alcohol Use Disorders Identification Test (AUDIT) [27] | 10 | Questions about frequency and amount plus possible negative consequences and regrets. Time frame: past year. | 0–40 | 16–19 = mild problem<br>≥20 = suggests need for treatment |
| **Coping Self-Efficacy Scale [28] | 13 | Measures perceived ability to cope effectively "when you're having problems." We used 13 of the original 26 items. Example: "Sort out what can be changed and what cannot be changed." No time frame. | 0–130 | None |
| Life Orientation Test (LOT) [29] | 12 | Designed to measure optimism versus pessimism. Example: "In uncertain times, I usually expect the best." No time frame. | 0–48 | ≥17 = optimism<br><17 = pessimism |
| **UCLA Loneliness Scale [30] | 10 | Ten of the original 20 items, including both negative ("I feel isolated from others") and positive ("There are people I can talk to") items, the latter scored in reverse. Time frame: past 2 weeks. | 10–40 | None |

*Note.* Higher scores represent a greater endorsement of the construct being measured. ***Note.* Score doubled to enable comparison with norms.

*2.3. Data Collection.* Interviews lasted about 90 minutes and took place between June 2013 and March 2015. Local participants were interviewed in person, while those outside New York City were interviewed by telephone. Interviews were audio-taped. Structured questions were coded, and open-ended queries were transcribed.

*2.4. Data Analysis.* Three open-ended queries were coded by question and theme. They inquired about "best things" about ACT UP, "worst things," and "sense of self." Three team members rated each and met to reach consensus on classification. We analyzed quantitative data using $t$-tests, chi-square for categorical variables, and Pearson's correlations. Fisher's Exact Test (FET) was used for analysis of categorical variables when cell size < 6. Three separate multiple regression analyses were performed, using total scores of each as the dependent variable to identify factors associated with depression, PTSD, and coping effectiveness. All predictors were included in the model simultaneously. Skewed data were log-transformed. Since this is an exploratory study, we did not correct for multiple comparisons but did not report statistical trends ($p$ > .05 – < .10). We defined statistical significance as $p \leq .05$, 2-tailed, in all analyses.

*2.5. Ethical Approvals.* The study was approved by the Institutional Review Board of New York State Psychiatric Institute-Columbia University. Participants signed consent forms after the consent process was conducted and all questions were addressed.

## 3. Results

*3.1. Sample Characteristics.* ACT UP members between 1987 and 1992 (102 men and 23 women) and 50 controls (non-ACT UP members) were study participants (Table 2). Seven continued to be ACT UP/New York members. Among members, 41 men and no women were HIV+. Nineteen of 50 controls were HIV+; all were male. Two-thirds of members and all controls were interviewed in New York City; the remaining 33 participants lived in 14 states and three foreign countries. Among members at the time of the interview, the mean age was 54 years (range: 37–74); 85% had completed college including 47% who completed graduate school. Thirty-six percent completed their education after leaving ACT UP. Three-quarters (76%) reported annual income of over \$30,000 and 40% earned over \$75,000 per year. Ninety-eight percent of participants were identified as gay/lesbian. Controls did not differ on these demographic measures.

TABLE 2: Demographic characteristics of ACT UP group and control group.

| | ACT UP group | | | | Control group N = 50 |
|---|---|---|---|---|---|
| | Male HIV+ N = 41 | Male HIV− N = 61 | Female* N = 23 | Total N = 125 | |
| Age, M (range) | 55 (45–73) | 54 (44–74) | 52 (37–68) | 54 (37–74) | 56 (44–68) |
| Ethnicity, N (%) | | | | | |
| White | 35 (85) | 51 (84) | 20 (87) | 106 (85) | 44 (88) |
| Black | 0 | 2 (3) | 3 (13) | 5 (4) | 3 (6) |
| Hispanic | 6 (15) | 7 (11) | 0 | 13 (10) | 1 (2) |
| Other | 0 | 1 (2) | 0 | 1 (1) | 2 (4) |
| Education (years), M (SD) | 17.2 (2.3) | 17.1 (2.3) | 17.7 (2.5) | 17.2 (2.3) | 16.9 (2.2) |
| Education, N (%) | | | | | |
| Less than college | 7 (17) | 9 (15) | 3 (13) | 19 (15) | 6 (12) |
| College | 15 (37) | 25 (38) | 7 (30) | 47 (38) | 24 (48) |
| Graduate training | 19 (46) | 27 (44) | 13 (57) | 59 (47) | 20 (40) |
| Income, N (%) | | | | | |
| Under $30,000 | 11 (28) | 13 (22) | 5 (22) | 29 (24) | 7 (14) |
| 30,000–75,000 | 14 (35) | 22 (37) | 9 (39) | 45 (36) | 4 (8) 9 (18) |
| 76,000–99,999 | 4 (10) | 11 (18) | 3 (13) | 18 (15) | 1 (2) |
| $100,000+ | 11 (27) | 14 (23) | 6 (26) | 31 (25) | 29 (58) |
| Major depression diagnosis, N (%) | 9 (22) | 1 (2) | 0 | 10 (8) | 1 (2) |

*All HIV−.

*3.2. Rates and Correlates of PTSD.* Twenty-one respondents (17%) reported current symptoms consistent with an approximate DSM-IV diagnosis of PTSD, including 20 men, of whom half were HIV-positive, and one woman. Comparing participants with and without PTSD (Table 3(a)), we found no differences in current age, income, education, or HIV serostatus. In addition, no differences were found in duration of ACT UP participation, number of demonstrations, arrests, frequency of attending, or other measures of activism. However, those with PTSD reported more deaths of friends ($p = .049$) and scored significantly worse on all self-reported measures of current adjustment and functioning (all $p$ values $< 0.002$) (Table 3(b)). In a regression analysis (Table 4(a)) using total PCL score as outcome, older age ($p = .02$) and committee membership during ACT UP ($p = .04$) were associated with lower scores, while those having intrusive thoughts and lacking future orientation were more likely to have higher scores (more PTSD symptoms, $p < .001$ and $p = .03$, respectively).

*3.3. Prevalence of Depression.* The depression measure, PHQ, provides both an *approximate* DSM-IV diagnosis of depressive disorders and a numerical indicator of symptom severity. HIV status is associated with current major depressive disorder (MDD), with nine HIV+ men and one HIV− man having a major depressive disorder. In a regression analysis using variables listed in Table 4(b), those with close friends (when interviewed) were 51% less likely to be depressed than others ($t = -3.92$, $p < .001$), adjusting for all covariates.

Of note, there was substantial overlap among participants with approximate diagnoses of depression (PHQ) and PTSD (PCL): for the entire sample, the correlation between scores on the PHQ and PCL was 0.74 ($p < .001$). We reanalyzed PCL scores after deleting three items (difficulty sleeping, problems with concentration, and loss of interest in formerly pleasurable events) that correspond to criteria for depressive disorders and prorated scores for the missing items. The correlation between the PHQ and adjusted PCL was 0.70 ($p < .001$), remaining essentially the same.

A small number of respondents (5 on the PCL and 1 on the PHQ) had high scores on these measures (over the cut-off on the PCL of 50 and on the PHQ of 14, used to signify a probable diagnosis). However, the distribution of their responses did not conform to the diagnostic algorithms of the respective measures, reflecting substantial distress without a diagnosis.

*3.4. The Role of Substance Use.* We asked respondents about current (past year) and historical use of recreational drugs and alcohol with open-ended questions. When reported, was there interference with social or occupational functioning? If yes, we defined this use as a "problem." Within the past year, 11 respondents (9%) reported problems with alcohol, methamphetamine, marijuana, and/or cocaine, in descending order of frequency. Of these, three had concurrent PTSD and/or depression.

Fifty-five respondents (44%) reported past substance use problems. The most common was alcohol, reported by 36 respondents (29%), including 11 HIV-positive men (27%), 20

TABLE 3: Comparisons of ACT UP study participants with and without PTSD diagnosis.

(a)

| Demographic variables and ACT UP experiences | PTSD diagnosis $N = 21$ | No diagnosis $N = 104$ | $t$ or $x^2$ | $p$ |
|---|---|---|---|---|
| Current age, *M (SD)* | 51.5 (4.9) | 54.1 (6.6) | −1.730 | .086 |
| Current annual income, *M (SD)* | $76,176 (67,780) | $81,400 (106,326) | −.216 | .829 |
| Education (years), *M (SD)* | 16.7 (2.5) | 17.3 (2.3) | −.982 | .328 |
| HIV status, *N (%)* | | | | |
| HIV+ | 10 (48) | 31 (30) | 2.326 | .127 |
| HIV− | 11 (52) | 73 (70) | | |
| Lost friends, *N (%)* | | | | |
| None | 1 (5) | 8 (8) | 6.051 | .049 |
| Some | 1 (5) | 29 (28) | | |
| Many | 19 (90) | 65 (63) | | |
| Lost partner, *N (%)* | 7 (33) | 19 (18) | 2.673 | .102 |
| Primary caregiver for sick friends, *N (%)* | 8 (38) | 29 (28) | .773 | .379 |
| Age when joined ACT UP, *M (SD)* | 27.1 (4.5) | 28.7 (6.1) | −1.155 | .250 |
| Number of years in ACT UP, *M (SD)* | 7.1 (7.9) | 5.0 (4.3) | 1.670 | .097 |
| Demonstrations, *N (%)* | | | | |
| None | - | 2 (2) | | |
| A few | 1 (5) | 1 (1) | 2.626 | .453 |
| Some | 1 (5) | 11 (11) | | |
| Many | 19 (90) | 88 (85) | | |
| Times arrested, *N (%)* | | | | |
| None | 7 (33) | 30 (29) | .201 | .904 |
| Once | 2 (10) | 12 (12) | | |
| More than once | 11 (52) | 57 (55) | | |
| Attended Monday meetings, *N (%)* | | | | |
| Rarely | - | 1 (1) | | |
| Occasionally | 1 (5) | 5 (5) | .385 | .943 |
| Often | 1 (5) | 3 (3) | | |
| Regularly | 19 (90) | 93 (89) | | |
| In a committee, *N (%)* | 14 (67) | 85 (82) | 3.080 | .079 |

(b)

| Self-reported measures | PTSD diagnosis $N = 21$ | No diagnosis $N = 104$ | $t$ or $x^2$ | $p$ |
|---|---|---|---|---|
| PHQ-9 [depression], *M (SD)* | 13.0 (5.7) | 3.8 (3.3) | 10.101 | <.001 |
| PHQ-9: DSM IV meets algorithm for major depression, *N (%)* | 7 (33) | 3 (3) | 21.536 | <.001 |
| PCL Checklist (PTSD), *M (SD)* | 54.7 (7.2) | 29.1 (9.5) | 11.633 | <.001 |
| PCL Checklist (PTSD): prorated total minus three depression items, *M (SD)* | 53.8 (7.8) | 28.4 (9.6) | 11.330 | <.001 |
| AUDIT: problematic alcohol use (scores ≥ 16), *N (%)* | 6 (29) | 14 (13) | 2.819 | .093 |
| Coping Self-Efficacy Scale, *M (SD)* | 57.9 (16.9) | 92.6 (18.4) | −7.980 | <.001 |
| LOT [optimism versus pessimism] | | | | |
| Optimistic (scores ≥ 17), *N (%)* | 7 (33) | 77 (74) | 13.134 | <.001 |
| Pessimistic (scores < 17), *N (%)* | 14 (67) | 27 (26) | | |
| UCLA Loneliness Scale, *M (SD)* | 49.5 (11.3) | 37.0 (8.8) | 5.634 | <.001 |

TABLE 4

(a) Independent variables included in regression analyses: PTSD (PCL total score)

| Independent variables | | Dependent variable PTSD (PCL total score) | | | |
|---|---|---|---|---|---|
| | | Estimate | Exponentiated estimate | $t$ | $p$ |
| Demographics | Age | −0.012 | 0.988 | −2.43 | .017 |
| | Gender | 0.062 | 1.064 | 0.72 | .472 |
| | Race | −0.098 | 0.907 | −1.00 | .318 |
| | HIV status | −0.098 | 1.053 | 0.72 | .475 |
| ACT UP | Years involved in ACT UP | 0.004 | 1.005 | 0.74 | .464 |
| | On a committee | −0.141 | 0.868 | −2.10 | .038 |
| | Arrested during demonstration | −0.117 | 0.889 | −1.11 | .270 |
| AIDS related | Friends died | −0.027 | 0.974 | −0.21 | .834 |
| | Partner died | 0.137 | 1.147 | 1.63 | .107 |
| Past year | Has intrusive thoughts | 0.295 | 1.344 | 3.71 | <.001 |
| | Lacks future orientation | 0.171 | 1.186 | 2.19 | .031 |
| | Feels AIDS is behind them | 0.005 | 1.005 | 0.06 | .952 |

(b) Independent variables included in 2 regression analyses: depression (PHQ total score) and coping (CESD total score)

| Independent variables | | Dependent variables | | | | | | |
|---|---|---|---|---|---|---|---|---|
| | | Depression (PHQ total score) | | | | Coping (CESD total score) | | |
| | | Estimate | Exponentiated estimate* | $t$ | $p$ | Estimate | $t$ | $p$ |
| Demographics | Age | −0.013 | 0.987 | −1.09 | .278 | 0.525 | 1.78 | .077 |
| | Gender | 0.003 | 1.003 | 0.01 | .989 | 2.015 | 0.39 | .694 |
| | Race | −0.278 | 0.758 | −1.27 | .205 | 13.769 | 2.49 | .014 |
| | HIV status | 0.122 | 1.130 | 0.74 | .462 | 5.725 | 1.36 | .176 |
| ACT UP | Years involved in ACT UP | 0.013 | 1.013 | 0.95 | .343 | −0.632 | −1.77 | .079 |
| | On a committee | −0.288 | 0.750 | −1.83 | .069 | 6.230 | 1.56 | .121 |
| AIDS related | Friends died | −0.133 | 0.876 | −0.44 | .658 | 14.275 | 1.88 | .062 |
| | Partner died | 0.334 | 1.396 | 1.82 | .071 | −0.688 | −0.15 | .882 |
| Past year | Has stable career | 0.019 | 1.019 | 0.08 | .936 | 1.697 | 0.28 | .780 |
| | Has close friends | −0.716 | 0.488 | −3.92 | <.001 | 12.265 | 2.64 | .009 |
| | In a relationship | −0.283 | 0.753 | −1.37 | .174 | 17.102 | 3.25 | .002 |
| | Part of a community | 0.153 | 1.166 | 0.72 | .474 | 2.155 | 0.40 | .691 |

*Regression for depression was run with log-normal data; therefore, exponentiated estimates are presented.

TABLE 5: Comparison of male ACT UP members by HIV serostatus.

(a)

| ACT UP experiences | HIV+ men N = 41 | HIV− men N = 61 | $t$ or $x^2$ | $p$ |
|---|---|---|---|---|
| Age when joined ACT UP, *M (SD)* | 29.0 (6.1) | 28.7 (5.3) | .292 | .771 |
| Number of years in ACT UP, *M (SD)* | 6.4 (6.1) | 5.1 (4.3) | 1.198 | .234 |
| Demonstrations, *N (%)* | | | | |
| None | 1 (2) | 1 (2) | | |
| A few | 0 (0) | 1 (2) | 3.594 | .309 |
| Some | 6 (15) | 3 (5) | | |
| Many | 34 (83) | 56 (92) | | |
| Times arrested, *N (%)* | | | | |
| None | 14 (34) | 18 (30) | 1.418 | .492 |
| Once | 5 (12) | 5 (8) | | |
| More than once | 19 (46) | 37 (61) | | |
| Attended Monday meetings, *N (%)* | | | | |
| Occasionally | 1 (2) | 2 (3) | .747 | .688 |
| Often | - | 1 (2) | | |
| Regularly | 40 (98) | 58 (95) | | |
| In a committee, *N (%)* | 36 (88) | 49 (80) | .987 | .320 |
| Lost partner, *N (%)* | 16 (39) | 11 (18) | 5.324 | .021 |
| Primary caregiver for sick friend(s), *N (%)* | 17 (41) | 16 (26) | 2.600 | .107 |

(b)

| Self-reported measures | | | | |
|---|---|---|---|---|
| PHQ-9 [depression], *M (SD)* | 6.93 (6.93) | 4.62 (3.77) | 2.205 | .03 |
| PHQ-9: DSM IV meets algorithm for major depression, *N (%)* | 9 (22) | 1 (2) | 16.3 | <.001 |
| PCL Checklist (PTSD), *M (SD)* | 35.3 (15.81) | 32.9 (11.4) | 1.321 | .190 |
| PCL Checklist (PTSD): prorated total minus three depression items, *M (SD)* | 34.5 (15.9) | 31.3 (11.3) | 1.178 | .242 |
| AUDIT: problematic alcohol use (scores ≥ 16), *N (%)* | 1 (2) | 5 (8) | 4.13 | .127 |
| Coping Self-Efficacy Scale, *M (SD)* | 90.5 (26.75) | 84.3 (18.7) | 1.353 | .179 |
| LOT [optimism versus pessimism], *N (%)* | | | | |
| Optimistic (Scores ≥ 17) | 26 (63) | 40 (66) | 3.911 | .141 |
| Pessimistic (Scores < 17) | 15 (37) | 21 (34) | | |
| UCLA Loneliness Scale, *M (SD)* | 19.36 (5.73) | 20.5 (4.92) | −.972 | .333 |

HIV-negative men (33%), and 5 women (22%). Two-thirds had started drinking heavily before they joined ACT UP. Of the 15 men (no women) who reported past methamphetamine problems, 11 were HIV-positive. Prior marijuana problems, reported by 14 respondents, and cocaine problems, reported by 12, did not differ by gender or HIV serostatus.

*3.5. Impact of HIV Serostatus.* When interviewed, 40% (41/102) of the men were HIV-positive. Ten (25%) had been diagnosed with HIV prior to ACT UP, and a total of 32 (78%) by 1995, when effective combination antiretroviral treatment became available. HIV-positive men did not differ from HIV seronegative men on demographic measures, scales assessing coping, loneliness, alcohol use, or optimism, nor did they differ in terms of ACT UP experiences, with one exception: more reported loss of a partner (Table 5). In terms of current psychological adjustment, they were more likely to have a current major depressive disorder (9/41 = 22% versus 1/61 = 2%, FET ≤ 0.003) and reports of past methamphetamine substance use disorder (11/15, FET ≤ .001).

*3.6. AIDS Survivor Syndrome.* Manifestations include depression, anger, anxiety, emotional numbness, behavior (e.g., sexual risk-taking, isolation), hopelessness, lack of future orientation, and social isolation. We identified 16 measurable symptoms for which we had data, excluding concepts such as "panic from unexpected older age" and "personality changes," and examined their distributions. The mean number of items affirmed by the entire sample was 2.4 (range: 0–13). For the 21 respondents with PTSD (PCL Scale), the mean number of ASS items endorsed was 6.8 (SD = 2.98), significantly greater than for the rest of the sample ($t = 7.77$, $p < .001$). For the 10 respondents classified as depressed (PHQ Scale), mean number was 8.7 (SD = 2.90) items endorsed, again greater than the rest of the sample ($t = -7.163$, $p < .001$). Looking at the symptom distribution for the sample ($N = 125$), the lowest quartile expressed no symptoms, while the mean for the top quartile was 6.4 (SD = 2.5).

*3.7. "Unit Cohesion".* When asked "In what ways was ACT UP a positive experience?," 99 respondents (79%) cited "social ties," the most commonly endorsed choice among 10 options provided (respondents could and usually did endorse more than one; see the Appendix). Other frequently endorsed (and overlapping) response options were "collective identity" ($N$ = 85, 68%) and "emotional support" ($N$ = 54, 43%).

When asked whether they missed anything after leaving ACT UP, with seven response options (see the Appendix), the most commonly endorsed was "loss of network." Finally, when asked to list the two "best things" about ACT UP in an open-ended format, the most commonly mentioned "best thing" was "sense of community, being part of something" ($N$ = 45, 37%). For example, one man said, "It was an all-encompassing sense of family and support. It was my family, my church, my sex life, where I got my optimism." Another said, "an incredible sense of camaraderie, being part of an army trying to change the world." When asked about the two "worst things," the most common responses were losses, "all the deaths that kept accelerating, without time for the grief process," and the infighting and arguments at meetings, "the acrimony, internal discord." Both weakened unit cohesion.

*3.8. Posttraumatic Growth: Change in Sense of Self.* In response to the open-ended query, "in what ways was ACT UP a positive experience?," 65% of the respondents described the theme of "empowerment." One respondent noted, "I was identified as an AIDS activist, a different identity that was strong and tough. I felt at the point of a spear." Another reflected, "I had agency. I could do something" and "the life and death context brought out the best in me. I could do something that was bigger than me and changed the world."

Respondents were asked, "Do you think your experience in ACT UP changed your sense of self, who you are as a person?" The overwhelming response was affirmative (93%), regardless of whether or not PTSD symptoms were present 25 years later. Table 6 presents a sample of responses for the three most common categories: agency ($N$ = 32), empowerment ($N$ = 28), and personal growth ($N$ = 29). Other themes, endorsed by less than 5% of respondents, were future life choices, a new identity, and finding meaning. One respondent illustrated parallel feelings of benefit and then loss: "I believe people in ACT UP experienced something really extraordinary and that people who have fought the good fight have the problem that when the fighting stops. . .there's a problem of finding meaning in ordinary life and rejoining the real world which really isn't compelling."

In a regression analysis (Table 4(b)), using the Coping Self-Efficacy Scale as the dependent variable, better coping was associated with minority status, having close friends, and those with partners, while holding all other covariates constant.

## 4. Discussion

Our findings support the notion of posttraumatic stress responses and posttraumatic growth as independent, parallel dimensions rather than endpoints in a single continuum. Taylor's [32] cognitive adaptation theory proposes that the adjustment to traumatic events includes three components: search for meaning (also cited in Folkman's expansion of her theory of stress and coping [21]), an attempt to regain control, and an effort to improve self-esteem. All three of these themes are expressed in responses (Table 6) to our query about the impact of ACT UP on sense of self.

We found somewhat elevated prevalence of both PTSD and depression in this sample of AIDS activists 25 years later, compared to rates found in general population-based studies, which range from 1% to 14% ([5], p. 426). Of note, the relationship of traumatic symptoms with ACT UP experiences is at best an estimate. While respondents were instructed to complete the PCL Checklist referring *only* to AIDS or ACT UP-related trauma, two-thirds reported traumatic events that were *not* specific to either.

The overall rate of major depressive disorder in our sample was 8%, with higher rates for HIV+ men. The prevalence of depression is known to be elevated among HIV+ men and women [33]. In national studies of HIV-positive adults, the observed rates of major depression range from 5.9% [34] to 22% [35], compared to 7% in the general population [36]. Although our finding for HIV+ men is at the high end of this range, it may be a measurement artifact: we relied only on self-report, while the cited studies used formal psychiatric evaluations which usually generate lower rates than self-report scales.

The overlap between depression and PTSD is substantial in our study, as is widely recognized in the literature. As Shalev et al. noted [37], the concurrence of depression and PTSD is up to 56%. The causal relationship between the two is unclear since each can be a risk factor for the other [38]. Neumeister [39] reported that PTSD appears to be "an umbrella diagnosis for a broad spectrum of symptoms ranging from chronic anxiety and panic disorder to emotional numbing and depression."

These diagnostic classifications did not include a subset of people who expressed stress-related or mood-related distress at a level below the diagnostic threshold. Since such findings are not formally reported, it is difficult to know whether the observed rates are common in other populations. Perhaps this is what is picked up by the ASS concept and may motivate some people to join support groups for long-term survivors.

Turning now to positive effects, participants found that ACT UP membership in 1987–1992 dramatically contributed to positive growth, which they still experience 25 years later. The vast majority reported an enhanced sense of self, confidence, belief in change, and their ability to influence

Table 6: Major categories of response to the question, "Do you think being in ACT UP changed your sense of self, who you are as a person?"

| Agency |
|---|
| I found my sense of agency in ACT UP. I found out who I was. I became who I could be because of ACT UP. It transformed me. I developed human skills and brain skills. It made me who I am. |
| Being in ACT UP changed the epidemic from something that was happening TO me, to something I could do about it. It was a really formative moment in my world framework. People I connected with inspired me to think anything is possible. I have political agency, can fight for beliefs. I was proud of being part of this group. |
| ACT UP was the most important thing I've ever done in my life. Those years were the least selfish, the most community-motivated. I also learned you never accept authority at the cost of discounting your own experience. It gave me a sense of purpose, of community, of hope - that something could be done. |
| After ACT UP, I felt able to change things |
| ACT UP made me step out of myself. I was shy and ACT UP gave me a voice. I felt I could make a change. I spoke from my heart, I did TV. I hadn't known I could organize and lead. |
| Empowerment |
| It enhanced my sense of self-worth. I feel compelled to do something when I see something wrong. I feel responsible. I feel I need to improve the lot of others |
| I found my voice. I learned to speak up for myself and what was right. For the first time I learned to think critically. It was a huge boost to my self-esteem. I felt really proud of what I was doing. Finding my voice, finding I had something to give and effect change and I had a part in doing something that changed the world. |
| It changed my feelings about myself. It made me more confident, more outgoing. I was really fearless back then in my 20's. Even if I never find it, I keep searching for the sense of purpose I had in ACT UP. |
| The experience changed my outlook, my sense of what I could accomplish, my view of the world, view of myself. It taught me I could do things I had no idea I could do. It taught me there were other people like me: smart, spiky, angry, fiercely committed. We had an effect. |
| It gave me confidence both socially and in my ability to motivate people. It felt empowering, being involved in something meaningful. I felt empowered we were going to save our friends' lives, inspired by the combination of street smarts and intelligence. |
| Personal growth |
| Being a member of a group working at a high level, knowing I could operate at that level. Discovering in myself powers I didn't know I had. |
| It made me much more confident and capable. I ended up more willing to try new things and try different directions. The skills I learned at ACT UP stayed with me. I believe in gay community and the importance of gay community, a bedrock belief that being gay matters, and I learned that at ACT UP. |
| It brought meaning to my life. It helped define, was part of my identity. I was proud to be part of ACT UP. It gave me a sense of purposefulness, feeling of use, self-worth. Now I can speak in front of a group of people and have the courage to say what I think. |
| It made me feel a better person, more serious, smarter, stronger. |
| Helped me define myself. I learned to respect that I have a voice, have my opinions, can work with others. Before, I didn't think people listened to me. I no longer felt like a contagious person. It changed my thinking about myself. |

events (agency). For some, there is also a sense of lingering, diffuse distress, not fully captured either by diagnoses of depression or PTSD: a sense of loss and echoes of distressing experiences. Loss refers not only to the deaths of friends and fellow ACT UP members, but also to loss of the spirit, the focus, and the support of ACT UP membership in its peak years. Respondents also spoke of loss of a sense of purpose, of relevance, of friendships and connection, the excitement and stimulation, the sense of community after the ACT UP years.

The concept of unit cohesion contributes to our understanding of the ability of ACT UP members to persevere in the face of unremitting AIDS losses, public and government indifference or outright hostility, and the intense confrontations including arrests that demonstrations entailed. In part, this cohesion derived from the organization within ACT UP, including committees and affinity groups that worked long hours together to plan and prepare for demonstrations and protests. In addition, standing Monday evening meetings, attended by all members, fostered a special identity and sense of belonging. Despite the grief, fear, anxiety and anger of the ACT UP years, the general sense of the 125 respondents is that these years were the highlight of their lives, the most important and influential experience they have had. Our findings suggest that group support is effective in achieving and maintaining well-being, with current implications for service interventions for long-term survivors of the epidemic generally, not only former ACT UP members.

More generally, activism in many contexts has been found to promote positive, increased self-esteem and well-being, as discussed by Klar and Kasser [3]. They suggest potential mediators such as the utilization of problem-focused coping [12] or heightened consistency between values and actions.

## 5. Study Strengths and Limitations

To our knowledge, this is the only study exploring the long-term impact of AIDS activism; its sample size and robust data collection make it a valuable contribution to the literature. Limitations include nonrandom sampling, although the demographics of our sample are roughly equivalent to those noted in a 1989 survey of 413 ACT UP/NY members conducted by Elbaz [40] in which 92% were white and 20% were women. Study participants may not represent the full spectrum of distress and disability since those who are doing better may be more likely to volunteer.

In conclusion, AIDS activists recalled their ACT UP years as "the best of times, the worst of times." Dramatic personal growth was often accompanied by lingering sadness, unresolved grief, and, for some, loss of perceived life purpose. However, the community bonds within ACT UP played a central and protective role, enabling most members to move forward and lead productive lives. As one man remembered, "ACT UP was exciting, joyous, a strange intersection of elation at the time, providing a scaffolding over this chasm of grief and sorrow."

## Appendix

Response options to the question, "In what ways was ACT UP a positive experience?"

(1) Sense of empowerment vis-à-vis AIDS
(2) New or stronger social ties (with others in ACT UP)
(3) Personal recognition, leadership role (limelight)
(4) Sense of collective identity, morale
(5) Fighting for one's life (or one's community's survival)
(6) Connecting with the gay community/confirming identity
(7) Sexual networking
(8) Emotional/psychological support
(9) Success in developing trials and treatments
(10) Stimulating/educational about HIV treatments

Response options to the question, "Since leaving ACT UP, do you miss anything?"

(1) Feelings of irrelevance
(2) Loss of direction
(3) Loss of a cause, or doing something that matters
(4) Loss of ACT UP limelight, early fame
(5) Loss of network
(6) Loneliness

## Conflicts of Interest

The authors declare that they have no conflicts of interest.

## Acknowledgments

This study was funded by amfAR, The Foundation for AIDS Research and Broadway Cares/Equity Fights AIDS. The authors would like to thank the participants for their time and willingness to share their experiences and memories of ACT UP years and also members of the Advisory Board. They also thank Erin Timperlake, Jennifer Scodes, and Madeline Finkel for their assistance with statistical work and tables.

## References

[1] D. Crimp and A. Rolston, *AIDS DemoGRAPHICS*, Bay Press, Seattle, Wash, USA, 1990.

[2] P. Reilly, *How to Survive a Plague*, Knopf, New York, NY, USA, 2016.

[3] M. Klar and T. Kasser, "Some benefits of being an activist: measuring activism and its role in psychological well-being," *Political Psychology*, vol. 30, no. 5, pp. 755–777, 2009.

[4] Y. Neria, L. DiGrande, and B. G. Adams, "Posttraumatic stress disorder following the September 11, 2001, terrorist attacks: a review of the literature among highly exposed populations," *American Psychologist*, vol. 66, no. 6, pp. 429–446, 2011.

[5] American Psychiatric Association, *Diagnostic and Statistical Manual of Mental Disorders (DSM-IV)*, American Psychiatric Publishing, Washington, D.C, USA, 1994.

[6] J. J. Vasterling, M. Aslan, S. P. Proctor et al., "Longitudinal examination of posttraumatic stress disorder as a long-term outcome of Iraq war deployment," *American Journal of Epidemiology*, vol. 184, no. 11, pp. 796–805, 2016.

[7] D.-M. Bichescu, M. Schauer, E. Saleptsi, A. Neculau, T. Elbert, and F. Neuner, "Long-term consequences of traumatic experiences: an assessment of former political detainees in Romania," *Clinical Practice and Epidemiology in Mental Health*, vol. 1, article 17, 2005.

[8] H. Tessems and T. Anderson, "Long-term survivors: kicking AIDS survivor syndrome," in *Proceedings of the 21st International AIDS Conference*, July 2016.

[9] T. Anderson, "What is AIDS Survivor Syndrome and why do you need to know?" 2017, https://letskickass.org.

[10] J. G. Rabkin, R. Remien, L. Katoff, and J. B. W. Williams, "Resilience in adversity among long term survivors of AIDS," *General Hospital Psychiatry*, vol. 44, no. 2, pp. 162–167, 1993.

[11] J. G. Rabkin, R. Remien, L. Katoff, and J. B. W. Williams, "Suicidality in AIDS long-term survivors: what is the evidence?" *AIDS Care*, vol. 5, no. 4, pp. 401–411, 1993.

[12] R. H. Remien, J. G. Rabkin, and J. B. W. Williams, "Coping strategies and health beliefs of aids longterm survivors," *Psychology & Health*, vol. 6, no. 4, pp. 335–345, 1992.

[13] S. Jue, "Psychosocial issues of AIDS long-term survivors," *Families in Society*, vol. 75, no. 6, p. 324, 1994.

[14] G. A. Bonanno and A. D. Mancini, "Beyond resilience and PTSD: Mapping the heterogeneity of responses to potential trauma," *Psychological Trauma: Theory, Research, Practice, and Policy*, vol. 4, no. 1, pp. 74–83, 2012.

[15] J. Du Preez, J. Sundin, S. Wessely, and N. T. Fear, "Unit cohesion and mental health in the UK armed forces," *Occupational Medicine*, vol. 62, no. 1, pp. 47–53, 2012.

[16] S. Junger, *Tribe: On Homecoming and Belonging*, Hachette, New York, NY, USA, 2016.

[17] L. M. Mcandrew, S. Markowitz, S.-E. Lu, A. Borders, D. Rothman, and K. S. Quigley, "Resilience during war: better unit cohesion and reductions in avoidant coping are associated with better mental health function after combat deployment," *Psychological Trauma: Theory, Research, Practice, and Policy*, vol. 9, no. 1, pp. 52–61, 2017.

[18] G. A. Bonanno, "Loss, trauma, and human resilience: have we underestimated the human capacity to thrive after extremely aversive events?" *American Psychologist*, vol. 59, no. 1, pp. 20–28, 2004.

[19] J. E. Milam, "Posttraumatic growth among HIV/AIDS patients," *Journal of Applied Social Psychology*, vol. 34, no. 11, pp. 2353–2376, 2004.

[20] M. E. Seligman and M. Csikszentmihalyi, "Positive psychology: an introduction," *American Psychologist*, vol. 55, no. 1, pp. 5–14, 2000.

[21] S. Folkman, "Stress, health, and coping: an overview," in *The Oxford Handbook of Stress, Health, and Coping*, S. Folkman, Ed., pp. 3–11, Oxford University Press, New York, NY, USA, 2011.

[22] J. Moskowitz, "Coping interventions and the regulation of positive affect," in *The Oxford Handbook of Stress, Health and Coping*, S. Folkman, Ed., pp. 407–427, Oxford University Press, New York, NY, USA, 2011.

[23] R. L. Spitzer, K. Kroenke, and J. B. W. Williams, "Validation and utility of a self-report version of PRIME-MD: the PHQ Primary Care Study," *Journal of the American Medical Association*, vol. 282, no. 18, pp. 1737–1744, 1999.

[24] U.S. Department of Veterans Affairs, "National Center for PTSD Using the PTSD Checklist for DSM-IV (PCL)," http://www.ptsd.va.gov.

[25] E. B. Blanchard, J. Jones-Alexander, T. C. Buckley, and C. A. Forneris, "Psychometric properties of the PTSD checklist (PCL)," *Behaviour Research and Therapy*, vol. 34, no. 8, pp. 669–673, 1996.

[26] K. J. Ruggiero, K. Del Ben, J. R. Scotti, and A. E. Rabalais, "Psychometric properties of the PTSD checklist—civilian version," *Journal of Traumatic Stress*, vol. 16, no. 5, pp. 495–502, 2003.

[27] T. Babor, J. Higgins-Biddle, J. Saunders, and M. Monteiro, *AUDT, The Alcohol Use Disorders Identification Test*, Bull World Health Organ, Geneva, Switzerland, 2nd edition, 2001.

[28] M. A. Chesney, T. B. Neilands, D. B. Chambers, J. M. Taylor, and S. Folkman, "A validity and reliability study of the coping self-efficacy scale," *British Journal of Health Psychology*, vol. 11, no. 3, pp. 421–437, 2006.

[29] M. F. Scheier, C. S. Carver, and M. W. Bridges, "Distinguishing optimism from neuroticism (and trait anxiety, self-mastery, and self-esteem): a reevaluation of the Life Orientation Test," *Journal of Personality and Social Psychology*, vol. 67, no. 6, pp. 1063–1078, 1994.

[30] D. W. Russell, "UCLA loneliness scale (version 3): reliability, validity, and factor structure," *Journal of Personality Assessment*, vol. 66, no. 1, pp. 20–40, 1996.

[31] C. Rimmerman, *ACT UP. Encyclopedia of AIDS*, R. A. Smith, Ed., Fitzroy Dearborn Publishers, Chicago, IL, USA, 1998.

[32] S. E. Taylor and J. D. Brown, "Illusion and well-being: a social psychological perspective on mental health," *Psychological Bulletin*, vol. 103, no. 2, pp. 193–210, 1988.

[33] M. Lopes, M. Olfson, J. Rabkin et al., "HIV status and psychiatric disorders: Results from the national epidemiologic study on alcohol and related conditions," *Journal of Clinical Psychiatry*, vol. 73, no. 3, pp. 384–391, 2011.

[34] D. L. Evans, D. S. Charney, L. Lewis et al., "Mood disorders in the medically ill: scientific review and recommendations," *Biological Psychiatry*, vol. 58, no. 3, pp. 175–189, 2005.

[35] M. Orlando, M. A. Burnam, R. Beckman et al., "Re-estimating the prevalence of psychiatric disorders in a nationally representative sample of persons receiving care for HIV: Results from the HIV cost and services utilization study," *International Journal of Methods in Psychiatric Research*, vol. 11, no. 2, pp. 75–82, 2002.

[36] R. C. Kessler, P. Berglund, O. Demler et al., "The epidemiology of major depressive disorder: results from the National Comorbidity Survey Replication (NCS-R)," *Journal of the American Medical Association*, vol. 289, no. 23, pp. 3095–3105, 2003.

[37] A. Y. Shalev, S. Freedman, T. Peri et al., "Prospective study of posttraumatic stress disorder and depression following trauma," *The American Journal of Psychiatry*, vol. 155, no. 5, pp. 630–637, 1998.

[38] M. L. O'Donnell, M. Creamer, and P. Pattison, "Posttraumatic stress disorder and depression following trauma: understanding comorbidity," *The American Journal of Psychiatry*, vol. 161, no. 8, pp. 1390–1396, 2004.

[39] A. Neumeister, "Deconstructing PTSD. NYU Physician," p. 7, Winter 2014-1015.

[40] G. Elbaz, "Beyond anger: the activist construction of the AIDS crisis," *Social Justice Research*, vol. 22, no. 4, pp. 43–76, 1995.

13

# Messaging Circumstances and Economic Pressures as Influences on Linkage to Medical Male Circumcision following Community-Based HIV Testing for Men in Rural Southwest Uganda

**Hannah N. Gilbert,[1] Monique A. Wyatt,[1,2] Stephen Asiimwe,[3] Bosco Turyamureeba,[3] Elioda Tumwesigye,[3] Heidi Van Rooyen,[4,5] Ruanne V. Barnabas,[6] Connie L. Celum,[6] and Norma C. Ware[1,7]**

[1] *Department of Global Health and Social Medicine, Harvard Medical School, Boston, MA, USA*
[2] *Harvard Global, Cambridge, MA, USA*
[3] *Integrated Community Based Initiatives, Kabwohe, Uganda*
[4] *Human Sciences Research Council, Durban, South Africa*
[5] *School of Clinical Medicine, Faculty of Health Sciences, University of the Witwatersrand, Johannesburg, South Africa*
[6] *Department of Global Health, School of Medicine and School of Public Health, University of Washington, Seattle, WA, USA*
[7] *Division of Global Health Equity, Department of Medicine, Brigham and Women's Hospital, Boston, MA, USA*

Correspondence should be addressed to Hannah N. Gilbert; hannah-gilbert@hms.harvard.edu

Academic Editor: Robert R. Redfield

Voluntary medical male circumcision (MMC) reduces risk of HIV infection, but uptake remains suboptimal among certain age groups and locations in sub-Saharan Africa. We analysed qualitative data as part of the Linkages Study, a randomized controlled trial to evaluate community-based HIV testing and follow-up as interventions promoting linkage to HIV treatment and prevention in Uganda and South Africa. Fifty-two HIV-negative uncircumcised men participated in the qualitative study. They participated in semistructured individual interviews exploring (a) home HTC experience; (b) responses to test results; (c) efforts to access circumcision services; (d) outcomes of efforts; (e) experiences of follow-up support; and (f) local HIV education and support. Interviews were audio-recorded, translated, transcribed, and summarized into "linkage summaries." Summaries were analysed inductively to identify the following three thematic experiences shaping men's circumcision choices: (1) intense relief upon receipt of an unanticipated seronegative diagnosis, (2) the role of peer support in overcoming fear, and (3) anticipation of missed economic productivity. Increased attention to the timing of demand creation activities, to who delivers information about the HIV prevention benefits of MMC, and to the importance of missed income during recovery as a barrier to uptake promises to strengthen and sharpen future MMC demand creation strategies.

## 1. Introduction

Linkage to antiretroviral treatment and effective prevention following widespread testing promises to reduce HIV incidence in Africa. A number of strategies to increase linkage are being evaluated, including integration and "streamlining" of services, point of care CD4 and viral load testing, economic incentives, and community-based testing with counselling and follow-up support [1–6]. Active linking to prevention services, such as voluntary medical male circumcision (MMC) is an important component of this comprehensive approach.

The efficacy of voluntary medical male circumcision (MMC) in reducing the risk of HIV infection has been demonstrated in three randomized controlled clinical trials (RCTs) in Africa. These RCTs revealed a nearly 60% reduction in female-to-male HIV transmission [7–9]. On the basis of this evidence, the World Health Organization and the Joint United Nations Program on HIV/AIDS (WHO/UNAIDS) recommended MMC as an effective component of combination prevention strategies in key countries with generalized heterosexual epidemics exhibiting both high rates of HIV and low rates of male circumcision [10].

Despite evidence of effectiveness, uptake of MMC has been suboptimal among African men in certain locations and age groups. According to 2015 figures, Uganda achieved 64% progress towards the 80% coverage target set by the WHO in 2011. The WHO has established a new 2020 Fast Track target of 90% MMC coverage. As funding gaps for MMC have increased across sub-Saharan Africa, the WHO has called for new and innovative approaches to make MMC programs more efficient [11]. MMC research priorities are increasingly oriented towards implementation, with a specific focus on how to generate interest and demand for the procedure [12–14]. Studies of MMC implementation programs have identified barriers associated with circumcision uptake; new analyses target incentives for men to pursue circumcision despite the obstacles they face [15].

The Linkages Study was a randomized controlled trial assessing the effectiveness of community-based HIV testing and counselling with follow-up support in linking HIV-positive individuals to HIV care and HIV-negative uncircumcised men to MMC. The trial was carried out in rural KwaZulu-Natal, South Africa, and in Kabwohe, Sheema District, in rural southwest Uganda. Based upon qualitative data collected as part of the Linkages Study, this paper describes key experiences impacting uncircumcised Ugandan men's interest in and ability to pursue MMC following a negative HIV test result. From these experiences, we draw inferences aimed at informing creation of demand for MMC services and strengthening strategies to promote linkage to HIV prevention in rural African settings.

## 2. Methods

*2.1. The Linkages Study.* Linkages Study participants received community-based HIV testing and counselling at home or via a mobile van. Individuals testing positive and not already prescribed antiretroviral therapy (ART) were randomized to one of two follow-up support interventions, or a control condition. Uncircumcised men testing negative were randomized to follow-up support interventions intended to stimulate demand for MMC: (1) home visits from lay counsellors at 1 and 3 months, (2) or text message reminders. The control condition was promotion of MMC at the testing visit. Men received text messages three weeks after testing, and follow-up calls at one month. Those reporting not having been circumcised received a second text message 6-7 weeks after testing, and a second follow-up call.

Uptake of circumcision in the Linkages Study was 42% (52/123) (RR = 2.37, 95% CI: 1.55, 3.63) for men receiving lay counsellor follow-up support, compared to 18% (23/129) for controls and 33% (52/156) for men receiving follow-up text messages compared to controls (RR = 1.87, 95% CI: 1.21, 2.88).

Table 1: Sampling of study participants.

| Time from enrollment to interview (in months) | |
|---|---|
| 1–3 | 11 (21.2%) |
| 7–12 | 15 (28.8%) |
| >12 | 26 (50%) |

Additional information on intervention results may be found elsewhere [5].

*2.2. Sampling and Recruitment for the Qualitative Research.* A purposeful sampling approach aims to maximize information-rich cases and capture variation in order to provide in-depth information about the topic under study [16]. To maximize variation, the qualitative study adopted a purposeful sampling approach that aimed to identify participants at different points across the trial follow-up period, targeting experiences of home HTC and follow-up support in linkage to HIV treatment, care, and MMC prevention services.

Potential participants were sampled at 1–3 months, 8–12 months, or >12 months following enrolment in the Linkages Study to ensure representation of perspectives from participants in both the first months and the later months of follow-up (see Table 1). The qualitative sample included two subgroups: 47 individuals testing HIV-positive and assigned to follow-up support or control for linkage to HIV treatment and care and 52 uncircumcised men testing negative and assigned to follow-up or control for linkage to MMC. This analysis draws exclusively on data from the subgroup of 52 uncircumcised Ugandan men.

Linkages experiences of the HIV-positive, treatment group in Uganda have been described by Ware and authors [17]. Qualitative and quantitative Linkages Study results from South Africa have been published elsewhere [18–20].

*2.3. Data Collection.* Data collection for the qualitative study included individual, semistructured interviews. These interviews relied on an interview guide consisting of open-ended questions that explored the following topics: (a) home HTC experience; (b) responses to test results; (c) plans to access HIV care or MMC prevention services; (d) outcomes of plans; (e) experiences of follow-up support; and (f) HIV education and support in local communities. Ugandan research assistants (RAs) trained in qualitative methods conducted the interviews in private settings, in the local language. Interviews took place from December 2013 through March 2015. They lasted 45–60 minutes and were audio-recorded. This analysis draws on interviews with 52 men who were seronegative and uncircumcised at the time of enrolment; it includes the experiences of men who ultimately went on to be circumcised and those who did not.

*2.4. Data Quality.* Audio-recordings were transcribed in English by the RAs. Transcripts were reviewed for quality as they were completed and used to provide continuous feedback on interview content and technique.

*2.5. Data Analysis.* Data analysis relied on an inductive, content analytic approach to develop thematic concepts [21]. Analysis began with data reduction. To reduce the data, two members of the research team read through the interview transcripts to create a "linkage summary" for each interviewee. These summaries recapitulated the interviewee's HIV testing and linkage experiences as they described them to highlight the individual trajectories involved and served in lieu of coding as a data reduction technique [16]. Summaries were subjected to thematic analysis. The documents were reviewed for repeated content to identify emergent patterns in interviewees' testing and linkage experiences. Employing an iterative process, these patterns were formulated as summary statements. The statements summarize themes resulting from the analysis, to represent key aspects of interviewees' experiences of HIV testing and perspectives on male circumcision, in terms of their impact upon subsequent linkage to services. As such, they constitute the key findings of the analysis. Summary statements appear as 1–3 in Results. Each is elaborated using descriptive content from the interviews and illustrated through quotes from interviewees.

*2.6. Ethical Statement.* The qualitative study was reviewed by the Committee on Human Studies at Harvard Medical School, the Human Subjects Division of the University of Washington, and the Uganda National Council for Science and Technology. Participants provided consent for the qualitative interviews as part of the Linkages Study consent process. Consent was reconfirmed verbally for the qualitative study.

## 3. Results

*3.1. Characteristics of Participants.* Median age of men taking part in the qualitative study was 26.5 (IQR 22.75–32.25) at Linkages Study enrolment. Slightly more than half (54%) were married. Forty percent ($N = 21$) had been randomized to counsellor follow-up for linkage to MMC services following home HIV testing; 54% were assigned to follow-up through text messages. Half were interviewed 12 months or more into follow-up. At exit, 42% ($N = 22$) of men taking part in the qualitative study had been circumcised.

*3.2. Qualitative Results.* The qualitative analysis revealed three themes in these men's experiences of linking (or not linking) to circumcision services, as described below.

*3.2.1. Relief at Unexpectedly Receiving a Negative HIV Test Result Created Strong Motivation to Link.* Many men reported entering the home HIV testing encounter convinced they would receive a seropositive diagnosis. Some believed they were HIV-positive because HIV was perceived as a ubiquitous, ever-present threat. Others felt at risk because they had engaged in unprotected sex with multiple partners, or with a partner presumed to be HIV-positive. Many offered persistent STI infections as presumed "proof" of seropositivity, with one many describing themselves as "a daily customer of gonorrhoea."

When provided with a negative test result, these men were shocked and elated. The experience was described as a "second chance" at life—*"like I had gone to heaven... received a new life,"* in the words of one. The intense relief associated with this "second chance" translated into a determination to preserve health for the future. One man described his experience this way.

> *I felt very happy and loved my life again. I loved my life and made good plans... you know, when you don't expect to be negative and you find you are negative you have all the reasons to love your life and make good plans. (Male, age 40)*

This surprise and delight instilled in participants a resolve to stay HIV-negative. Following the Linkages Study protocol, counsellors who delivered test results immediately followed up with messages about HIV prevention benefits of circumcision. With newfound determination to avert future infection, men were eager to take steps towards preserving their health. Circumcision presented an immediate and feasible means of enacting "good plans" to remain uninfected. The following quotes illustrate:

> *When the counsellor tested me and I found that I don't have HIV I became happy. When they convinced me that I should circumcise because the cover can keep viruses after having sex, [then] I decided to circumcise as one way of protecting myself against HIV. (Male, 38 years old)*

> *When he [counsellor] finished testing, he told me that I don't have HIV virus in my blood and I praised God. He told me that I have to make sure to protect myself against the HIV virus. Now that I know I am HIV-negative, I shouldn't do wrong things. At that time I told him that I want to circumcise. (Male, age 49)*

*3.2.2. Hearing Circumcision Success Stories from Peers Helps Overcome Fear of the Procedure.* Fear emerged as a barrier to circumcision in this study. Some men feared physical pain—what one participant called *"the pain inflicted by the circumcision knife."* Expected invasiveness of the surgery was particularly concerning for others.

> *Me, I thought they would cut me deeply... Like cutting the whole penis. I thought that they were going to cut like a part and throw it away. (Male, age 24)*

The emotional and marital impact of refraining from sexual intercourse during convalescence was a circumcision-related fear for many. Still others worried that the procedure might permanently compromise their sexual health.

> *I am worried that if I circumcise I will be sexually weak... because they will cut some parts of my manhood which God created with me [sic]. And I think that will make me sexually weak in the future. (Male, age 19)*

Some men were able to overcome their fears and follow through on their resolve to circumcise. Support from peers who had successfully completed the procedure emerged as the lynchpin enabling men to act upon their initial receptivity to circumcision. Peer support included reminders, transport, and accompaniment to the clinic. The most widely acknowledged form of support, however, was positive reports from circumcised peers, whose experiences counteracted circumcision fears. One young man described his brother's influence.

> *Since he was already circumcised, he told me that circumcision prevents you from many diseases, especially STDs. He also told me that the pain is not much and even said he would volunteer to take me to the Health Centre. (Male, age 24)*

Another man explained that he often bathes in the river with his friends, where the topic of circumcision is frequently raised.

> *We do the same work so sometimes, we may be discussing and such topics come [up], and they tell me [about circumcision]. We even bathe from the same river here in the village, so I see them... They like it [circumcision] and they encourage me to do it...like telling me to go and circumcise and telling me their experiences. (Male, age 49)*

The effectiveness of these success stories as a circumcision driver was dependent upon identifying relevant "peers." Peers were local friends, neighbours, or family members, who, importantly, were similar in age.

> *Our people here... you see if one is not of your age, he can't listen to you. The person you can tell is someone of your age. Someone who is in the same age bracket as you. But for people who are older, at times, they don't even need your advice. For them, they don't want that. (Male, age 30)*

*3.2.3. Anticipation of Missed Economic Productivity Was an Insurmountable Barrier to Linkage for Many Men.* Many men who emerged from the testing encounter keen to pursue circumcision explained that they were unable to follow through because they anticipated a healing period that could last weeks. The economic consequences of this period of missed work were particularly significant for men who performed agricultural or day labour for income. They explained that their work consisted of planting, cutting, and carrying grasses or transporting bananas on bicycles; they relied entirely upon their physical strength for survival. The unrelenting schedule of agricultural labour afforded no "down time" to recover, as the following examples illustrate:

> *I dig; okay, the most important thing is digging. I use my hands, so because I have to work to eat, you find that I have no time to get circumcised. (Male, age 22)*

> *I do manual work with my hands, which means if I don't work I will not be having what to eat. That's what I fear... but I like circumcision. (Male, age 39)*

The significance of missed productivity was compounded by men's positions as family providers. Men with multiple dependents faced a formidable set of daily responsibilities that forced them to weigh the long-term health benefit of increased HIV protection against the immediate food and economic needs of their families. In such a calculus, circumcision was simply not an option.

> *I realized that if I go and circumcise and sit home without working, my family will starve. I will not be having money since I will not be working. If I spend time at home not working during the recovery period, my family cannot survive, because they will need home items yet I will not be having money. (Male, age 27)*

The few men who overcame this economic barrier had more flexibility in their social and economic lives. These men held jobs outside of the agricultural sector and could shift their workload to accommodate recovery time. For example, a policeman scheduled his circumcision between demanding "special assignments" when he could do light deskwork.

> *As I was not doing a lot of work, I would wake up, bathe, put on my uniform, go and sit at the bank where I was working as a security personnel and work. (Male, age 38)*

These men were also often unmarried and thus not financially responsible for a family. Their expenses were straightforward and predictable, allowing them to calculate precisely how much money would be required to support themselves during their convalescence

> *Okay, I had prepared in advance because I knew that I was going to get circumcised. They had said you can get a problem and spend days without working. Because of that, I kept some money aside to use while waiting to recover. (Male, age 25)*

## 4. Discussion

Many men in this study entered the home testing encounter expecting a positive diagnosis; the unanticipated news that they were HIV-negative created a strong motivation to preserve health. Some men then simply went on to be circumcised. For others, initial motivation was stymied by fears about the procedure. Circumcision success stories, a set of informal communications in which circumcised men described positive experiences of the procedure, helped some men overcome their fear. Others, while motivated to circumcise, were unable to act because of the economic challenges posed by missed work. These men were unable to reconcile the long-term health benefits of circumcision with the short-term imperatives of providing for their families in an economy based on agricultural labour. These men saw missed productivity during the MMC recovery period as an insurmountable barrier.

A number of lessons may be drawn from these findings to inform demand creation for MMC. One such lesson has to do with the timing of demand creation activities. For men participating in this study, relief and joy at learning their HIV test result was negative quickly evolved into new determination to remain free of HIV. We propose this new determination represented a moment of particular receptivity to receipt of education and counselling about the HIV prevention benefits of circumcision, suggesting both that the timing of demand creation interventions makes a difference and that optimal timing coincides with "moments" when men may be predisposed to hearing and acting on HIV prevention information. One such moment, this study teaches us, is immediately after receiving a negative HIV test result.

A second lesson for MMC demand creation that may be drawn from these study results speaks to the question of who should deliver information about the prevention benefits of circumcision. Our study and others [22, 23] suggest that peers who have been through the procedure are in particularly strong positions to influence the thinking of age-similar uncircumcised men. Related research points to other categories of persons whose opinions and advice men may hold in especially high regard, such as mothers [24], wives, and other female sexual partners [25–27], and cultural authorities, for example, religious leaders [28]. MMC demand creation messages may be more effective when delivered by important others in men's lives.

Finally, concern over gaps in income associated with recovery from the circumcision procedure highlights the importance of missed work as a barrier to uptake in low resource settings. Elsewhere, unemployed men and informal wage earners have expressed concern about missed work [29]. Our data shows that men with families and agricultural day labourers who rely on their physical strength to generate income are particularly vulnerable to this barrier. The significance of concern over income gaps helps to explain the effectiveness of financial compensation as a demand creation tool [30–32]. Qualitative research investigating how compensation influenced the decision to be circumcised for a Kenyan cohort indicates it (at least partially) offsets lost income as a circumcision barrier, rather than appealing to a motive for financial gain [33]. Our findings corroborate these results.

Qualitative studies have identified barriers and facilitators of MMC uptake across sub-Saharan Africa, including anticipated pain and medical complications [25, 34, 35] cost [36, 37], and perceptions of circumcision's effects on male sexuality [20, 38–42]. Perceived association between circumcision and increased sexual capacity was a concern for some men [40, 41, 43] as was age [34, 44]. These perceptions of MMC also appeared in our data. However, they were overshadowed by predominant themes of expectation of seropositivity and relief at testing, peer support as a mechanism to overcome fear, and concern over income gaps resulting from time away from work.

This study has the following limitations. First, while we believe the insights represented here will be relevant in other settings, as a qualitative study, the results are not formally generalizable. Second, members of support networks were not interviewed as part of the study, precluding an analysis of peer support as a linkage mechanism from the points of view of the peers themselves. Finally, these qualitative data were examined using an inductive, thematic analysis approach. A strength of this approach is that it represents salient aspects of linkage experiences from the points of view of the study participants. A potential disadvantage, in this instance, is that its results largely targeted factors outside the Linkages Study intervention. This limited our ability to evaluate intervention components.

## 5. Conclusions

In addition to the content of MMC demand creation interventions, attention to their circumstances—the "when" and "who" of intervention delivery—may improve effectiveness. The need to sustain income during recovery from circumcision for many men living in settings of economic scarcity must be addressed in order for circumcision targets to be met.

## Conflicts of Interest

The authors declare that they have no conflicts of interest.

## Authors' Contributions

Jacqueline Karuhanga, Justine Abenaitwe, Robert Baijuka, and John Bosco Tumuhairwe collected the interview data. Melanie Tam and Emily E. Pisarski coordinated data collection and provided supervision to the Ugandan research assistants. Meighan Krows, Justin Brantley, and Torin Schaafsma helped coordinate the qualitative study and the Linkages Study intervention trial.

## Acknowledgments

The authors extend their thanks to the men who participated in the qualitative interviews for their essential contributions. Financial support for the research was provided by a grant from the National Institute of Allergy and Infectious Disease (NIAID) of the US National Institutes of Health (NIH; RC4 AI092552).

## References

[1] S. Rosen, M. Maskew, and MP. Fox, "Correction: initiating antiretroviral therapy for HIV at a patient's first clinic visit: the RapIT randomized controlled trial," *PLOS Medicine*, vol. 13, no. 6, 2016.

[2] S. Rosen, M. Maskew, M. P. Fox et al., "Initiating Antiretroviral Therapy for HIV at a Patient's First Clinic Visit: The RapIT Randomized Controlled Trial," *PLoS Medicine*, vol. 13, no. 5, Article ID e1002015, 2016.

[3] A. Van Rie, M. R. Patel, M. Nana et al., "Integration and task shifting for TB/HIV care and treatment in highly resource-scarce settings: one size may not fit all," *Journal of Acquired Immune Deficiency Syndromes*, vol. 65, no. 3, pp. e110–e117, 2014.

[4] M. Faal, N. Naidoo, D. K. Glencross, W. D. F. Venter, and R. Osih, "Providing immediate CD4 count results at HIV testing improves ART initiation," *Journal of Acquired Immune Deficiency Syndromes*, vol. 58, no. 3, pp. e54–e59, 2011.

[5] R. V. Barnabas, H. van Rooyen, E. Tumwesigye et al., "Uptake of antiretroviral therapy and male circumcision after community-based HIV testing and strategies for linkage to care versus standard clinic referral: A multisite, open-label, randomised controlled trial in South Africa and Uganda," *The Lancet HIV*, vol. 3, no. 5, pp. e212–e220, 2016.

[6] S. Asiimwe, J. M. Ross, A. Arinaitwe et al., "Expanding HIV testing and linkage to care in southwestern Uganda with community health extension workers," *Journal of the International AIDS Society*, vol. 20, Article ID 21633, 2017.

[7] B. Auvert, D. Taljaard, E. Lagarde, J. Sobngwi-Tambekou, R. Sitta, and A. Puren, "Randomized, controlled intervention trial of male circumcision for reduction of HIV infection risk: the ANRS 1265 trial," *PLoS Medicine*, vol. 2, no. 11, article e298, 2005.

[8] R. C. Bailey, S. Moses, C. B. Parker et al., "Male circumcision for HIV prevention in young men in Kisumu, Kenya: a randomised controlled trial," *The Lancet*, vol. 369, no. 9562, pp. 643–656, 2007.

[9] R. H. Gray, G. Kigozi, D. Serwadda et al., "Male circumcision for HIV prevention in men in Rakai, Uganda: a randomised trial," *The Lancet*, vol. 369, no. 9562, pp. 657–666, 2007.

[10] World Health Organization and UNAIDS, *New data on male circumcision and HIV prevention: Policy and programme implications*, WHO/ UNAIDS technical consultation on male circumcision and HIV prevention: Research implications for policy and programming, Montreaux, Switzerland.

[11] World Health Organization, *Voluntary medical male circumcision for HIV prevention in 14 priority countries in East and Southern Africa*, WHO Progress Brief, Geneva, Switzerland, 2016.

[12] L. W. Chang, D. Serwadda, T. C. Quinn, M. J. Wawer, R. H. Gray, and S. J. Reynolds, "Combination implementation for HIV prevention: Moving from clinical trial evidence to population-level effects," *The Lancet Infectious Diseases*, vol. 13, no. 1, pp. 65–76, 2013.

[13] M. Katisi and M. Daniel, "Safe male circumcision in Botswana: Tension between traditional practices and biomedical marketing," *Global Public Health*, vol. 10, no. 5-6, pp. 739–756, 2015.

[14] S. K. Sgaier, J. B. Reed, A. Thomas, and E. Njeuhmeli, "Achieving the HIV Prevention Impact of Voluntary Medical Male Circumcision: Lessons and Challenges for Managing Programs," *PLoS Medicine*, vol. 11, no. 5, Article ID e1001641, 2014.

[15] K. E. Wirth, B.-W. Semo, C. Ntsuape et al., "Triggering the decision to undergo medical male circumcision: A qualitative study of adult men in Botswana," *AIDS Care Psychological and Socio-medical Aspects of AIDS/HIV*, vol. 28, no. 8, pp. 1007–1012, 2016.

[16] M. Q. Patton, *Qualititative Research and Evaluations Methods*, Thousand Oaks: Sage Publications, 2002.

[17] N. C. Ware, M. A. Wyatt, S. Asiimwe et al., "How home HIV testing and counselling with follow-up support achieves high testing coverage and linkage to treatment and prevention: A qualitative analysis from Uganda," *Journal of the International AIDS Society*, vol. 19, no. 1, Article ID 20929, 2016.

[18] H. van Rooyen, R. V. Barnabas, J. M. Baeten et al., "High HIV testing uptake and linkage to care in a novel program of home-based HIV counseling and testing with facilitated referral in KwaZulu-Natal, South Africa," *Journal of Acquired Immune Deficiency Syndromes*, vol. 64, no. 1, pp. e1–e8, 2013.

[19] L. C. Knight, H. Van Rooyen, H. Humphries, R. V. Barnabas, and C. Celum, "Empowering patients to link to care and treatment: Qualitative findings about the role of a home-based HIV counselling, testing and linkage intervention in South Africa," *AIDS Care Psychological and Socio-medical Aspects of AIDS/HIV*, vol. 27, no. 9, pp. 1162–1167, 2015.

[20] H. Humphries, H. van Rooyen, L. Knight, R. Barnabas, and C. Celum, "'If you are circumcised, you are the best': understandings and perceptions of voluntary medical male circumcision among men from KwaZulu-Natal, South Africa," *Culture, Health and Sexuality*, vol. 17, no. 7, pp. 920–931, 2015.

[21] H. F. Hsieh and S. E. Shannon, "Three approaches to qualitative content analysis," *Qualitative Health Research*, vol. 15, no. 9, pp. 1277–1288, 2005.

[22] L. Muhamadi, M. Ibrahim, F. Wabwire-Mangen, S. Peterson, and S. J. Reynolds, "Perceived medical benefit, peer/partner influence and safety and cost to access the service: Client motivators for voluntary seeking of medical male circumcision in Iganga District Eastern Uganda, a qualitative study," *Pan African Medical Journal*, vol. 15, article no. 117, 2013.

[23] J. E. Price, L. Phiri, D. Mulenga et al., "Behavior change pathways to voluntary medical male circumcision: Narrative interviews with circumcision clients in Zambia," *PLoS ONE*, vol. 9, no. 11, Article ID e111602, 2014.

[24] H. Osaki, G. Mshana, M. Wambura et al., ""If You Are Not Circumcised, i Cannot Say Yes": The role of women in promoting the uptake of voluntary medical male circumcision in Tanzania," *PLoS ONE*, vol. 10, no. 9, Article ID e0139009, 2015.

[25] N. Westercamp and R. C. Bailey, "Acceptability of male circumcision for prevention of HIV/AIDS in sub-Saharan Africa: A review," *AIDS and Behavior*, vol. 11, no. 3, pp. 341–355, 2007.

[26] A. Obure, E. O. Nyambedha, and B. O. Oindo, "Interpersonal influences in the scale-up of male circumcision services in a traditionally non-circumcising community in rural western Kenya," *Global Journal of Community Psychology Practice*, vol. 1, no. 3, pp. 1–11, 2011.

[27] E. H. Layer, S. W. Beckham, R. B. Momburi, M. Peter, E. Laizer, and C. E. Kennedy, "'He is proud of my courage to ask him to be circumcised': experiences of female partners of male circumcision clients in Iringa region, Tanzania," *Culture, Health and Sexuality*, vol. 16, no. 3, pp. 258–272, 2014.

[28] J. A. Downs, A. H. Mwakisole, A. B. Chandika et al., "Educating religious leaders to promote uptake of male circumcision in Tanzania: a cluster randomised trial," *The Lancet*, vol. 389, no. 10074, pp. 1124–1132, 2017.

[29] E. Odoyo-June, K. Agot, J. M. Grund et al., "Predictors of voluntary medical male circumcision prevalence among men aged 25-39 years in Nyanza region, Kenya: Results from the baseline survey of the TASCO study," *PLoS ONE*, vol. 12, no. 10, Article ID e0185872, 2017.

[30] H. Thirumurthy, S. H. Masters, S. Rao et al., "The effects of providing fixed compensation and lottery-based rewards on uptake of medical male circumcision in Kenya: A randomized trial," *Journal of Acquired Immune Deficiency Syndromes*, vol. 72, pp. S309–S315, 2016.

[31] N. Wilson, S. Frade, D. Rech, and W. Friedman, "Advertising for demand creation for voluntary medical male circumcision," *Journal of Acquired Immune Deficiency Syndromes*, vol. 72, pp. S293–S296, 2016.

[32] E. Marshall, R. Rain-Taljaard, M. Tsepe et al., "Obtaining a male circumcision prevalence rate of 80% among adults in a short time: An observational prospective intervention study in the Orange Farm township of South Africa," *Medicine*, vol. 96, no. 4, p. e5328, 2017.

[33] E. Evens, M. Lanham, C. Hart, M. Loolpapit, I. Oguma, and W. Obiero, "Identifying and addressing barriers to uptake of voluntary medical male circumcision in Nyanza, Kenya among men 18-35: A qualitative study," *PLoS ONE*, vol. 9, no. 6, Article ID e98221, 2014.

[34] K. Hatzold, W. Mavhu, P. Jasi et al., "Barriers and motivators to voluntary medical male circumcision uptake among different age groups of men in Zimbabwe: Results from a mixed methods study," *PLoS ONE*, vol. 9, no. 5, Article ID e85051, 2014.

[35] M. Sabone, M. Magowe, L. Busang, J. Moalosi, B. Binagwa, and J. Mwambona, "Impediments for the uptake of the botswana government's male circumcision initiative for HIV prevention," *The Scientific World Journal*, vol. 2013, Article ID 387508, 2013.

[36] J. Chinkhumba, S. Godlonton, and R. Thornton, "The demand for medical male circumcision," *American Economic Journal: Applied Economics*, vol. 6, no. 2, pp. 152–177, 2014.

[37] P. Lissouba, D. Taljaard, D. Rech et al., "Adult male circumcision as an intervention against HIV: an operational study of uptake in a South African community (ANRS 12126)," *BMC Infectious Diseases*, vol. 11, article 253, 2011.

[38] A. Herman-Roloff, N. Otieno, K. Agot, J. Ndinya-Achola, and R. C. Bailey, "Acceptability of medical male circumcision among uncircumcised men in Kenya one year after the launch of the national male circumcision program," *PLoS ONE*, vol. 6, no. 5, Article ID e19814, 2011.

[39] E. Lagarde, T. Dirk, A. Puren, R.-T. Reathe, and A. Bertran, "Acceptability of male circumcision as a tool for preventing HIV infection in a highly infected community in South Africa," *AIDS*, vol. 17, no. 1, pp. 89–95, 2003.

[40] K. Lundsby, T. Dræbel, and D. Wolf Meyrowitsch, "'It brought joy in my home as in the area of my wife.' How recently circumcised adult men ascribe value to and make sense of male circumcision," *Global Public Health*, vol. 7, no. 4, pp. 352–366, 2012.

[41] T. H. Riess, M. M. Achieng, S. Otieno, J. O. Ndinya-Achola, and R. C. Bailey, ""when I was circumcised I was taught certain things": Risk compensation and protective sexual behavior among circumcised men in Kisumu, Kenya," *PLoS ONE*, vol. 5, no. 8, Article ID e12366, 2010.

[42] R. Ssekubugu, E. Leontsini, M. J. Wawer et al., "Contextual barriers and motivators to adult male medical circumcision in Rakai, Uganda," *Qualitative Health Research*, vol. 23, no. 6, pp. 795–804, 2013.

[43] L. M. Albert, A. Akol, K. L'Engle et al., "Acceptability of male circumcision for prevention of HIV infection among men and women in Uganda," *AIDS Care Psychological and Socio-medical Aspects of AIDS/HIV*, vol. 23, no. 12, pp. 1578–1585, 2011.

[44] M. Plotkin, D. Castor, H. Mziray et al., ""Man, what took you so long?" Social and individual factors affecting adult attendance at voluntary medical male circumcision services in Tanzania," *Global Health Science and Practice*, vol. 1, no. 1, pp. 108–116, 2013.

14

# HIV-Stigma in Nigeria: Review of Research Studies, Policies, and Programmes


**Clifford O. Odimegwu,[1] Joshua O. Akinyemi,[1,2] and Olatunji O. Alabi[1,3]**

[1]*Demography and Population Studies Programme, Schools of Public Health and Social Sciences, University of the Witwatersrand, Johannesburg, South Africa*
[2]*Department of Epidemiology and Medical Statistics, Faculty of Public Health, College of Medicine, University of Ibadan, Ibadan, Nigeria*
[3]*Department of Demography and Social Statistics, Federal University, Birnin Kebbi, Nigeria*

Correspondence should be addressed to Joshua O. Akinyemi; odunjoshua@gmail.com



Academic Editor: Robert R. Redfield



Nigeria has about 3.8 million people living with HIV, the second largest globally. Stigma and discrimination are major barriers to testing, treatment uptake, and adherence. In this review, we synthesized information on research studies, policies, and programmes related to HIV-stigma in Nigeria. This was with a view to identify critical areas that research and programmes must address in order to accelerate the progress towards zero (new infections, discrimination, and death) target by year 2030. Existing studies were mostly devoted to stigma assessment using varieties of measures. Research, policies, and programmes in the past two decades have made very useful contributions to stigma reduction. We identified the need for a consistent, valid, and objective measure of stigma at different levels of the HIV response. Nigeria does not lack relevant policies; what needs to be strengthened are design, planning, implementation, monitoring, and evaluation of context-specific stigma reduction programmes.


## 1. Introduction

One of the successes recorded in the Millennium Development Goals was target 6A which aimed to halt HIV by 2015 and begin to reverse its spread. As of 2014, the number of new HIV infections and AIDS-related deaths has declined by 40% and 42%, respectively [1]. Sub-Saharan Africa region was not left behind in this achievement despite the fact that the region is home to 70.0% of persons living with HIV globally [1]. This progress has been attributed to massive improvement in funding which enhanced wider coverage of antiretroviral treatment, innovative approaches to treatment, and prevention interventions [1]. Some challenges still remain which include the need to attain universal treatment coverage and eliminate new infections; treatment of comorbidities; stigma; and discrimination [2]. To confront these challenges and build on the laudable progress so far recorded, one of the health targets under the new Sustainable Development Goals (SDG) is to end the AIDS epidemic by 2030. In pursuit of this, the Joint United Nations Program on HIV/AIDS (UNAIDS) has proposed a global strategy whose target is reducing the number of new HIV infections by 90% and number of AIDS-related deaths by 80% of the level at year 2010 [1]. In fact, UNAIDS has a new vision of "zero new HIV infections, zero discrimination, and zero AIDS-related deaths" [3].

Meanwhile, recent statistics shows that 36.7 million persons were living with HIV as of the end of 2015 of which about 46% have access to treatment [3]. Of these, Nigeria has the second highest number, 3.8 million with adult prevalence of 3.1% [4]. About 44% of adults and children living with HIV have access to ART based on the eligibility criteria of CD4 count of 350 cells/mm$^3$. With the largest population in SSA, only 26% of its people have ever done HIV testing [4]. HIV epidemiology in Nigeria indicates that infections are higher among women while prevalence varied across the six geopolitical regions with the highest rate in the South South (5.5%). One of the main factors driving the infection in Nigeria includes low risk perception, concurrent sexual partnerships, and inadequate access to quality healthcare services [4]. At the centre of these factors is the challenge of HIV-stigma and discrimination which are a major barrier militating against the national response to the epidemic.

According to UNAIDS 2015 guidelines on terminologies, stigma refers to beliefs and/or attitudes marking or staining a person or group of people as unworthy or discreditable [5]. Discrimination results from stigma when any form of distinction, exclusion, or restriction is displayed against an individual because of an attribute or a personal characteristic. For operational and programmatic purposes, HIV-related stigma is described as "negative beliefs, feelings, and attitudes towards people living with HIV (PLHIV), groups associated with PLHIV and other key populations at higher risk of HIV infection" [2]. HIV-related discrimination is the "unfair and unjust treatment (act or omission) of an individual based on his or her real or perceived HIV status." Stigma Stigma and discrimination are formidable threats to the success of HIV care and treatment programs. Several studies have shown stigma and discrimination to affect HIV testing [6], disclosure of serostatus [7], retention, and adherence to treatment [8]. Meta-analysis of 64 studies conducted in different settings demonstrated significant effects of HIV-stigma on mental health, quality of life, use of health services, and physical health of PLHIV [9]. Manifestations or expression of stigma is influenced by sociocultural, political, and economic factors all of which translates into different forms of inequalities in access to HIV care, treatment, and support [10]. The consequence of these multilevel influences is that HIV-stigma operates at individual, family, community, and institutional levels and many of these factors also varied across cultures, thereby necessitating context-specific strategies to address the phenomena.

In congruence with the advancement in the global response, research and programmes on HIV-related stigma have witnessed improvement since the entrance of HIV into public health discourse. For instance, beyond the initial complexities associated with definition, measurement, impact assessment, and reduction of HIV-stigma [11], empirical measures for different domains of stigma have been proposed and validated in some sub-Saharan African countries [12]. Systematic reviews and other forms of research studies have provided evidence on various interventions to reduce HIV-stigma [13–15]. Examples of these interventions which have dominated the HIV-stigma reduction efforts include information-based approaches such as behaviour change communications; capacity building (training of healthcare providers and other allied workers); counselling and support for PLHIV (support groups and network); and involvement of PLHIV in different activities as a way of humanizing the infection such that it is seen as any other chronic health condition.

Nigeria as one of the countries with the largest number of PLHIV has strived to combat HIV-stigma and discrimination to curtail the epidemic. The early (1990s) and peak years (mid-2000s) of the epidemic in Nigeria were characterised by various forms of stigma and discrimination at different levels of human interaction [16]. A review of studies on HIV-related stigma in Nigeria between 1987 and 2008 found eight peer-re viewed articles [17]. The main findings include the following: HIV-stigma manifests mostly as negative attitudes against PLHIV by individuals and community members and unwillingness to treat PLHIV by healthcare workers. The potential of educational interventions to reduce HIV-related stigma was also demonstrated among secondary school pupils, students in nursing schools, and practicing healthcare workers. Some critical gaps identified by the review were absence of coherent and consistent measure of stigma across studies and near absence of intervention studies on stigma reduction [17]. An obvious gap in the previous review of HIV-stigma in Nigeria was the lack of evidence on the experiences of stigma among PLHIV. Furthermore, almost one decade after the review, the national response to HIV in Nigeria has experienced positive shifts in diverse ramifications. For instance, information and awareness about HIV are almost universal; political will and stakeholder involvement have become more robust [4]. It is also expected that research work on HIV-stigma must have advanced beyond the level it was in 2007. Therefore, this paper is aimed at reviewing studies, policies, and programmes related to HIV-stigma in Nigeria. We synthesized data and information on these issues and identified critical areas that research and programmes must address to accelerate progress towards zero (new infections, discrimination, and death) target set by UNAIDS.

## 2. Methods

In March 2017, we searched electronic databases for articles on HIV-stigma in Nigeria between 1999 and 2016. The databases were PubMed, African Journal Online, and JSTOR. Search terms involved different combination of the following: HIV, AIDS, Stigma, Discrimination, and Nigeria. The word "attitude" was also used as a search term because many of the related articles used it to connote stigma or discrimination. Abstracts of each article in the search results were reviewed to determine whether they met criteria for inclusion in the review. For an article to be included in the review, it must address HIV/AIDS stigma or discrimination as a dependent or independent variable. Inclusion was not restricted to any study design; therefore, both quantitative and qualitative studies that addressed HIV-stigma and/or discrimination in Nigeria were selected. Full text of articles that met the inclusion criteria were retrieved and reviewed. For each reviewed article, information was extracted on authorship and year of publication; objective; research design; how stigma was measured (and whether as a dependent or independent variable); and the main findings. These details were summarised in a Table 1. Since this review also includes policies and programmes related to HIV-stigma in Nigeria, we searched the website of relevant organisations for documents related to the subject of interest. Such organisations included the National AIDS Control Agency (NACA), Federal Ministry of Health and Joint United Nations Programme on HIV/AIDS (UNAIDS), Network of People Living with HIV in Nigeria (NEPWHAN). References of retrieved articles, policy documents, and programme reports were also physically scrutinized.

## 3. Results

Compared to the previous review by Monjok et al. [17], we found greater number of research articles related to

Table 1: Literature matrix of studies on HIV-stigma in Nigeria: 2002–2016.

| SN | Ref: author (year) | Study design | Study population and location | Objectives |
|---|---|---|---|---|
| (1) | 1999: Fawole et al. | Quasi-experimental study | Secondary students in South West Nigeria | To assess the effect of educational intervention on attitudes of students to people living with HIV/AIDS |
| (2) | 2000: Uwakwe | Quasi-experimental study | Student nurses in SW Nigeria | To investigate the effect of educational program on attitudes and behaviour regarding HIV/AIDS |
| (3) | 2002: Alubo et al. | Qualitative study | Community members in southern part of Benue State, North Central Nigeria | To document the perceptions of PLHIV, family, and community members about HIV stigma |
| (4) | 2002: Ezedinachi et al. | Quasi-experimental study | Facility-based among health workers in South South Nigeria | To assess the effect of educational intervention on knowledge and attitudes of workers to PLHIV |
| (5) | 2003: Adebajo et al. | Cross-sectional survey | Nurses and medical lab scientists in public health facilities in Lagos, South West, Nigeria | To document attitudes to PLHIV |
| (6) | 2005: Adedigba et al. | Cross-sectional study | Oral health workers in Osun State, South West Nigeria | Assessed KAP of infection control in managing HIV-infected patients |
| (7) | 2005: Reis et al. | Cross-sectional survey | Health workers at a tertiary facility in 4 states of Nigeria | To assess the extent of discrimination against PLHIV |
| (8) | 2006: Adeokun et al. | HIV surveillance project | Market women in Ibadan and Ogbomosho, South West Nigeria | To assess the effect of behavioural change intervention on HIV stigma and discrimination |
| (9) | 2007: Babalola | Cross-sectional survey | Population-based sample, Bauchi (North East) and Kano (North West), Nigeria | To assess the relationship between individual perceived stigma, community stigma (social norm), and attitude to VCT. Male and females were analysed separately Stigma was used as main IV |
| (10) | 2008: Bukar et al. | Cross-sectional study among | Dental professionals in one state in each region of Nigeria | To investigate discrimination against PLHIV among dental professionals |
| (11) | 2008: Lapinski and Nwulu | Field experiment: Group 1 exposed to a film versus another group not exposed | Community-based study, Abuja, North Central Nigeria | The assess the efficacy of an education-entertainment intervention (film) on HIV risk perceptions and perceived stigma |
| (12) | 2009: Adewuya et al. | Cross-sectional study | PLHIV at a private HIV/AIDS care centre in South West Nigeria | Determine prevalence and factors associated with PTSD induced by a stigmatising event among PLHIV |
| (13) | 2009: Babalola et al. | Secondary analysis of cross-sectional survey-National HIV/AIDS and Reproductive Health Survey (NARHS) 2005 | Population-based nationally representative sample | To determine the relationship between media exposure, community media saturation, and accepting attitudes to PLHIV in Nigeria |
| (14) | 2009: Sadoh et al. | Cross-sectional study | Healthcare workers at a facility in South Eastern Nigeria | To document the attitude of health workers to colleagues infected with HIV |
| (15) | 2010: Fakolade et al. | Secondary analysis of NARHS 2003, 2005, and 2007 data | Population-based nationally representative sample | Assess the impact of mass media exposure on HIV stigma and discrimination |
| (16) | 2010: Mbonu et al. | Qualitative method: in-depth interview (IDI) | Community members, healthcare workers and PLHIV in Port-Harcourt, South South Nigeria | To explore power-related differences between men and women in their reactions to people living with HIV/AIDS at family, community, and societal (institutional) level |
| (17) | 2010: Smith and Mbakwem | IDI and observation in 2004, 2006, and 2007 | PLHIV selected from a tertiary treatment facility in Owerri, South East Nigeria | To explore the reproductive life of HIV-positive men and women and understand how they balance medical advice with societal expectations about marriage and reproduction |

Table 1: Continued.

| SN | Ref: author (year) | Study design | Study population and location | Objectives |
|---|---|---|---|---|
| (18) | 2011: Adebayo et al. | Secondary analysis of NARHS 2003, 2005, and 2007 data | Population-based nationally representative sample | Explore levels, trends, and geographical variations in accepting attitude to PLHIV (stigma measure) |
| (19) | 2011: Winskell et al. | Textual analysis of narratives from a writing contest on HIV stigma | Youth participants, Enugu, South East Nigeria | Compare social representation of symbolic stigma (moralistic blaming and shaming of those infected) across 6 countries |
| (20) | 2012: Owolabi et al. | Cross-sectional study | PLHIV at a tertiary treatment facility in Ilorin North Central, Nigeria | Describe the level of stigma and discrimination faced by ART patients |
| (21) | 2013: Blessed and Ogbalu | Cross-sectional study | PLHIV at a tertiary facility in SE Nigeria | Describe the forms of stigma experienced by PLHIV |
| (22) | 2013: Kavanaugh et al. | Cross-sectional study | Community-based sample; Lagos (South West), Benue (North Central), Kaduna (North West), and Enugu (South West) | Describe community attitudes towards possible outcomes of pregnancy by HIV-positive women (abortion or birth) |
| (23) | 2013: Odimegwu et al. | Mixed-method cross-sectional study | Community-based; Osogbo (South West) and Orlu (South East) Nigeria | Describe attitude of community members to PLHIV and how this affects VCT uptake |
| (24) | 2013: Okoror et al. | Qualitative exploration (FGD and IDI) | Community-based organisation in South West Nigeria | Explore how stigma affects ART adherence and the effect of ART on perceived stigma |
| (25) | 2013: Sekoni and Owoaje | Cross-sectional study | Healthcare workers at Primary Healthcare Centres in Kwara State, North Central Nigeria | To investigate stigma and discrimination against PLWHA among PHC workers |
| (26) | 2014: Aransiola et al. | Qualitative study | PLHIV at a secondary health facility in South West Nigeria | To explore stigma and other survival challenges among ART patients |
| (27) | 2014: Olalekan et al. | Qualitative study | PLHIV at a facility in Lagos, South West Nigeria | To explore the perceptions of PLHIV about societal stigma associated with HIV |
| (28) | 2014: Omosanya et al. | Cross-sectional study | PLHIV, tertiary facility in South West Nigeria | To investigate the relationship between HIV stigma and ART adherence |
| (29) | 2014: Onyebuchi-Iwudibia and Brown | Cross-sectional study | PLHIV; treatment facility in Enugu, South East Nigeria | To determine prevalence of depression and its association with HIV-related stigma |
| (30) | 2015: Dahlui et al. | Secondary analysis of Nigeria Demographic and Health Survey 2013 data | Population-based nationally representative sample | Describe the level of stigma against PLHIV in Nigeria |
| (31) | 2015: Schwartz et al. | Longitudinal study among | MSM at a secured clinic setting in Abuja, North Central Nigeria | To investigate the effect of the same-sex prohibition act on stigma and discrimination against MSM in Nigeria |
| (32) | 2016: Olley et al. | Cross-sectional study | PLHIV, tertiary treatment facility in Akure, South West, Nigeria | To investigate the mediating or moderating role of anticipated discrimination in the relationship between HIV-related stigma and status disclosure |

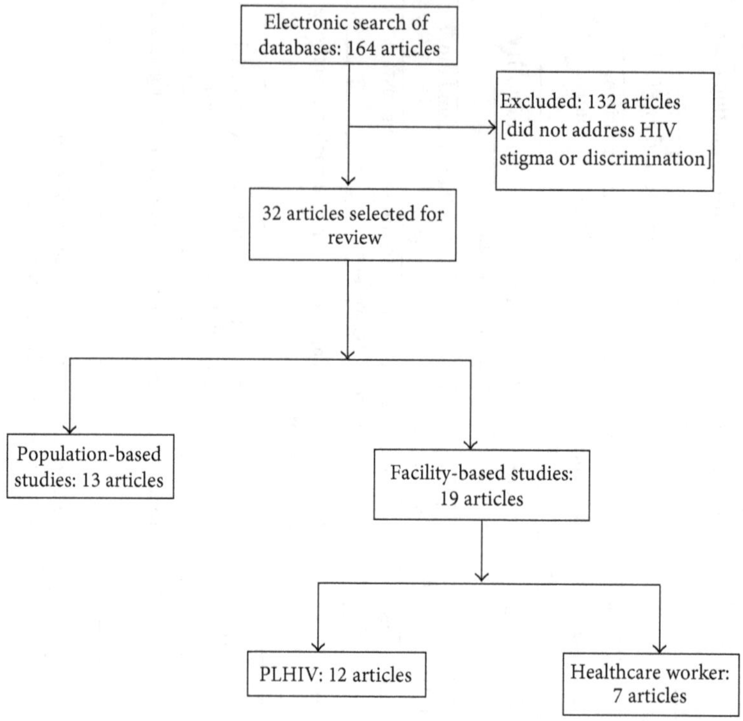


FIGURE 1: Flow chart of articles selected for review.

HIV-stigma in Nigeria. Figure 1 shows the search results, exclusions, and the number of articles eventually included in the review. Of the 32 articles reviewed, 13 were population-based studies. The remaining 19 articles were based in health facilities (11 among PLHIV; 1 among men who have sex with men [MSM]; and 7 among health workers). Apart from 6 articles with national representation, majority of the others (especially those that utilised qualitative techniques) were based in the Southern regions of Nigeria. About 60% of all articles used quantitative techniques while qualitative papers constituted 21.9%. Substantive findings from review of research articles are summarised according to the study population: general population (community members); healthcare workers; and people living with HIV (PLHIV).

*3.1. Population-Based Studies of HIV-Stigma.* Many population-based studies in Nigeria have attempted to measure HIV-related stigma using attitudinal questions as proxy. A tenuous challenge that emanates from many of these studies was that the attitudinal questions used to represent stigma were rarely the same across different studies. One of the earliest community-based research on HIV-stigma in Nigeria was a mixed-method study conducted in South West and South East Nigeria in the early 2000s [18] but published in 2013 [19]. Seven dimensions of HIV-stigma were measured using questions about attitudes of community members towards anyone living with HIV. These dimensions were negative feelings, coercive attitudes, attribution of blame, avoidant behaviours, symbolic contact, interaction with PLHIV, and attitude to an infected partner. Results showed that there was a high prevalence of stigma and discrimination across these domains and stigma was also found to be associated with low uptake of voluntary counselling and testing. It was as high as 85% for avoidant behaviours. Participants from the South Eastern region exhibited stigma more than those from the South West [19]. Negative relationship between HIV-stigma and VCT was also documented among youths in North Eastern and North Western part of Nigeria [20]. Adopting the collectivity of behaviour model, the authors investigated three dimensions of perceived stigma (labelling, relationship, and status disclosure) at individual and community levels. High level of stigma was associated with lower odds of VCT and the effect was even stronger at the community level. There were also gender differences with females showing greater level of stigma. Other population-based studies of HIV-stigma in Nigeria have used accepting attitude as indicator [21, 22]. Incidentally, these were based on nationally representative samples of men and women aged 15–59 and 15–49 years, respectively, with higher prevalence of stigma among women. Analysis of the 2005 National HIV/AIDS and Reproductive Health Survey (NARHS) data revealed that exposure to media information about HIV/AIDS was associated with increased knowledge about the infection and ultimately translated to better accepting attitude [22]. Regional differences in HIV-stigma were also observed despite adjustment for individual characteristics and community media exposure. Adebayo et al. [21] analysed data from the NARHS 2003–2007 to provide evidence on improvement in the level of accepting attitude in Nigeria over this period. In a recent analysis of Nigeria Demographic and Health Survey (NDHS) 2013 data, Dahlui et al. [23] showed that about half of Nigerians still exhibited stigmatizing attitude against PLHIV. This was found associated with younger age, urban residence, lack of formal education, and poor household wealth quintile. The measure of stigma was two attitudinal questions which focused on blaming and shaming of persons living with HIV.

Fertility desires among people living with HIV have attracted attention of researchers especially with improved quality of life offered by ART [24]. To fill important gap about the attitude of people to reproductive decisions of HIV-positive women, a community-based study was conducted in Nigeria and Zambia to describe attitudes towards abortion or childbirth by HIV-positive pregnant women [25]. The Nigeria arm of the study was conducted in selected enumeration areas in Lagos (South west), Enugu (South east), Benue (North Central), and Kaduna (North West). Findings revealed that the level of stigma against birth or abortion by HIV-positive pregnant women was low and similar between men and women. Lack of formal education was the main factor independently associated with stigmatizing attitude towards abortion or childbirth by HIV-positive woman [25]. Analysis was not stratified by state because of the multicountry nature of the study. Therefore, it is not known whether there were variations across the four states (regions) where the study was conducted in Nigeria.

Few of the population-based studies of HIV-stigma in Nigeria have some semblance of interventions to assess the effectiveness of health educational intervention on stigma reduction. All the three studies in this category utilised a quasi-experimental design and showed that stigma reduction can be achieved using educational interventions. Although the interventions were conducted among market women [16], secondary school students [26], and student nurses [27], the efficacy of this approach in the larger population has been demonstrated in a field experiment [28] and analysis of repeated cross-sectional data [29].

Very few community-based qualitative studies of HIV-stigma were found in the course of the review. Incidentally, these were mostly based in Southern parts of Nigeria. Evidence from the south west revealed that social constructions of HIV-stigma are deeply rooted in cultural beliefs and perceptions about the lifestyle of those infected [16, 19]. A cross-national textual analysis of narratives from a writing contest among youths was conducted to compare social representation of symbolic stigma in six SSA countries including Nigeria [30]. The findings pointed to the fact that social representation of stigmatizing attitudes often pertained to the circumstances around the process of HIV infection though there were variations across the six sociocultural contexts analysed. Negative views about PLHIV were more predominant in low HIV prevalence settings. The study further revealed that Nigerian participants who were selected from the South Eastern part displayed the highest cases of symbolic stigma [30]. To shed more light on the gender differences in HIV-stigma, Mbonu et al. [31] adopted Cornell's theory of gender and power to explore power-related differences between men and women in their reactions to PLHIV at family, community, and institutional level. In-depth interviews were conducted among community members, healthcare providers, and PLHIV. The study also showed that stigmatizing behaviour was worst against women and was a reflection of the subsisting power imbalance that exists in patriarchal societies such as Nigeria. This imbalance manifested in forms of financial inequality, authority, and structural norms.

*3.2. Facility-Based Studies of HIV-Stigma in Nigeria.* The second group of studies on HIV-stigma found to be common in Nigeria were those conducted in health facilities. As expected, the study population were either healthcare providers or PLHIV who receive care and treatment from the facilities. An important observation about many of these studies was that they were domiciled mostly in facilities providing specialist or tertiary care and as such were in urban areas. Findings from the review of these studies are summarised according to the study population, healthcare workers and PLHIV.

*3.2.1. Healthcare Workers.* Majority of the studies among healthcare workers were conducted around early and mid-2000s. This was a time that could be referred to as the peak of the HIV epidemic in Nigeria. Virtually all of them were aimed at accessing attitudes towards care and treatment of PLHIV. The earliest among these studies was a quasi-experimental study in South South Nigeria by Ezedinachi et al. [32]. They documented unwillingness to treat, fear, and avoidance of PLHIV among clinicians. Following educational interventions, data collected one year later showed there was significant decline in stigmatization and discriminatory behaviour towards PLHIV [32]. Preponderance of stigma against PLHIV was very common in all the other studies found in this category and this was similar among clinicians [33], dental and oral health professional [34–36], nurses, and medical lab scientists [37]. In anticipation of the potential roles of primary healthcare workers in care and treatment of PLHIV, a study in North Central Nigeria showed similar findings of a high level of stigma which often manifest in form of fear of casual transmission, shaming and blaming, discrimination, and status disclosure [38].

*3.3. Stigmatization Experiences among People Living with HIV.* The second group of facility-based studies are those that documented stigmatization and discrimination experiences among PLHIV. Prevalence of stigmatizing experiences varied widely, ranging from 8% to 60%. This wide variation is due to the diverse indices/measures used for stigma. In fact, no two studies defined or measured HIV-stigma in the same manner. This posed limitations to study comparisons and generalisation from one study setting to another. As observed earlier, majority of the studies in this category were conducted at tertiary health facilities in Southern Nigeria except one at a Teaching Hospital in North Central region by Owolabi et al. [39]. In the paper, 25% of ART patients reported that they had experienced stigma or discrimination at family, hospital, and community levels and at the workplace. Forms of stigma experienced included blaming for being HIV-positive and name calling (prostitute, skeleton, and unfaithful person among others). Examples of discriminatory practices against PLHIV were hospital (selective use of gloves, poor quality care, and isolation from other patients); community (social isolation, restriction in family events, and hostility); family (not sharing of cutleries and toilet facilities, breach of confidentiality); workplace (threat of employment termination, isolation by coworkers). Adapting the Berger stigma scale [40], forms of stigma experienced by PLHIV were also documented in a cross-sectional study conducted at another tertiary facility in South East Nigeria [41]. These were personalised/internalised stigma, status disclosure, negative self-image, and concerns about public attitude. Females were found to experience higher degree of the first three dimensions. A weakness of the paper was that the stigma scale was treated as a continuous measure and scores were generated for analyses. It was therefore difficult to estimate the magnitude or prevalence of stigma in the four domains examined.

The burden of stigma among PLHIV may be higher than documented in quantitative studies as findings from FGD participants in Lagos, Nigeria, showed that almost 75% reported that life has become very traumatic due to stigmatization from friends, family members, healthcare workers, and workplace [42]. Studies have shown that stigma was associated with ART adherence and mental health status of PLHIV. For instance, low stigma level was found to be associated with good ART adherence among participants in a cross-sectional study at a tertiary facility in South West Nigeria [43]. Regarding the consequences of HIV-related stigma, Adewuya et al. [44] found that 27.3% of patients who had experienced stigmatizing events such as isolation and blaming had post-traumatic stress disorder (PTSD). The study was conducted at a private HIV/AIDS care facility in South West Nigeria. It is suspected that the situation could be worst in public health facility where there are larger patient population and therefore greater pressure on healthcare providers. Evidence from another study in South East region suggests that the prevalence of depression was 33.3% and this was associated with negative self-image domain on the Berger HIV scale [45]. Personalised or internalised stigma was also associated with lesser likelihood of status disclosure among PLHIV [46]. These limit the self-esteem and confidence among PLHIV with a negative consequence on their overall mental health status.

Quite a few qualitative studies have also explored the experiences of stigma and discrimination among PLHIV. Results from focus group discussion in Southern parts of Benue State in North Central region of Nigeria highlighted the high level of rejection and discrimination of PLHIV in the late 1990s [47]. Isolation and avoidance of those infected by HIV were a common practice fuelled by fear of being infected by "a disease without cure." Community members believed that caring for anyone infected by HIV was waste of resources because HIV was more like a death sentence [47]. With better awareness and availability of ART, the negative perception has waned over time such that PLHIVs also desire to fulfil social expectations about marriage and reproduction [48]. Ethnographic case studies from South East Nigeria actually showed that marriage and reproduction by HIV-positive men and women are strategies used to confront the problem of HIV-stigma [48].

Drawing on Deacon's framework [49], a qualitative exploration of stigma before and after ART initiation revealed very interesting findings about the dynamic nature of stigma [50]. The central argument of the Deacon's framework was that stigma is a dynamic sociocultural phenomenon that changes in response to different situations [49]. Based on this premise, stigma could be classified as self-stigma, anticipated stigma, and enacted stigma. Before ART, there were experiences of self-isolation, fear of death, family withdrawal, rejection, and abandonment [50]. After ART commencement, with better or healthier physical appearance, family and community members began to accept PLHIV and status disclosure also improved. In sum, stigma was a motivator for treatment adherence which in turn reduced self-stigma, enacted stigma, and anticipated stigma [50]. This evidence needs to be further substantiated because participants in the study were recruited from a community-based organisation. If participants had been recruited from a public health facility, could the findings be different? Another exploratory study of stigma and survival challenges among ART patients at a secondary health facility in South West Nigeria revealed that stigmatizing experiences were low among family members but high from nonfamily members including health workers [51]. The study also showed that some well-intentioned social interventions (such as packaged food parcels for nutritional supplementation) for PLHIV ended up stigmatizing them. In the face of these daunting challenges of stigma and discrimination, a study in Lagos, South West Nigeria, documented the coping strategies that have been deployed by PLHIV. The most common were maintaining a low public profile by avoiding public functions, avoiding seeking care in public health facilities, and nondisclosure of serostatus [42]. Of course, these approaches do not augur well for universal coverage of care, treatment, or support and it is a serious threat to secondary prevention of HIV infection.

We found a study conducted among MSM in North Central Nigeria which investigated the impact of the law prohibiting such relationship in Nigeria [52]. The authors argued that there was increased fear of stigma and discrimination among this key population and as a result, access to care was affected.

*3.4. Policies Related to HIV-Stigma in Nigeria.* In Nigeria, policies and programmes for the national HIV response are coordinated by the National AIDS Control Agency (NACA). Other key partners include the Federal Ministry of Health (FMoH) as well as the State AIDS Control Agency (SACA) and Ministries of Health in the 36 states of the Federation. Policies are usually formulated at the national level and domesticated by the states. Though the administrative structure in Nigeria stipulates that states are federating units with autonomy to develop their own policies and programmes on issues such as health and education, there is a lot of synergy and cooperation among the federal and state government agencies. In this review, only policies and programmes enacted by the national government are reviewed because they apply across the entire country. Also, in order not to lose sight of the aim of this paper, we focused on the policy and programme components related to HIV-stigma.

*3.4.1. National HIV/AIDS Policy.* The current HIV/AIDS policy in Nigeria was launched in 2009 [53]. Prior to that, similar policies have been formulated in 1997 and 2001. The 2009 policy document adopted a multisectoral approach to the fight against HIV in Nigeria. Therefore, its formulation involved extensive stakeholder engagement across public sector, private sector, and international development partners. Among the guiding principles of the 2009 policy was protection of rights of PLHIV and reduction of stigma and discrimination. The six strategic thrusts of the policy were (1) behaviour change and prevention of new infections; (2) treatment; (3) care and support for infected and affected persons; (4) institutional architecture and resourcing; (5) advocacy, legal issues, and rights; (6) monitoring and evaluation; (7) research and knowledge management. Stigma and discrimination were part of several policy objectives under strategic thrusts 1, 2, 3, and 5. The policy document clearly stated that "the rights of PLHIV include freedom from stigma and discrimination." Stakeholders with stigma related responsibilities were national and state legislative assemblies (promoting policy dialogue and leading advocacy to reduce stigma and discrimination); faith-based organisations (advocacy for care and support; promoting stigma and discrimination reduction); traditional and religious leaders (supporting HIV/AIDS programmes and advocate for stigma reduction). Surprisingly, the policy document was silent on specific strategies to reduce stigma and discrimination under treatment, care, and support services.

*3.4.2. The 2010–2015 HIV/AIDS National Strategic Plan (NSP).* This was the third in a series of plans to combat HIV epidemic in Nigeria. The first plan captioned HIV/AIDS Emergency Action Plan (HEAP) 2001–2003 was developed in early 2001 and targeted at public awareness about the epidemic. Its successor was the National Strategic Framework for Action 2005–2009 developed in 2004/2005. It served as blueprint on implementation for different stakeholders. The 2010–2015 NSP [54] which has already completed its lifespan at the time of this review had six thematic areas which were lifted directly from the strategic thrust in the 2009 HIV/AIDS policy document. In the NSP, stigma and discrimination featured as an objective under care and support services. The strategic aim was "to reduce stigma and discrimination (S and D) against PLHIV and PABA by at least 60% of the baseline value by 2015." Though the baseline year was 2010, the value is unknown. Thus, it is difficult to assess whether the target of 60% reduction has been met or not. Furthermore, S and D reduction was also listed among the activities to be carried out under policies, rights, and legal issues. Perhaps, the revision and eventual publication of the National HIV/AIDS Workplace policy in 2014 is an evidence of achievement on this note. Related to this are the passing and signing into law of the Nigeria's HIV/AIDS Antidiscrimination bill.

*3.4.3. National Workplace Policy on HIV and AIDS.* The Nigeria National Workplace Policy on HIV and AIDS was first developed in 2005 to address the workplace response to the epidemic. The latest review was adopted and published in 2013 [55]. Such a policy became necessary because the population most affected by HIV in Nigeria are youths and those who are in the reproductive age groups. These also constitute the workforce of the country. Latest review was necessitated by three factors: changing epidemiology of HIV in the country; revision of the national HIV/AIDS policy which was its parent document; and implementation of the International Labour Organisation (ILO) recommendation 200 on HIV and AIDS in the workplace [56]. Nigeria is a signatory to several ILO recommendations and conventions. Guided by the 2009 National Policy on HIV and AIDS, the workplace policy document showed linkages with several other documents and legislations in Nigeria. One of the eight specific objectives of the policy focused on *"eliminating discrimination and stigmatization in the workplace based on real or perceived HIV status including dealing with HIV testing, confidentiality, and disclosure."* The scope of the policy includes both public and private sectors including the uniformed services. Its guiding principles also conspicuously included *"nondiscrimination"* alongside nine others. To ensure that majority of Nigerians remain HIV-negative, the strategies itemised to achieve the objectives of the policy include prevention, HIV testing, treatment, care, and support, and promotion and protection of workers' rights. Responsibilities for the following stakeholders were also spelt out: Federal Ministry of Labour and Productivity, employers, workers, and their organisations, National Agency for Control of AIDS, State Agency for Control of AIDS, and National Steering Committee for HIV Workplace Issues. Curiously, implementation and action plans which were to be developed by different stakeholders are still being awaited.

*3.4.4. Nigeria's HIV and AIDS Antidiscrimination Act, 2014.* First introduced to the National Legislature in 2005, the bill was passed and signed into law in April and November 2014, respectively. It serves a significant milestone in the national response to HIV/AIDS in Nigeria. This is because the nonpassage of the bill was a recurrent comment in the PLHIV stigma index and gender assessment report which are both reviewed in the next sections. The antidiscrimination act was very clear on rights of individuals [57]; their responsibilities; institutional obligations; and penalties for violations. It stipulates that PLHIV have rights to privacy about their serostatus, employment, welfare benefits, compensation, appeal, and recourse to courts as well as occupational safety. All Nigerians have responsibility to prevent stigma and discrimination. The responsibilities of PLHIV were disclosure of status to partner, demand for their right, and reporting of violations. Obligations of institutions, employers, and communities include protecting rights of PLHIV; providing equal opportunities to PLHIV; confidentiality of information; development of HIV/AIDS workplace policy; compensation for occupational HIV infection. Penalties for violations of the laws in the antidiscrimination act could be fines and/or imprisonment. Available information from the legal unit of NACA is that the act has been domesticated in 17 states across Nigeria. Two years after the law became active, there is a need for empirical evidence on the level of awareness; compliance; and the impact of the law on different aspects of the national HIV response in Nigeria. This is very crucial for the development of the next strategic response plan. Anecdotal evidence shows that lack of laws is not the main problem.

*3.5. National HIV/AIDS Stigma Reduction Strategy, 2016.* In response to the formidable threats posed by stigma and discrimination to the success of HIV prevention and treatment programmes, NACA in collaboration with other stakeholders developed the stigma reduction strategy for Nigeria [58].

Launched in November 2016, the goal of the strategy document was to "eliminate all forms of stigma and discrimination against people infected and affected by HIV in Nigeria by the year 2020." It has nine strategic objectives with one contributing to the goal from different operational perspectives cutting across community-based organisations, faith-based organisations, media, entertainment and art industry, health and education institutions, and employers of labour (private and public), PLHIV and PABA. In other words, it was designed to achieve synergy among different players working with responsibilities to reduce/eliminate HIV-stigma with each entity leveraging on its comparative strengths in their jurisdictions, domains of coverage, and influence. Several strategic actions were listed including survey on behavioural, biomedical, and structural drivers of stigma and discrimination at different levels, increasing awareness about related laws. This national stigma reduction strategy actually integrated many of the UNAIDS suggestions on programmes and initiatives to promote stigma reduction at individual, community, structural, and institutional levels [2, 59].

*3.6. Programmes Related to HIV-Stigma in Nigeria.* Country annual report on the global response to HIV usually submitted to UNAIDS provides a comprehensive description of programmes implemented as part of the national response to HIV in Nigeria [4]. The commonest programme targeted at HIV-stigma and discrimination reduction in Nigeria is media and awareness campaigns aimed at educating the populace about HIV and ultimately reduce stigma and discrimination. Other approaches include the strategies deployed for universal counselling, testing, and treatment. The main philosophy of the approach was that if HIV is seen as a chronic condition just like hypertension or any other, then the infection would be better humanized thereby reducing stigma and discrimination against those infected and affected by HIV. Two other programmes related to HIV-stigma in Nigeria were the PLHIV stigma index measurement [60] and the Legal Environment Assessment in the HIV response [61].

*3.6.1. The PLHIV Stigma Index.* The stigma index was designed to collect data on stigma, discrimination, and rights of people living with HIV. It was also aimed at serving as an advocacy tool and a way to operationalize the principle of Greater Involvement of People Living with HIV (GIPA). As of September 2013, it has been used in more than 50 countries including Nigeria. Further details on the development and processes involved in using the index are available on its dedicated website (www.stigmaindex.org).

In Nigeria, the index was applied by Networks of People Living with HIV and AIDS in Nigeria (NEPWHAN) in late 2009. Data was collected from 706 persons living with HIV selected from support groups in 12 states of the federation. The interviewers were also PLHIV. Report from the assessment documented several experiences of stigma and discrimination across three themes: exclusion, access to work, health, and educational services; internalised stigma; and fears [60]. Nearly one-third of respondents reported that they have been excluded from family and religious or other social functions due to their HIV status. A similar percentage also reported that they have experienced denial to health and educational services. Internalised stigma in form of shame, feeling of low self-esteem, and blaming oneself was reported by about 63%. In a nutshell, the index showed that stigma and discrimination experiences were prevalent among PLHIV in Nigeria. It is noted that the stigma assessment was done before the enactment of antidiscrimination law. Also, several programmes and initiatives have been implemented which must have influenced the narratives about HIV S and D in Nigeria. A repeat application of the stigma index is necessary to empirically assess the impacts of these various interventions.

*3.7. Legal Environment Assessment for HIV/AIDS Response (LEA) in Nigeria.* There has been a drive at international and regional levels to use laws as tools for HIV elimination. Particularly, to improve equity in access to services among key populations, law and regulatory environment must not be prohibitive. For instance, in Nigeria, HIV prevalence is higher among brothel-based female sex workers (19.4%), non-brothel-based female sex workers (8.6%), and men having sex with men (22.9%) [62]. Incidentally, there is a law prohibiting same-sex relationships in Nigeria. Empirical investigation of the effect of this law showed that it increased the incidence of stigma and discrimination against MSM such that they are afraid of accessing HIV care and treatment from public health facilities [52].

Stigma and discrimination are a main driver of inadequate access to care and treatment among these key populations. This would constitute a weak link in the HIV prevention efforts if an enabling environment is not created to protect this group against marginalisation and stigma.

The LEA in Nigeria was therefore designed to identify and review existing laws, regulations, and policies that could impact the national HIV response. Varieties of qualitative research methodologies (desk review, focus group discussion, in-depth interview, and key informant interview) were employed for the exercise. Findings showed that the legal environment in Nigeria is weak for effective human rights based response to HIV/AIDS [61]. Even though the 1999 constitution (amended) guaranteed rights of individuals against stigma and discrimination in any form, the institutional mechanisms for seeking redress could be easily exploited to the disadvantage of those in lower socioeconomic strata. Some of the legal provisions under different laws such as the criminal codes (which operates in Southern regions), penal codes (in the Muslim dominated northern regions), and same-sex marriage laws were found inconsistent [61]. While advocating for review of many of the existing laws related to stigma and discrimination, the LEA report also called for legal literacy among key populations and stakeholders in the justice sector.

## 4. Discussion

Although the measures used have not been consistent, there is evidence to show that the level of HIV-stigma in Nigeria has declined in the past two decades. This is demonstrated in results from analysis of attitudinal questions about people living with HIV in nationally representative surveys such as the NARHS 2003, 2005, 2007, and 2012 and NDHS 2013 [21, 23, 29, 63]. At least, early stories of isolation, abandonment, avoidance, and so forth have reduced drastically while uptake of HIV counselling and testing have improved [4]. HIV-stigma exists beyond the individual level and persists in families, communities, workplace, and other institutional contexts. Forms of HIV-stigma and discriminatory practices vary from one setting to another and this contextual difference is driven by economic and sociocultural diversity characteristic of Nigeria. At the base of this is the problem of power and inequality which visibly manifests as gender differences in HIV-stigma. Apart from the effect of stigma on testing, treatment uptake, adherence, care, and support, there is emerging evidence of a negative effect on treatment outcomes (quality of life and mental health). This review also found that PLHIVs have devised different positive and negative responses to stigma. Example of a positive response is by choosing to maintain good adherence so that physical health and overall quality of life can be like that of HIV-negative individuals. Another one is their family formation behaviour which is strongly motivated by a desire to demystify the misconceptions that fuel HIV-stigma and discrimination.

This review also revealed that the Government of Nigeria with support from development partners have done a lot to confront HIV-stigma. National policies and strategic plans have been revised about three times to align with international best practices as well as respond to the epidemiological and structural dynamics of the HIV epidemic in the country. A robust multisectoral approach with stakeholders involvement, political will, and policy advocacy at national and state levels have all contributed to general awareness about the urgent need to eliminate stigma and curtail HIV spread. To further improve on the successes recorded so far, some recommendations are made which could strengthen the stigma reduction programmes in the country.

There is a need for reliable, validated empirical measures of HIV-stigma. Even though the Berger HIV-stigma scale was applied at a facility in SW Nigeria [46], its internal consistency (reliability) was just average. Measures already validated in other SSA settings [12] can be revalidated in the country. Availability of reliable and validated measures will facilitate objective assessment which is very important for the monitoring of the recent stigma reduction strategy in the country. The need to monitor the impact of the 2014 antidiscrimination law also makes this necessary.

Another reason for new measures of stigma stems from the scale-up of ART services to secondary and primary healthcare facilities. It is expected that a deeper population penetration of ART would help correct the wrong belief that HIV is a death sentence. This misconception has been responsible for abandonment in the early 2000s. It also heightened the fear of casual transmission via mere physical contact. Now that treatment is closer to the grassroots, it ought to have indirectly mitigated some of the stigma. Operational research studies need to be undertaken to explore this proposition.

Much of what is known about HIV-stigma in Nigeria have come largely from research studies in North Central, South East, South West, and South South regions. Considering the evidence about the dynamic sociocultural nature of stigma, there is need for complimentary evidence from the North East and North West regions. The case for the North East is even more sacrosanct because of the internal population displacement occasioned by the Boko Haram insurgency. There is anecdotal evidence of increased new HIV infections in internally displaced persons (IDP) camps. Although some of these internally displaced persons are being resettled in their communities, the level of HIV-stigma in IDP camps must have been enormous. The experiences of those affected and how they coped with the challenges would provide useful lessons for stigma reduction programmes in Nigeria.

Another implication of the preponderance of HIV-stigma studies in Nigeria being domiciled in tertiary health facilities is that they also provide information about urban areas. Could stigma be higher in rural areas? Evidence from population-based surveys suggests that stigmatizing attitudes towards PLHIV was associated with lower education, poverty, and poor knowledge of HIV [23, 63]. These features are characteristic of rural settings in Nigeria. In addition, the only facility-based study among health workers in primary health centres also showed that stigma was high among this cadre of health workforce [38]. These are kinds of facilities that exist in most rural areas. Therefore, it can be expected that stigma will be higher in rural areas.

The legislative environment in Nigeria is not favourable to key populations at risk of HIV such as MSM. This may also explain why investigation of HIV-stigma in this population is rare. The only study among this group showed that enactment of the law prohibiting same-sex partnership in Nigeria has contributed to higher level of fear [52], although, prior to the legislation, the existing social environment cannot be claimed to be conducive to MSM. Therefore, it is difficult to draw a definitive conclusion about the effect of the new law.

## 5. Conclusion

Without prejudice to other strategies aimed at eliminating HIV by year 2030, stigma and discrimination reduction is a priority. Research, policies, and programmes in the past decade have made tremendous contributions to this drive. Newer approaches tailored to the epidemiological and social contexts of individual countries would continue to evolve. In this regard, this paper reviewed research studies, policies, and programmes related to HIV stigma in Nigeria, the country with the second largest number of people living with HIV in the world. This review identified the need for a consistent valid and objective measure of stigma at different levels of the HIV response. Empirical evidence on the awareness and effect of anti-HIV discrimination law and other interventions are urgently needed. Nigeria is not lacking in policies as this review shows that the country is nearly up to date in compliance with UNAIDS guidelines on several policy requirements. What need to be strengthened are programmes design, planning, monitoring, and evaluation. It is necessary to intensify advocacy, awareness, and enforcement of the anti-HIV discrimination law. It is also very important to develop systems for evaluating the impact of stigma and discrimination reduction programmes at national and subnational levels.

## Conflicts of Interest

The authors declare that there are no conflicts of interest regarding the publication of this paper.

## Acknowledgments

The authors are grateful to CODESRIA African Academic Diaspora Support for Diaspora Research Partnership Network/Visiting Professorship to African Universities, for the financial support to implement this study. They appreciate Yomi Olatunji and Adeoluwa Aiyewumi of the National Agency for the Control of AIDS in Abuja, Nigeria, for helping with some policy documents used for this review.

## References

[1] WHO, *Health in 2015: From MDG to SDG*, World Health Organization, Geneva, Switzerland, 2015.

[2] UNAIDS, *Reduction of HIV-related stigma and discrimination: Guidance note*, Joint United Nations Programme on HIV/AIDS, Geneva, Switzerland, 2014.

[3] UNAIDS, *Global HIV Statistics Fact Sheet*, Joint United Nations Programme on HIV/AIDS, Geneva, Switzerland, 2016.

[4] National Agency for the Conrol of AIDS, *Global AIDS Response Country Progress Report, 2015*, NACA, Abuja, Nigeria, 2015.

[5] UNAIDS, *UNAIDS Terminologies Guidelines*, Joint United Nations Programme on HIV/AIDS, Geneva, Switzerland, 2015.

[6] L. A. Yahaya, A. A. Jimoh, and O. R. Balogun, "Factors hindering acceptance of HIV/AIDS voluntary counseling and testing (VCT) among youth in Kwara State, Nigeria.," *African Journal of Reproductive Health*, vol. 14, no. 3, pp. 159–164, 2010.

[7] O. T. Okareh, O. M. Akpa, J. O. Okunlola, and T. A. Okoror, "Management of Conflicts Arising From Disclosure of HIV Status Among Married Women in Southwest Nigeria," *Health Care for Women International*, vol. 36, no. 2, pp. 149–160, 2015.

[8] I. Okoronkwo, U. Okeke, A. Chinweuba, and P. Iheanacho, "Nonadherence Factors and Sociodemographic Characteristics of HIV-Infected Adults Receiving Antiretroviral Therapy in Nnamdi Azikiwe University Teaching Hospital, Nnewi, Nigeria," *ISRN AIDS*, vol. 2013, pp. 1–8, 2013.

[9] S. Rueda, S. Mitra, S. Chen et al., "Examining the associations between HIV-related stigma and health outcomes in people living with HIV/AIDS: a series of meta-analyses," *BMJ Open*, vol. 6, no. 7, p. e011453, 2016.

[10] J. E. Ehiri, J. Iwelunmor, T. Iheanacho et al., "Using a cultural framework to understand factors influencing HIV testing in Nigeria," *International Quarterly of Community Health Education*, vol. 37, no. 1, pp. 33–42, 2016.

[11] A. P. Mahajan, J. N. Sayles, V. A. Patel et al., "Stigma in the HIV/AIDS epidemic: a review of the literature and recommendations for the way forward," *AIDS*, vol. 22, supplement 2, pp. S67–S79, 2008.

[12] L. Nyblade, A. Jain, M. Benkirane et al., "A brief, standardized tool for measuring HIV-related stigma among health facility staff: results of field testing in China, Dominica, Egypt, Kenya, Puerto Rico and St. Christopher & Nevis.," *Journal of the International AIDS Society*, vol. 16, no. 3, Article ID 18718, 2013.

[13] L. Brown, K. Macintyre, and L. Trujillo, "Interventions to reduce HIV/AIDS stigma: what have we learned?" *AIDS Education and Prevention*, vol. 15, no. 1, pp. 49–69, 2003.

[14] S. Sengupta, B. Banks, D. Jonas, M. S. Miles, and G. C. Smith, "HIV interventions to reduce HIV/AIDS stigma: A systematic review," *AIDS and Behavior*, vol. 15, no. 6, pp. 1075–1087, 2011.

[15] A. L. Stangl, J. K. Lloyd, L. M. Brady, C. E. Holland, and S. Baral, "A systematic review of interventions to reduce HIV-related stigma and discrimination from 2002 to 2013: how far have we come?" *Journal of the International AIDS Society*, vol. 16, no. 3, Article ID 18734, 2013.

[16] L. A. Adeokun, P. Okonkwo, and O. Ladipo, "The stigmatization of people living with HIV/AIDS," in *AIDS in Nigeria: A Nation on the Threshold*, O. Adeyi, Ed., Harvard University Press, Boston, Mass, USA, 2006.

[17] E. Monjok, A. Smesny, and E. J. Essien, "HIV/AIDS-related stigma and discrimination in Nigeria: review of research studies and future directions for prevention strategies.," *African Journal of Reproductive Health*, vol. 13, no. 3, pp. 21–35, 2009.

[18] C. O. Odimegwu, *Prevalence and predictors of HIV-related stigma and knowledge in Nigeria: Implications for HIV/AIDS prevention initiatives*, Harvard School of Public Health, Boston, Mass, USA, 2003.

[19] C. Odimegwu, S. A. Adedini, and D. N. Ononokpono, "HIV/AIDS stigma and utilization of voluntary counselling and testing in Nigeria," *BMC Public Health*, vol. 13, no. 1, article 465, 2013.

[20] S. Babalola, "Readiness for HIV testing among young people in northern Nigeria: The roles of social norm and perceived stigma," *AIDS and Behavior*, vol. 11, no. 5, pp. 759–769, 2007.

[21] S. B. Adebayo, R. Fakolade, J. Anyanti, B. Ekweremadu, O. Ladipo, and A. Ankomah, "Modelling level, trend and geographical variations in stigma and discrimination against people living with HIV/AIDS in Nigeria," *Sahara J*, vol. 8, no. 3, pp. 115–127, 2011.

[22] S. Babalola, A. Fatusi, and J. Anyanti, "Media saturation, communication exposure and HIV stigma in Nigeria," *Social Science & Medicine*, vol. 68, no. 8, pp. 1513–1520, 2009.

[23] M. Dahlui, N. Azahar, A. Bulgiba et al., "HIV/AIDS related stigma and discrimination against PLWHA in Nigerian population," *PLoS ONE*, vol. 10, no. 12, Article ID e0143749, 2015.

[24] D. A. Adekanle, S. A. Olowookere, A. D. Adewole, N. A. Adeleke, E. A. Abioye-Kuteyi, and M. Y. Ijadunola, "Sexual experiences of married HIV positive women in Osogbo, southwest Nigeria: Role of inappropriate status disclosure," *BMC Women's Health*, vol. 15, no. 1, article no. 6, 2015.

[25] M. L. Kavanaugh, A. M. Moore, O. Akinyemi et al., "Community attitudes towards childbearing and abortion among HIV-positive women in Nigeria and Zambia," *Culture, Health and Sexuality*, vol. 15, no. 2, pp. 160–174, 2013.

[26] I. O. Fawole, M. C. Asuzu, S. O. Oduntan, and W. R. Brieger, "A school-based AIDS education programme for secondary school students in Nigeria: A review of effectiveness," *Health Education Research*, vol. 14, no. 5, pp. 675–683, 1999.

[27] C. B. U. Uwakwe, "Systematized HIV/AIDS education for student nurses at the University of Ibadan, Nigeria: Impact on knowledge, attitudes and compliance with universal precautions," *Journal of Advanced Nursing*, vol. 32, no. 2, pp. 416–424, 2000.

[28] M. K. Lapinski and P. Nwulu, "Can a short film impact HIV-related risk and stigma perceptions? Results from an experiment in Abuja, Nigeria," *Health Communication*, vol. 23, no. 5, pp. 403–412, 2008.

[29] R. Fakolade, S. B. Adebayo, J. Anyanti, and A. Ankomah, "The impact of exposure to mass media campaigns and social support

on levels and trends of HIV-related stigma and discrimination in Nigeria: tools for enhancing effective hiv prevention programmes," *Journal of Biosocial Science*, vol. 42, no. 3, pp. 395–407, 2010.

[30] K. Winskell, E. Hill, and O. Obyerodhyambo, "Comparing HIV-related symbolic stigma in six African countries: Social representations in young people's narratives," *Social Science & Medicine*, vol. 73, no. 8, pp. 1257–1265, 2011.

[31] N. C. Mbonu, B. Van Den Borne, and N. K. De Vries, "Gender-related power differences, beliefs and reactions towards people living with HIV/AIDS: An urban study in Nigeria," *BMC Public Health*, vol. 10, article 334, 2010.

[32] E. Ezedinachi, M. Ross, M. Meremiku et al., "The impact of an intervention to change health workers' HIV/AIDS attitudes and knowledge in Nigeria: A controlled trial," *Public Health*, vol. 116, no. 2, pp. 106–112, 2002.

[33] A. E. Sadoh, W. E. Sadoh, W. E. Sadoh, A. O. Fawole, A. Oladimeji, and O. Sotiloye, "Attitude of health care workers to patients and colleagues infected with human immunodeficiency virus," *Journal of Social Aspects of HIV/AIDS*, vol. 6, no. 1, pp. 17–23, 2009.

[34] M. A. Adedigba, E. O. Ogunbodede, B. A. Fajewonyomi, O. O. Ojo, and S. Naidoo, "Gender differences among oral health care workers in caring for HIV/AIDS patients in Osun state, Nigeria," *African Health Sciences*, vol. 5, no. 3, pp. 182–187, 2005.

[35] C. Reis, M. Heisler, L. L. Amowitz et al., "Discriminatory attitudes and practices by health workers toward patients with HIV/AIDS in Nigeria," *PLoS Medicine*, vol. 2, no. 8, pp. 743–752, 2005.

[36] A. Bukar, R. Gofwen, O. A. Adeleke, O. O. Taiwo, I. S. Danfillo, and P. H. Jalo, "Discriminatory attitudes towards patients with HIV/AIDS by dental professionals in Nigeria.," *Odontostomatologie tropicale = Tropical dental journal*, vol. 31, no. 122, pp. 34–40, 2008.

[37] S. B. Adebajo, A. O. Bamgbala, and M. A. Oyediran, "Attitudes of health care providers to persons living with HIV/AIDS in Lagos State, Nigeria," *African Journal of Reproductive Health*, vol. 7, no. 1, pp. 103–112, 2003.

[38] O. O. Sekoni and E. T. Owoaje, "HIV/AIDS stigma among primary health care workers in Ilorin, Nigeria.," *African Journal of Medicine and Medical Sciences*, vol. 42, no. 1, pp. 47–57, 2013.

[39] R. S. Owolabi, M. O. Araoye, G. K. Osagbemi, L. Odeigah, A. Ogundiran, and N. A. Hussain, "Assessment of stigma and discrimination experienced by people living with HIV and AIDS receiving care/treatment in University of Ilorin Teaching Hospital (UITH), Ilorin, Nigeria," *Journal of the International Association of Physicians in AIDS Care*, vol. 11, no. 2, pp. 121–127, 2012.

[40] B. E. Berger, C. E. Ferrans, and F. R. Lashley, "Measuring stigma in people with HIV: psychometric assessment of the HIV stigma scale," *Research in Nursing & Health*, vol. 24, no. 6, pp. 518–529, 2001.

[41] N. O. Blessed and A. I. Ogbalu, "Experience of HIV-related stigma by people living with HIV/AIDS at Federal Medical Center, Owerri, Nigeria," *Journal of Public Health and Epidemiology*, vol. 5, no. 11, pp. 435–439, 2013.

[42] A. Olalekan, A. Akintunde, and M. Olatunji, "Perception of Societal Stigma and Discrimination Towards People Living with HIV/AIDS in Lagos, Nigeria: a Qualitative Study," *Materia Socio Medica Journal*, vol. 26, no. 3, p. 191, 2014.

[43] O. E. Omosanya, O. T. Elegbede, S. M. Agboola, A. O. Isinkaye, and O. A. Omopariola, "Effects of stigmatization/discrimination on antiretroviral therapy adherence among HIV-infected patients in a rural tertiary medical center in Nigeria," *Journal of the International Association of Providers of AIDS Care*, vol. 13, no. 3, pp. 260–263, 2014.

[44] A. O. Adewuya, M. O. Afolabi, B. A. Ola et al., "Post-traumatic stress disorder (PTSD) after stigma related events in HIV infected individuals in Nigeria," *Social Psychiatry and Psychiatric Epidemiology*, vol. 44, no. 9, pp. 761–766, 2009.

[45] O. Onyebuchi-Iwudibia and A. Brown, "HIV and depression in Eastern Nigeria: The role of HIV-related stigma," *AIDS Care Psychological and Socio-medical Aspects of AIDS/HIV*, vol. 26, no. 5, pp. 653–657, 2014.

[46] B. O. Olley, M. J. Ogunde, P. O. Oso, and A. Ishola, "HIV-related stigma and self-disclosure: The mediating and moderating role of anticipated discrimination among people living with HIV/AIDS in Akure Nigeria," *AIDS Care Psychological and Socio-medical Aspects of AIDS/HIV*, vol. 28, no. 6, pp. 726–730, 2016.

[47] O. Alubo, A. Zwandor, T. Jolayemi, and E. Omudu, "Acceptance and stigmatization of PLWA in Nigeria," *AIDS Care Psychological and Socio-medical Aspects of AIDS/HIV*, vol. 14, no. 1, pp. 117–126, 2002.

[48] D. J. Smith and B. C. Mbakwem, "Antiretroviral therapy and reproductive life projects: mitigating the stigma of AIDS in Nigeria," *Social Science & Medicine*, vol. 71, pp. 345–352, 1982.

[49] H. Deacon, I. Stephney, and S. Prosalendis, *Understanding HIV/AIDS stigma: A theoretical and methodological analysis*, Human Sciences Research Council, Capetown, South Africa, 2005.

[50] T. A. Okoror, C. O. Falade, A. Olorunlana, E. M. Walker, and O. T. Okareh, "Exploring the cultural context of HIV stigma on antiretroviral therapy adherence among people living with HIV/AIDS in Southwest Nigeria," *AIDS Patient Care and STDs*, vol. 27, no. 1, pp. 55–64, 2013.

[51] J. Aransiola, W. Imoyera, S. Olowookere, and C. Zarowsky, "Living well with HIV in Nigeria? Stigma and survival challenges preventing optimum benefit from an ART clinic," *Global Health Promotion*, vol. 21, no. 1, pp. 13–22, 2014.

[52] S. R. Schwartz, R. G. Nowak, I. Orazulike et al., "The immediate eff ect of the Same-Sex Marriage Prohibition Act on stigma, discrimination, and engagement on HIV prevention and treatment services in men who have sex with men in Nigeria: Analysis of prospective data from the TRUST cohort," *The Lancet HIV*, vol. 2, no. 7, pp. e299–e306, 2015.

[53] National Agency for the Conrol of AIDS, *National Policy on HIV/AIDS*, NACA, Abuja, Nigeria, 2009.

[54] National Agency for the Conrol of AIDS, *National HIV/AIDS Strategic Plan 2010-2015*, NACA, Abuja, Nigeria, 2010.

[55] National Agency for the Conrol of AIDS, *National Workplace Policy on HIV and AIDS*, NACA, Abuja, Nigeria, 2013.

[56] International Labour Organisation (ILO), *Recommendation concerning HIV and AIDS and the World of Work, 2010 (No. 200)*, ILO, Geneva, Switzerland, 2010.

[57] *A Popular Version of Nigeria's HIV and AIDS Anti-Discrimination Act, 2014: Individual Rights and Responsibilities*, Institutional Obligations! And Penalties, 2015.

[58] National Agency for the Conrol of AIDS, *Stigma and Discrimination Reduction in the National HIV/AIDS Response*, NACA, Abuja, Nigeria, 2016.

[59] UNAIDS, *Key programmes to reduce stigma and discrimination and increase access to justice in national HIV responses*, Joint United Nations Programme on HIV/AIDS, Geneva, Switzerland, 2012.

[60] *HIV Leadership through Accountability Programme: GNP+; NEPWHAN. PLHIV Stigma Index Nigeria Country Assessment. Amsterdam: GNP+*, 2011.

[61] National Agency for the Conrol of AIDS., *Legal Environment Assessment for HIV/AIDS Response in Nigeria*, NACA, Abuja, Nigeria, 2015.

[62] National HIV/AIDS & STIs Control Programme, *Integrated Biological and Behavioural Surveillance Survey (IBBSS) 2014 Report*, Federal Ministry of Health, Abuja, Nigeria, 2015.

[63] M. A. Shodimu, O. B. Yusuf, J. O. Akinyemi, A. F. Fagbamigbe, E. A. Bamgboye, E. Ngige et al., "Determinants of perceived stigmatizing and discriminating attitudes towards people living with HIV/AIDS among women of reproductive age in Nigeria," *Journal of AIDS and HIV Research*, vol. 9, no. 6, pp. 139–151, 2017.

15

# The Palatability of Lopinavir and Ritonavir Delivered by an Innovative Freeze-Dried Fast-Dissolving Tablet Formulation

**David W. Pittman,[1] Alexandra M. Brantly,[1] Alexandra L. Drobonick,[1] Hannah T. King,[1] Daniel C. Mesta,[1] Caroline G. Richards,[1] Manjari Lal,[2] and Manshun Lai[2]**

[1]*Department of Psychology, Wofford College, 429 North Church Street, Spartanburg, SC 29303, USA*
[2]*PATH, 2201 Westlake Avenue, Suite 200, Seattle, WA 98121, USA*

Correspondence should be addressed to David W. Pittman; pittmandw@wofford.edu

Academic Editor: David Katzenstein

Negative hedonic sensory qualities of HIV antiretroviral drugs often reduce patient adherence particularly in pediatric populations requiring oral consumption. This study examines the palatability of an innovative delivery mechanism utilizing a freeze-drying-in-blister approach to create fast-dissolving tablets (FDTs) containing a fixed-dose combination of lopinavir and ritonavir (LPV/r). Consumption patterns of solutions during brief-access and long-term testing and baby foodstuff consumption were analyzed to evaluate the orosensory detection and avoidance of placebo FDTs containing no LPV/r (FDT−) and FDTs containing LPV/r (FDT+). Rats showed no change in consumption patterns for the placebo FDT− compared with control solutions. Rats can detect but do not avoid FDT+ at body-weight-adjusted dosages in both brief-access (30-s) and long-term (23 h) consumption tests. There is an aversive response to concentrated doses of FDT+ during brief-access tests that cannot be masked by 25% sucrose. However, the strongest FDT+ concentration was not rejected when mixed with 50 g of applesauce, banana sauce, or rice cereal baby foodstuffs. The averseness of the FDT+ was associated with the presence of LPV/r and not the FDT− formulation itself. The novel FDT formulation appears to be a palatable delivery mechanism for oral antiretroviral pharmaceuticals especially when mixed with baby foodstuffs.

## 1. Introduction

As of 2015, there were an estimated 1.8 million children under the age of fourteen living with HIV, and only half of those children were receiving medical treatment [1]. One of the most common and successful treatments for HIV is antiretroviral therapy through pharmaceuticals such as the protease inhibitors lopinavir and ritonavir (LPV/r) [2]. LPV/r effectively reduces circulating HIV which in turn has been shown to reduce the risk of opportunistic infections in a pediatric population [3]. Despite a recommended twice-daily dosing regimen of LPV/r for patients as young as 14 days old [4], and even with recently approved LPV/r pellet formulation, poor palatability still exists, posing a challenge in patient compliance [5]. Furthermore, the current oral liquid formulation of LPV/r contains 42% ethanol (EtOH) and 15% propylene glycol which elicits an aversive response. In children under the age of four, taste and the inability to swallow were the most commonly reported problems with the adherence for either liquid or minitablet formulations of LPV/r [6, 7].

The feasibility of an innovative formulation developed using water soluble excipients to effectively deliver combination hydrophobic drugs LPV/r to newborns and infants was recently reported by PATH [8]. Using a freeze-drying-in-blister approach to create a fast-dissolving tablet (FDT) containing LPV/r, PATH was able to reconstitute a single dose of LPV/r with less than 1 mL of water. This small quantity of liquid allows for easier oral consumption of the antiretroviral drugs or the ability to add the drug to a small amount of baby foodstuff for consumption. In addition, the FDTs are heat and humidity stable eliminating the necessity for cold-chain transportation and storage required for the current oral liquid LPV/r medication.

Although ultimately of greatest interest, the use of a human taste panel to screen pharmaceutical drugs for palatability is not cost-effective or feasible in a timely manner. Furthermore, screening drug palatability in a human pediatric population presents even more challenges. The Sprague-Dawley rat is an invaluable model for examining taste perception as there is vast background knowledge of the rodent gustatory system with considerable evidence of similarities to the human gustatory system and taste perceptions [9–14]. The rat behavioral avoidance taste model has been validated as a useful surrogate test to quickly screen compounds that may produce bitter taste and masking agents that may increase the palatability of the drugs [15]. The goal of this study was to assess patterns of consumption related to the palatability of FDTs containing LPV/r when presented in brief-access gustatory palatability tests, long-term solution consumption tests, and foodstuff consumption tests. Given that the LPV/r within the freeze-dried FDTs may still elicit a bitter taste, additional goals of this study sought to identify concentrations of the bitter tastant quinine-HCl that match the licking behavior to the FDTs containing LPV/r and identify potential taste-masking agents to reduce any averseness associated with the drug or comparable quinine concentrations.

## 2. Materials and Methods

*2.1. Subjects.* Adult, male Sprague-Dawley rats, average body weight 264.6 ± 8.4 g (Charles River Laboratories, Raleigh, NC) were individually housed in transparent plastic cages in a temperature-controlled colony room on a 12-12-h light-dark cycle with lights out 30 minutes prior to the start of daily test sessions. Unless otherwise noted, rats had ad libitum access to Teklad 8604 rodent chow and deionized water. All experiments were conducted in accordance with the National Institutes of Health *Guide for the Care and Use of Laboratory Animals*, and all procedures were approved by the Institutional Animal Care and Use Committee of Wofford College.

*2.2. Chemical Stimuli.* All experimental stimuli were mixed daily immediately prior to each test session. In the brief-access gustatory palatability experiment, licking was assessed to four concentrations of LPV/r fast-dissolving tablets (FDT+) prepared as previously described [8]. Each FDT contains 80 mg lopinavir (LPV) and 20 mg ritonavir (r). The concentrations of FDT+ listed in order of increasing concentration were FDT 1 : 30 (1 tablet per 30 mL deionized water); FDT 1 : 3 (1 tablet per 3 mL deionized water), FDT 1 : 2 (1 tablet per 2 mL deionized water), and FDT 1 : 1 (1 tablet per 1 mL deionized water). The dilution of the FDT containing LPV/r at a ratio of 1 tablet to 30 mL solution is a body-weight-adjusted (BW) dosage for the rat (266 g) comparable to a 6-month-old human male at the 50 percentile of growth (8 kg). In addition to the FDT+, a placebo condition of a fast-dissolving tablet containing no LPV/r (FDT−) was also assessed. Three concentrations of the bitter taste stimulus quinine-HCl (1.5, 2.0 and 2.5 mM) were tested alone and with the addition of either 250 mM (8% w/w) or 750 mM (25% w/w) sucrose as taste-masking stimuli. Deionized water was always included as a test stimulus.

In the 23-h fluid consumption experiment, the placebo condition of an FDT− was tested along with the body-weight-adjusted dosage of LPV/r in FDTs (1 FDT+ : 30 mL water ratio) by dissolving 3 FDT+ or 3 FDT− in 3 mL of deionized water and adding 87 mL of either deionized water or whole milk to produce the following stimuli: water alone, water with FDT−, water with FDT+, milk alone, milk with FDT−, and milk with FDT+. The current liquid oral formulation of LPV/r added to 42% EtOH (42% EtOH LPV/r) and a vehicle 42% EtOH alone (42% EtOH) were also tested along with a body-weight-adjusted dosage of 3 mL of 42% EtOH with or without LPV/r added to 87 mL deionized water.

In the foodstuff consumption experiment, one FDT+ or one FDT− was dissolved in 1 mL deionized water and mixed thoroughly into 50 g samples of one of three baby foodstuffs: applesauce (Gerber 2nd Foods, Sitter, Walmart), banana sauce (Gerber 2nd Foods, Sitter, Walmart), or rice cereal single grain (10 g Gerber Rice Cereal, Supported Sitter, Walmart, plus 40 mL whole milk) to produce the following test stimuli: applesauce (AS), AS with FDT−, AS with FDT+, banana sauce (BS), BS with FDT−, BS with FDT+, rice cereal (RC), RC with FDT−, and RC with FDT+.

*2.3. Brief-Access Gustatory Palatability Tests.* Behavioral responses to taste solutions were assessed in an MS-160 contact lickometer (DiLog Instruments, Tallahassee FL). The MS-160 measures rat licking behavior at a resolution of 1 ms during the controlled presentation of up to 16 taste stimuli, as previously described [16, 17]. The MS-160 is housed within an acoustic isolation chamber with 7 dB of white noise. An intake fan and an exhaust fan are mounted on either side of the chamber to produce constant airflow along the axis of the stimulus delivery tray thus diluting and mixing potential olfactory cues during stimulus presentations. Rats ($n = 13$) were placed on a 23-h water restriction schedule during two training days and the duration of testing. Access to 1 h of supplemental water was given 15 minutes after the conclusion of each daily test session. The test stimuli were grouped into four stimulus sets which were presented in a single daily test session in the following order: quinine-HCl concentrations, FDT− and FDT+ concentrations, quinine-HCl plus sucrose-masking solutions, and FDT+ plus sucrose-masking solutions. Each test session consisted of three blocks of randomly ordered test stimuli, including deionized water with stimulus durations of 30 s, a wait time for the first lick of 30 s, and 10-s intervals in between trials.

The total number of licks, latency until first lick, and average interlick interval (ILI) per stimulus were averaged across the three presentations of each stimulus within each daily test session. Consumption of palatable taste solutions results in maximal licking rates with consistently brief ILIs. As taste solutions become less palatable and more aversive the number of licks decreases and the length of ILIs increases. All rats sampled at least one trial of each stimulus during each daily test session. All licking data were converted to a standardized lick ratio [18, 19], which accounts for individual differences in local lick rates independent of motivational state by dividing the licks for each stimulus by the subject's maximum potential lick rate. The maximum potential lick rate was determined by dividing the duration of the stimulus trial by the average ILI (in the range of 125 to 211 ms) during water training tests. This number represents the greatest number of licks each individual rat could perform in a 30-s-duration trial. By dividing the average licks per stimulus by the maximum possible number of licks, the standardized lick ratio becomes a ratio where 1.0 equals the maximum number of licks possible for each individual rat, 0.5 represents half of the maximal number of licks, and 0.0 represents no licks. The latency until the first lick is a measurement of stimulus control and the ability or lack thereof for nonoral cues, such as olfaction, to influence licking behavior. If the rat can detect the stimulus prior to licking the stimulus through either visual or olfactory cues, then the time to approach the spout and initiate the first lick will be longer for that stimulus. Rats had a wait time of 30 s to approach and initiate the trial (30 s duration) with their first lick. Consistent latencies to the first lick that are less than 10 s provide good evidence that rats are motivated to sample each solution with no influence of external cues. An omnibus repeated measures analysis of variance (ANOVA) was performed for all solutions. Post hoc ANOVAs were performed for each set of fluid type with pairwise comparisons (Bonferroni correction) identifying sources of significant ANOVA effects.

*2.4. 23-h Fluid Consumption Tests.* Consumption of solutions during 23-h test sessions was measured by an AC-108 single-spout contact lickometer (DiLog Instruments, Tallahassee, FL). The AC-108 measures licking behavior of up to eight spout lickometers simultaneously at a resolution of 1 ms for up to 23-h periods as previously described [20]. Three days prior to testing, rats ($n = 8$) were trained to lick in the AC-108 using a 23-h water restriction period followed by a 60-minute presentation of 200 mM sucrose in the AC-108. After training, rats were returned to ad libitum water access. Testing was conducted in two replicated phases. Using a within-subject design, each phase consisted of ten consecutive daily 23-h test sessions from 1500 to 1400 the following day. Between each test session from 1400 to 1500 the solutions were changed, chow consumption was measured, rats were weighed, and cages were cleaned. For the first eight test sessions, rats were given solutions in a counterbalanced design (Table 1). Due to the aversive nature of 42% EtOH and 42% EtOH + LPV/r, these stimuli were tested on days 9 and 10. Rats consumed very little of these aversive solutions, essentially inducing a water deprivation state during each 23-h test session. After each of these test sessions rats were given ad libitum water access during the 1-h break in testing from 1400 to 1500 to ensure the rats did not begin the next 23-h test session in a water-restricted state. After completion of test phase 1, rats were returned to their home cages with ad libitum water and food access for 14 days before test phase 2, which replicated phase 1 to provide a total of 16 data points for each condition.

Licks for each rat during the 23-h test sessions were grouped into meals initiated by 5 licks within 1 s and terminated by a pause of 600 s or greater. Consumption behaviors during the 23-h test session were quantified by total licks per session, latency until the first lick of the session, number of meals per session, chow consumption, and change in body weight. The pattern of licking within each meal of the test session was characterized through a microstructure analysis of licking behavior as previously described [20–23]. This analysis identifies whole-meal measures (meal lick count and meal duration) and intrameal licking patterns (number of bursts, size of bursts, mean burst duration, mean pause duration, and average lick rate in licks/s) in order to characterize taste-guided behaviors and behaviors influenced by postingestive feedback. Oromotor coordination was assessed by analysis of interlick intervals (ILIs) and the duration of tongue contact with the fluid spout. Licking bursts were defined by a 1-s pause in licking. Mean burst duration is the average length of time for each licking burst within the meal. Mean pause duration is the average length of time from the termination of a burst to the initiation of the next licking burst. Average lick rate was calculated by dividing the meal licks by the meal duration to determine the average number of licks per second. Contact duration was the duration in which the tongue made contact with the spout sufficient to provide electrical bridging. The number of ILIs in the 250–1,000-ms range was divided by the total number of ILIs from 50 ms to 1,000 ms, to yield an ILI ratio (%) reflecting the number of ILIs in the 250–1,000-ms range relative to the majority of ILIs in the meal. The meal pattern analysis variables were averaged across all meals within a single test session. An omnibus repeated measures ANOVA was performed using solutions and phases 1 and 2 as experimental variables for the 16 test sessions. There were no significant differences between phase 1 and phase 2 for any of the dependent variables; therefore the results were combined and post hoc repeated measures ANOVA was performed for each set of stimulus type with post hoc pairwise comparisons (Bonferroni correction) identifying sources of significant ANOVA effects.

*2.5. Foodstuff Consumption Tests.* All training and testing were conducted in 1 h sessions in standard transparent plastic cages. Foodstuffs (50-g samples) were placed in a heavy circular glass container (10 cm diameter) in the corner of the otherwise empty cage. All test sessions were videotaped in high-definition (1020 × 720) for offline behavioral analysis. Seven days prior to testing, rats ($n = 9$) were exposed to each foodstuff (AS, BS, and RC) in a 1-h training session to reduce neophobic responses during testing. Rats ($n = 9$) were given each foodstuff condition once in a counterbalanced design across nine consecutive days, as described in Table 2.

Feeding behavior was quantified through video analysis by experimenters who were blind to the test condition. Total food consumption (g) was used to calculate total calories consumed. Latency to first consumption, time spent feeding, time spent not feeding, number of feeding bouts (defined by a pause of feeding greater than 1 s), and the length of each feeding bout were measured. An omnibus repeated measures ANOVA was performed for all foodstuffs. Post hoc repeated measures ANOVA was performed for each set of food type with post hoc pairwise comparisons (Bonferroni correction) identifying sources of significant ANOVA effects.

TABLE 1: Schedule for the 23-h consumption test sessions of water (W) and milk (MS) alone, with placebo FDT− and with FDT+ and body-weight-adjusted (BW) and full-strength 42% ethanol (EtOH) with and without LPV/r.

| | Day 1 | Day 2 | Day 3 | Day 4 | Day 5 | Day 6 | Day 7 | Day 8 | Day 9 | Day 10 |
|---|---|---|---|---|---|---|---|---|---|---|
| Rat 1 | W | W + FDT+ | W + FDT− | MS | MS + FDT− | MS + FDT+ | BW 42% EtOH + LPV/r | BW 42% EtOH | 42% EtOH + LPV/r | 42% EtOH |
| Rat 2 | W + FDT+ | W + FDT− | MS | MS + FDT− | MS + FDT+ | BW 42% EtOH + LPV/r | BW 42% EtOH | W | 42% EtOH | 42% EtOH + LPV/r |
| Rat 3 | W + FDT− | MS | MS + FDT− | MS + FDT+ | BW 42% EtOH + LPV/r | BW 42% EtOH | W | W + FDT+ | 42% EtOH + LPV/r | 42% EtOH |
| Rat 4 | MS | MS + FDT− | MS + FDT+ | BW 42% EtOH + LPV/r | BW 42% EtOH | W | W + FDT+ | W + FDT− | 42% EtOH | 42% EtOH + LPV/r |
| Rat 5 | MS + FDT− | MS + FDT+ | BW 42% EtOH + LPV/r | BW 42% EtOH | W | W + FDT+ | W + FDT− | MS | 42% EtOH + LPV/r | 42% EtOH |
| Rat 6 | MS + FDT+ | BW 42% EtOH + LPV/r | BW 42% EtOH | W | W + FDT+ | W + FDT− | MS | MS + FDT− | 42% EtOH | 42% EtOH + LPV/r |
| Rat 7 | BW 42% EtOH + LPV/r | BW 42% EtOH | W | W + FDT+ | W + FDT− | MS | W + FDT− | MS + FDT+ | 42% EtOH + LPV/r | 42% EtOH |
| Rat 8 | BW 42% EtOH | W | W + FDT+ | W + FDT− | MS | MS + FDT− | MS + FDT+ | BW 42% EtOH + LPV/r | 42% EtOH | 42% EtOH + LPV/r |

TABLE 2: Schedule for daily 1-h consumption tests of applesauce (AS), banana sauce (BS), and rice cereal (RC), with placebo FDT− and with FDT+.

| | Day 1 | Day 2 | Day 3 | Day 4 | Day 5 | Day 6 | Day 7 | Day 8 | Day 9 |
|---|---|---|---|---|---|---|---|---|---|
| Rat 1 | AS | AS + FDT+ | AS + FDT− | RC | RC + FDT+ | RC + FDT− | BS | BS + FDT+ | BS + FDT− |
| Rat 2 | BS | BS + FDT+ | BS + FDT− | AS | AS + FDT+ | AS + FDT− | RC | RC + FDT+ | RC + FDT− |
| Rat 3 | RC | RC + FDT+ | RC + FDT− | BS | BS + FDT+ | BS + FDT− | AS | AS + FDT+ | AS + FDT− |
| Rat 4 | AS + FDT+ | AS + FDT− | AS | RC + FDT+ | RC + FDT− | RC | BS + FDT+ | BS + FDT− | BS |
| Rat 5 | BS + FDT+ | BS + FDT− | BS | AS + FDT+ | AS + FDT− | AS | RC + FDT+ | RC + FDT− | RC |
| Rat 6 | RC + FDT+ | RC + FDT− | RC | BS + FDT+ | BS + FDT− | BS | AS + FDT+ | AS + FDT− | AS |
| Rat 7 | AS + FDT− | AS | AS + FDT+ | RC + FDT− | RC | RC + FDT+ | BS + FDT− | BS | BS + FDT+ |
| Rat 8 | BS + FDT− | BS | BS + FDT+ | AS + FDT− | AS | AS + FDT+ | RC + FDT− | RC | RC + FDT+ |
| Rat 9 | RC + FDT− | RC | RC + FDT+ | BS + FDT− | BS | BS + FDT+ | AS + FDT− | AS | AS + FDT+ |

## 3. Results

*3.1. Brief-Access Gustatory Palatability Tests.* There was a significant main effect ($F_{[5,60]} = 664.270$, $p < .001$) of increasing the LPV/r FDT+ concentration on the standardized lick ratio during 30-s trials (Figure 1(a)) with post hoc pairwise comparisons revealing no difference between water, the FDT− placebo, and the body-weight-adjusted dosage of FDT 1:30 ratio (tablet to mL water). All three of these solutions elicited significantly higher licking than the remainder of increased FDT+ concentrations (1:3, 1:2, 1:1; all $p < .001$). Lastly, the strongest concentration of FDT+ (1:1) had significantly fewer licks than all of the other stimuli (all $p < .01$). As shown in Figure 1(b), a significant main effect of concentration

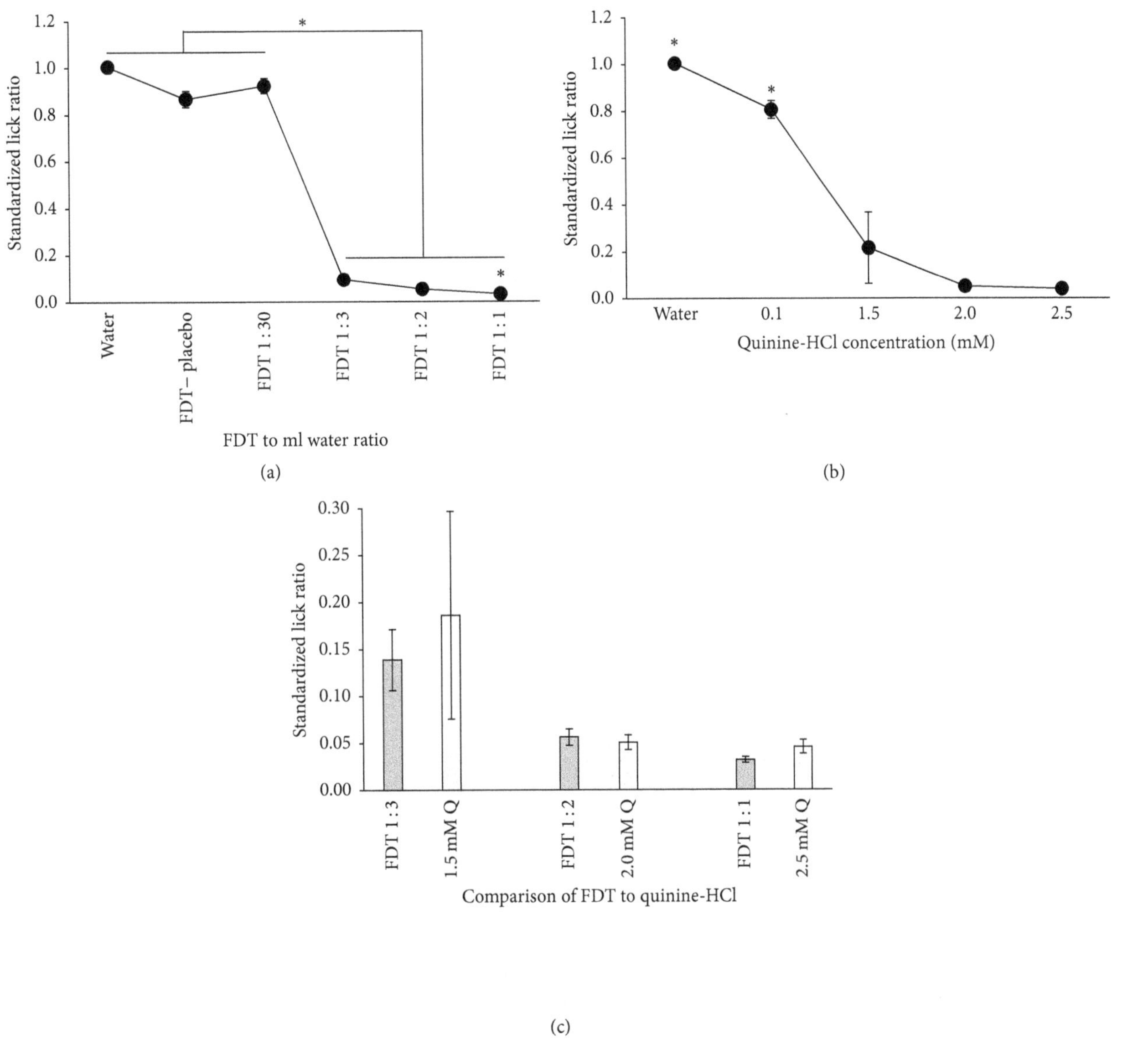


FIGURE 1: Average licks to stimuli normalized to licks to water in water-restricted rats ($n = 13$) with SEM represented in errors bars. (a) Stars represent significant differences ($p < .01$) in licking to water and body-weight-adjusted FDT+ (FDT 1:30) compared with concentrated FDT+ ratios of tablets dissolved in mL water with FDT 1:1 having significantly less licks than all stimuli. (b) Stars represent significant differences ($p < .01$) in licking to water and increasing concentrations of quinine-HCl. (c) A comparison of licking to concentrated FDT+ and high concentrations of quinine (Q).

($F_{[4,48]} = 41.288$, $p < .001$) revealed that moderate to high concentrations of the prototypical bitter tastant, quinine-HCl, evoked reductions in licking compared with water and a low quinine concentration (0.1 mM). Figure 1(c) compares the reduced licking for the three highest concentrations of FDT+ to the moderate to high quinine concentrations. Pairwise comparisons reveal no difference in licking between the three matched concentrations of FDT+ and quinine shown in Figure 1(c).

In an attempt to reduce the averseness of the concentrated FDT+ and quinine, either 250 mM sucrose (8% w/w) or 750 mM sucrose (25% w/w) was added to each concentration of the aversive stimuli. While the addition of sucrose did not significantly increase the licking to FDT+ (Figure 2(a)), there was a main effect of FDT+ concentration ($F_{[2,24]} = 6.780$, $p = .005$) with pairwise comparisons showing FDT 1:3 > FDT 1:2 > FDT 1:1 (all $p < .01$). As shown in Figure 2(b), sucrose was effective at masking the averseness of quinine ($F_{[2,24]} = 33.491$, $p < .001$) with pairwise comparisons showing the addition of 250 mM sucrose significantly increased licking for 2.0 mM and 2.5 mM quinine (both $p < 0.5$) and the addition of 750 mM sucrose increased licking across all three quinine concentrations (all $p < 0.01$) compared with the quinine alone stimuli.

The ILI (duration between each lick in ms) is a measurement of the rate of licking during a trial and can be associated

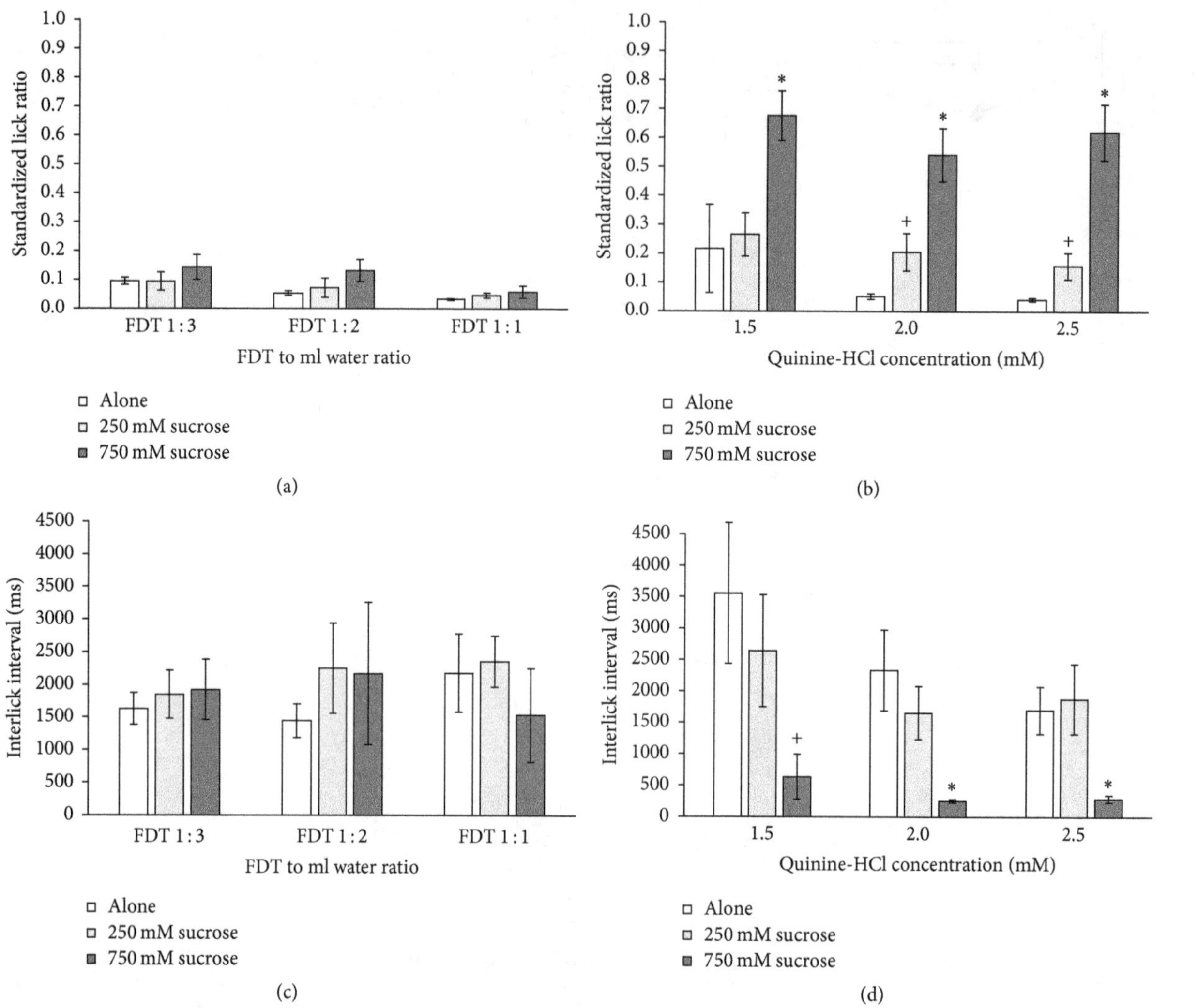


Figure 2: Average licks (a and b) and interlick intervals (c and d) to FDT (a and c) and quinine (b and d) with and without 250 mM or 750 mM sucrose as a masking agent with SEM represented in errors bars. (a) Sucrose did not increase licking to FDT+. (b) Star ($p < .01$) and plus ($p < .05$) symbols represent significant increases in licking when sucrose was added to quinine-HCl. (c) Sucrose did not affect the interlick intervals for FDT+. (d) Star ($p < .01$) and plus ($p < .05$) symbols represent significant decreases in the interlick interval when 750 mM sucrose was added to quinine-HCl.

with the palatability of a taste solution. When rats encounter appetitive stimuli, they tend to produce very consistent ILIs in the range of 150–200 ms in duration. When encountering a negative hedonic stimulus, rats will perform stereotypical oromotor responses such as gaping and tongue protrusions in response to the aversive taste stimulus [10]. These gapes and tongue protrusions cause a lengthening of the ILI to the range of 1,000–3,000 ms, as shown in Figures 2(c) and 2(d). In Figure 2(c), it is evident that the two sucrose concentrations did not mask the aversive quality of the FDT+ and there was virtually no change in the long-duration ILIs; however, in Figure 2(d), there is a significant ($F_{[2,24]} = 9.779$, $p = .001$) shortening of the ILI when 750 mM sucrose was added to the quinine concentrations compared with quinine alone (1.5 mM $p = .047$; 2.0 mM $p = .017$; 2.5 mM $p = .012$). This is evidence that 750 mM sucrose effectively suppressed the stereotypical aversive oromotor responses normally elicited by strong concentrations of quinine.

There were no significant effects on the latency to approach and lick the spout for any of the stimuli. Across all trials and stimuli, rats consistently approached and licked the spout within the first 10 s of the trial, demonstrating equivalent motivation to sample the stimuli with no influence of external guiding cues.

*3.2. 23-h Fluid Consumption Test.* There was a slight decrease in the normal consummatory behavior when LPV/r in a fast-dissolving tablet (FDT+ 1 : 30 BW) was added to either water ($F_{[2,28]} = 10.702$, $p < .001$) or milk ($F_{[2,28]} = 19.395$, $p < .001$). As shown in Figure 3(a), the total number of licks in a 23-h test session was slightly lower for both water containing FDT+ and milk containing FDT+ compared with either solution alone or when the placebo FDT− was added

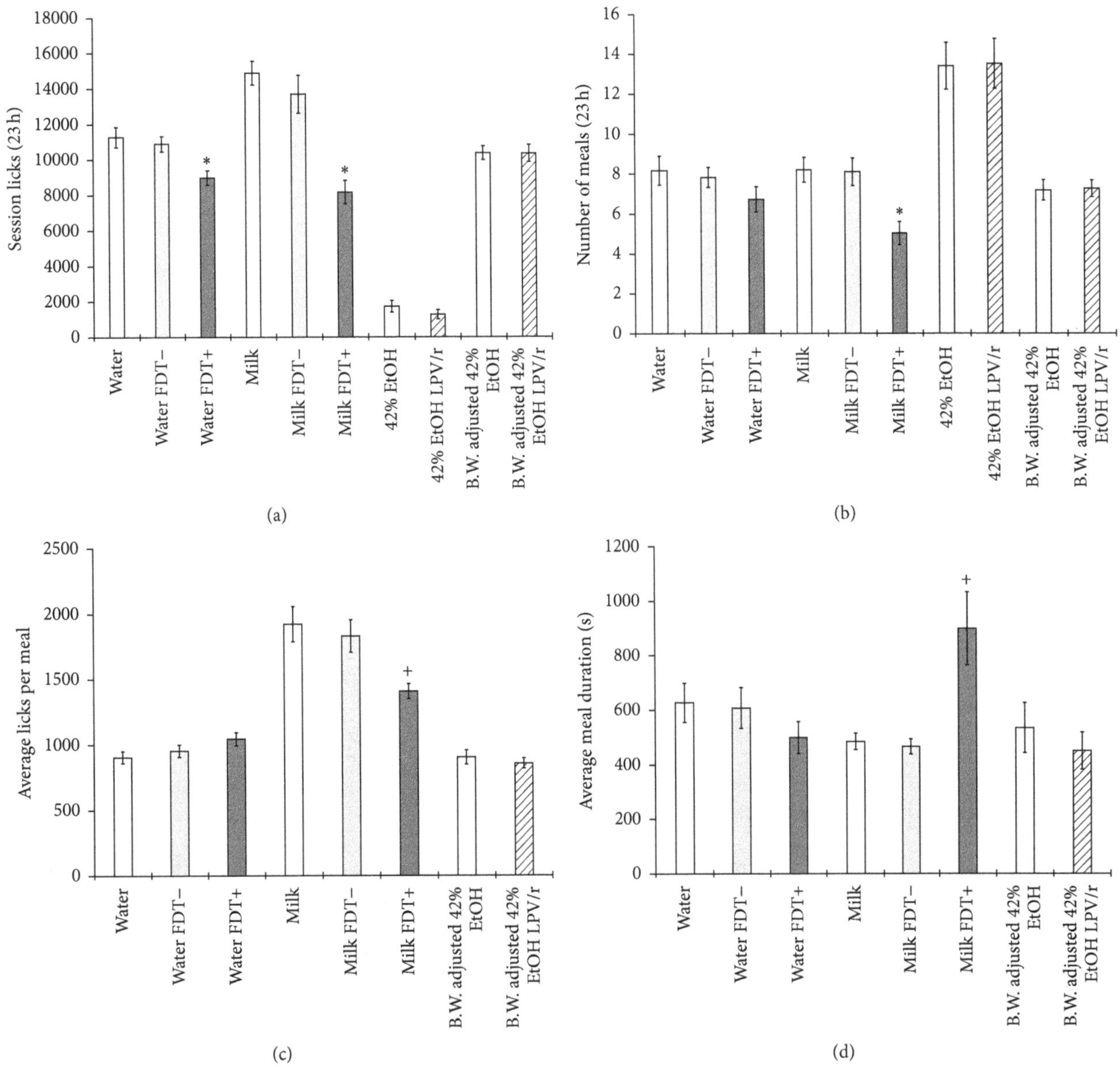


FIGURE 3: Meal ingestion analysis during 23-h consumption tests with bars representing the means with SEM error bars. Stars represent significant differences ($p < .01$) between solutions containing FDT+ (dark bars) and control solutions (open bars). (a) Total licks to single test solutions. (b) The number of meals defined by pauses greater than 10 minutes. (c) Licks per meal averaged across the test session. (d) Duration of meals averaged across the test session.

to the solutions. Rats showed a strong aversion to both 42% EtOH and 42% EtOH containing LPV/r, failing to consume sufficient fluid in 23 h to meet their daily hydration need. As shown in Figure 4, this water-deprived state significantly reduced chow consumption ($F_{[9,126]} = 82.090$, $p < .001$) and body weight ($F_{[9,126]} = 47.755$, $p < .001$) during the EtOH test sessions (all $p < .01$ compared with all other solutions except each other). There were insufficient licks during the ethanol sessions to allow any meal pattern analysis and therefore the two EtOH solutions were excluded from further meal pattern analyses (Figures 3(c) and 3(d)).

A meal pattern analysis examining the number, duration, and licks per meal during the 23-h test session can identify the source of decreased licking to water with FDT+ and milk with FDT+. While there was a significant decrease in total licks to water with FDT+ compared with the control stimuli, the decrease was so subtle that there were no significant differences in the number of meals, duration of meals, or licks per meal. There was a slight decrease in both the number and duration of meals that likely underlies the overall decrease in total licks to water with FDT−. In contrast, the greater decrease in total licks for milk with FDT+ is reflected in both a significant decrease in the number of meals (Figure 3(b), $F_{(2,28)} = 9.083$, $p = .001$) and the average licks per meal (Figure 3(c), $F_{(2,28)} = 6.440$, $p = .005$). Interestingly there was also a large significant increase in average meal duration

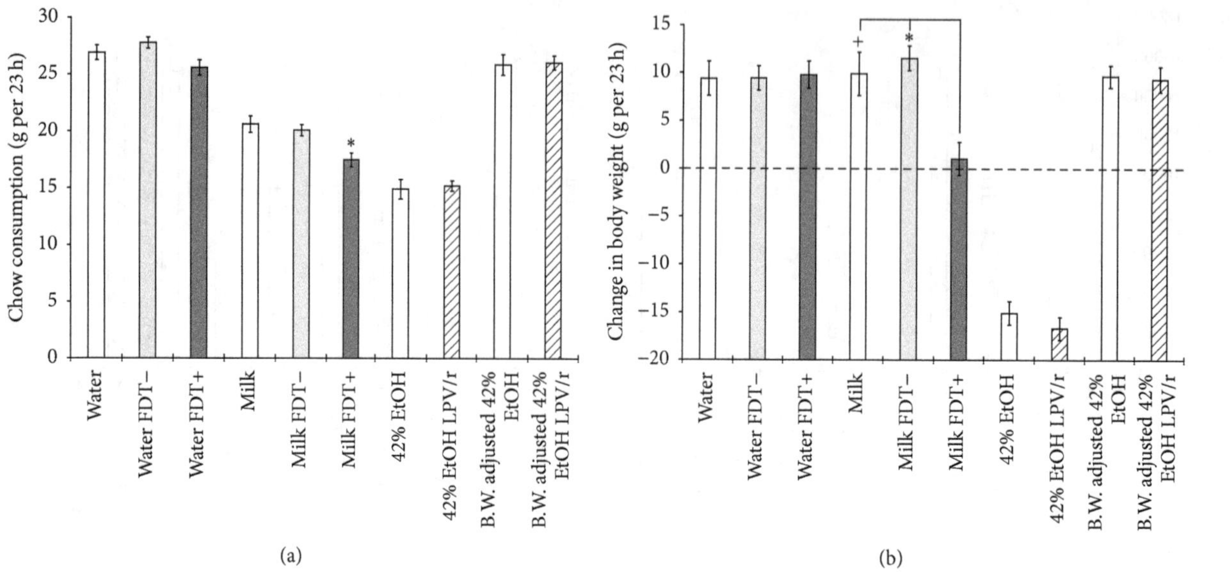

FIGURE 4: Solid food consumption (a) and changes in body weight (b) during the 23-h solution test sessions. Star ($p < .01$) and plus ($p < .05$) symbols represent significant decreases for the FDT+ compared with control solutions.

(Figure 3(d), $F_{(2,28)} = 9.835$, $p = .001$), indicating a slower rate of ingestion during the meal possibly due to negative postingestive effects produced by milk containing FDT+. Another potential indicator of negative postingestive actions of milk containing FDT+ is a reduction in the ad libitum chow consumed and decreased body weight during the 23-h test session.

Figure 4(a) shows a significant reduction in chow consumption for all of the milk solutions and the two 42% EtOH solutions ($F_{[9,126]} = 82.090$, $p < .001$). The reduction of chow during the EtOH test sessions is likely due to the water/fluid deprivation state while the reduction of chow for milk alone and milk with FDT− is likely due to the extra calories consumed in the milk itself; however, compared with milk alone and milk with FDT−, there was also a further significant decrease in chow consumption, specifically for milk containing FDT+ ($F_{[2,28]} = 22.666$, $p < .001$). The reduction in chow consumption combined with lowering the milk consumption during the test containing FDT+ resulted in a net weight gain of zero over the 23-h test session (Figure 4(b)) compared with a normal gain of 10 g for milk and milk with FDT− ($F_{[2,28]} = 22.666$, $p < .001$).

Within each meal, rats consumed the test solutions in a stereotypical manner with bursts of licking separated by pauses greater than 1 s. The number of bursts within a meal significantly increased for both water ($F_{[2,28]} = 11.363$, $p < .001$) and milk ($F_{[2,28]} = 8.494$, $p = .001$) containing FDT+ compared with the control solutions (Figure 5(a)). As each burst is defined by a pause, an increase in the number of bursts directly corresponds to an increase in the number of pauses. The duration of pauses within a meal is related to the palatability of, or motivation to consume, a taste solution. As palatability decreases and the averseness of a taste solution increases the pause durations between licking bursts will increase. The smaller the pause duration is, the more motivated the rat is to consume the solution. As shown in Figure 5(b), both milk alone and milk plus FDT− have very low pause durations, indicating that once rats initiated licking in a meal, their consummatory behavior was very driven, which resulted in fewer and shorter breaks. When FDT+ was added to water, there was no effect on pause duration, indicating that FDT+ alone does not produce a change in the hedonic value of water; however, the addition of FDT+ to milk appears to produce an interaction that results in significantly longer pause durations ($F_{[2,28]} = 14.798$, $p < .001$). This interaction between milk and FDT+ appears to produce a negative hedonic value (demonstrated by more frequent and longer pauses) that decreases normal motivation to consume milk or milk with FDT−.

Licking within the first minute of each meal is presumably under the influence of orosensory cues rather than postingestive cues or motivational state. Figure 6(a) reveals consistent licking at near-maximal rates for all stimuli except water and milk containing FDT+. The addition of FDT+ to water significantly reduced the licks in the first minute of each meal ($F_{[2,28]} = 12.758$, $p < .001$) compared with water alone ($p = .001$) and water plus FDT− ($p = .004$), and the addition of FDT+ to the milk solution also significantly reduced the licks in the first minute of each meal ($F_{[2,28]} = 70.053$, $p < .001$) compared with milk alone ($p < .001$) and milk plus FDT− ($p < .001$). Bursts of licking are the result of a central pattern generator that produces reflexive licking with consistent ILIs between 150 and 170 ms in duration [24–27]. As shown in Figure 6(b), these ILIs have extremely low variability and are consistent across all test stimuli, indicating no impairment or influence on the motor system. Typically less than 5% of the ILIs within a burst exceed 250 ms in duration except when rats encounter an aversive taste stimulus. In that case, rats exhibit stereotypical oromotor behaviors of gaping (wide stretches of the mouth)

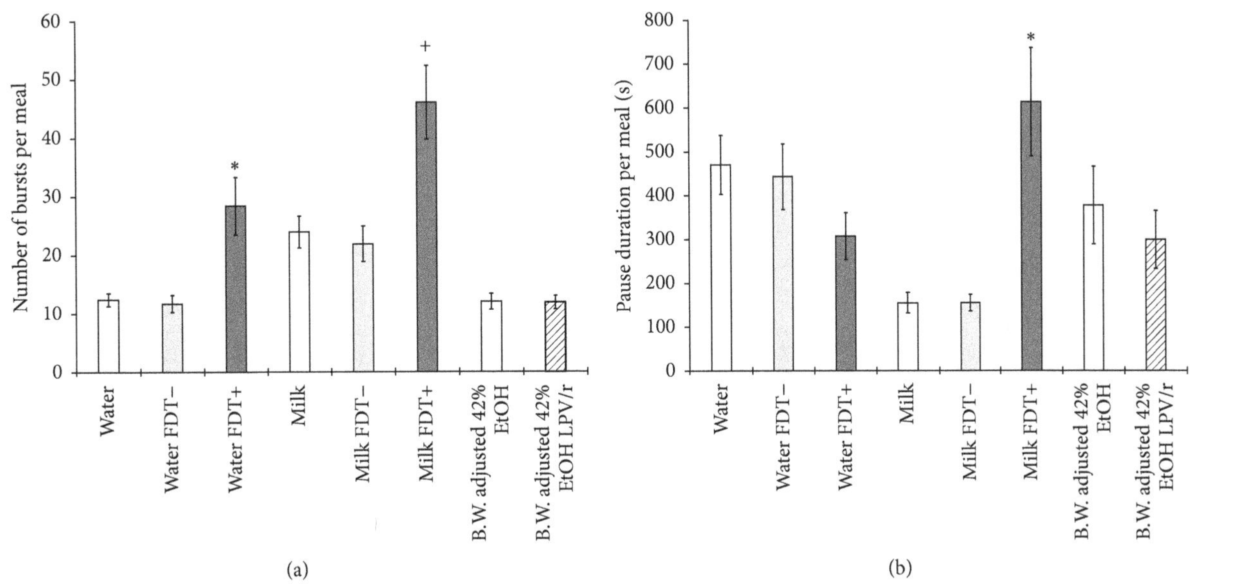


FIGURE 5: Analyses of licking patterns within meals with bars representing means and SEM error bars. (a) The average number of licking bursts defined by a pause ≥ 1 second. Star ($p < .01$) and plus ($p < .05$) symbols represent significant increases in bursts of licking for FDT+. (b) Cumulative time spent not licking during a meal. The star ($p < .01$) represents a significant increase in time spent paused for FDT+ in milk.

and lateral tongue protrusions between licks, increasing the percentage of ILIs in the range of 250 to 1,000 ms. As shown in Figure 6(c), the addition of FDT+ to both water ($F_{[2,28]} = 24.453$, $p < .001$) and milk ($F_{[2,28]} = 11.857$, $p < .001$) significantly increases the percentage of ILIs greater than 250 ms compared with water and milk control solutions.

*3.3. Foodstuffs Consumption.* Overall, the consumption of foodstuffs was significantly different ($F_{[2,16]} = 16.420$, $p < .001$), with increasing consumption from AS < BS < RC, which was the most palatable foodstuff. Figure 7(a) shows the consumption of the three foodstuffs with and without FDT− and FDT+. There was a significant main effect of condition for all three foodstuffs: AS ($F_{[2,16]} = 8.113$, $p = .004$), BS ($F_{[2,16]} = 7.431$, $p = .005$), and RC ($F_{[2,16]} = 4.377$, $p = .030$), indicating that the pattern of food consumption varied across conditions. However, post hoc pairwise comparisons yield no significant differences between the foodstuff conditions for AS or RC, meaning that no comparisons between any two conditions could account for the significant main effect. There were significant pairwise comparisons for the BS, revealing significantly more consumption of BS with FDT− compared with BS alone ($p = .041$) or BS with FDT+ ($p = .030$).

The latency until first consumption can be a measure of palatability with more palatable foods having a shorter latency until first consumption. A significant main effect of foodstuffs ($F_{[2,16]} = 4.377$, $p = .030$) indicated that RC was more palatable with pairwise comparisons, showing that RC had shorter latencies (20.2 s) than both AS (163.0 s, $p = .017$) and BS (105.3 s, $p = .039$). There was no effect of FDT− or FDT+ condition on the latency to consumption within each foodstuff.

Within the meal, feeding bouts were defined by pauses in consumption greater than 1 s. There was a significant effect ($F_{[2,16]} = 9.014$, $p = .002$) to increase the number of feeding bouts when adding FDT− ($p = .039$) or FDT+ ($p = .002$) to RC compared with RC alone (Figure 7(b)). However, there was no effect of adding FDT− or FDT+ on the length of the feeding bouts within each foodstuff (Figure 7(c)). There was a main effect ($F_{[2,16]} = 7.854$, $p = .004$) of foodstuffs on feeding bout length for RC compared with AS ($p = .10$), again indicating a greater palatability and increased motivation to consume the RC foodstuff. There were no significant effects of FDT− or FDT+ on the calories consumed or the total time spent feeding for any of the foodstuffs.

## 4. Discussion

In the present study, avoidance of LPV/r (FDT+) during brief-access tests demonstrated an aversive orosensory component that was attributed to the LPV/r component and not the FDT formulation (FDT−) and furthermore this averseness could not be masked by sucrose. Long-term solution consumption of a body-weight-adjusted LPV/r (FDT+) dosage was mildly aversive in water and interacted with milk to produce a negative hedonic quality but was significantly more palatable than the body-weight-adjusted standard formulation of LPV/r in 42% EtOH. Finally, small quantities of baby food sufficiently masked any negative sensory components of LPV/r (FDT+), suggesting delivery of the drug in food is the most successful method for patient adherence.

*4.1. Palatability of FDT with and without LPV/r.* Licking during brief-access-duration trials is governed by sensory

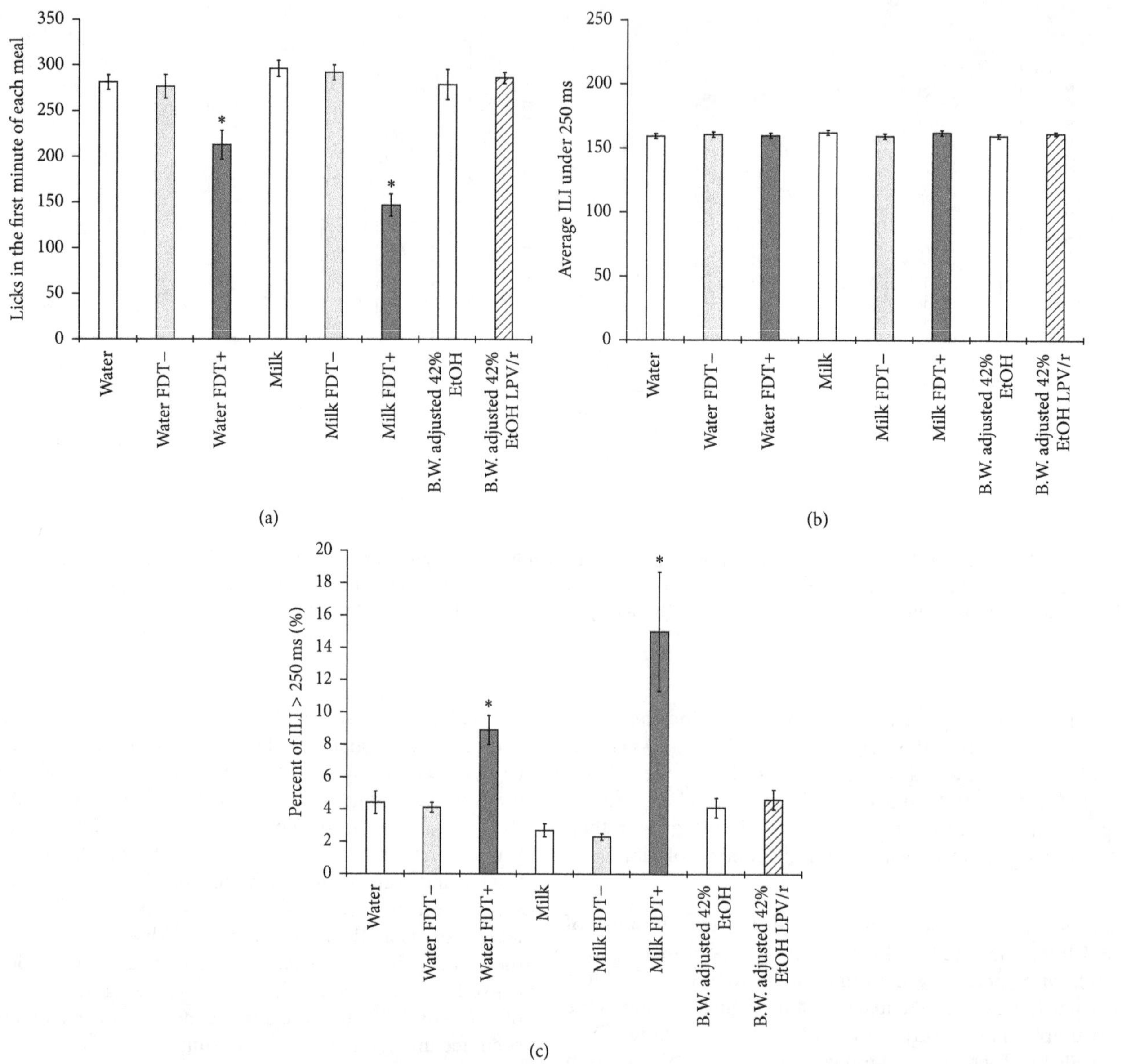


FIGURE 6: Analyses of intrameal licking patterns associated with palatability with bars representing means and SEM error bars. (a) Licks in the first 60 s of each meal. Stars represent significant ($p < .01$) decreases in licking to the FDT+ solutions. (b) The average interlick interval (ILI) when less than 250 ms. (c) The percentage of interlick intervals in the range of 250–1,000 ms with stars representing significant ($p < .01$) increases in longer ILI for FDT+.

cues from the oral cavity as opposed to postingestive feedback. When motivated to lick by water restriction, rats will decrease from a maximal lick rate when a stimulus elicits sufficient negative hedonic orosensory cues. Rats did not avoid FDT+ at a body-weight-adjusted dosage but showed strong avoidance of concentrated FDT+ doses. Licking to quinine at high concentrations could be matched to the FDT+ doses providing an index of the potential averseness of the FDT+. When rats consume an aversive tastant, such as quinine, they perform reflexive oromotor responses known as taste reactivity [10]. Grill and Norgren [10] classically defined the taste reactivity rejection responses to strong quinine concentrations as a series of gapes and lateral tongue movements that interrupt a rat's stereotypical rhythmic licking behavior. Gape series typically include 2 to 6 gapes of 166 ms in duration with 85–115-ms intergape intervals followed by singular lateral tongue protrusions (85–215 ms), producing a total interruption in the ILI ranging from 600 to 1,800 ms. Rats motivated by water restriction consistently demonstrate ILIs ranging from 150 to 170 ms when licking neutral or appetitive stimuli; however, as shown in Figures 2(c) and 2(d), there is a substantial increase in the ILIs for the strong quinine and concentrated FDT+ ratios. Negative taste reactivity responses (gapes and lateral tongue movements) likely account for the increased ILI durations in both cases. The similarity between the strong quinine and concentrated

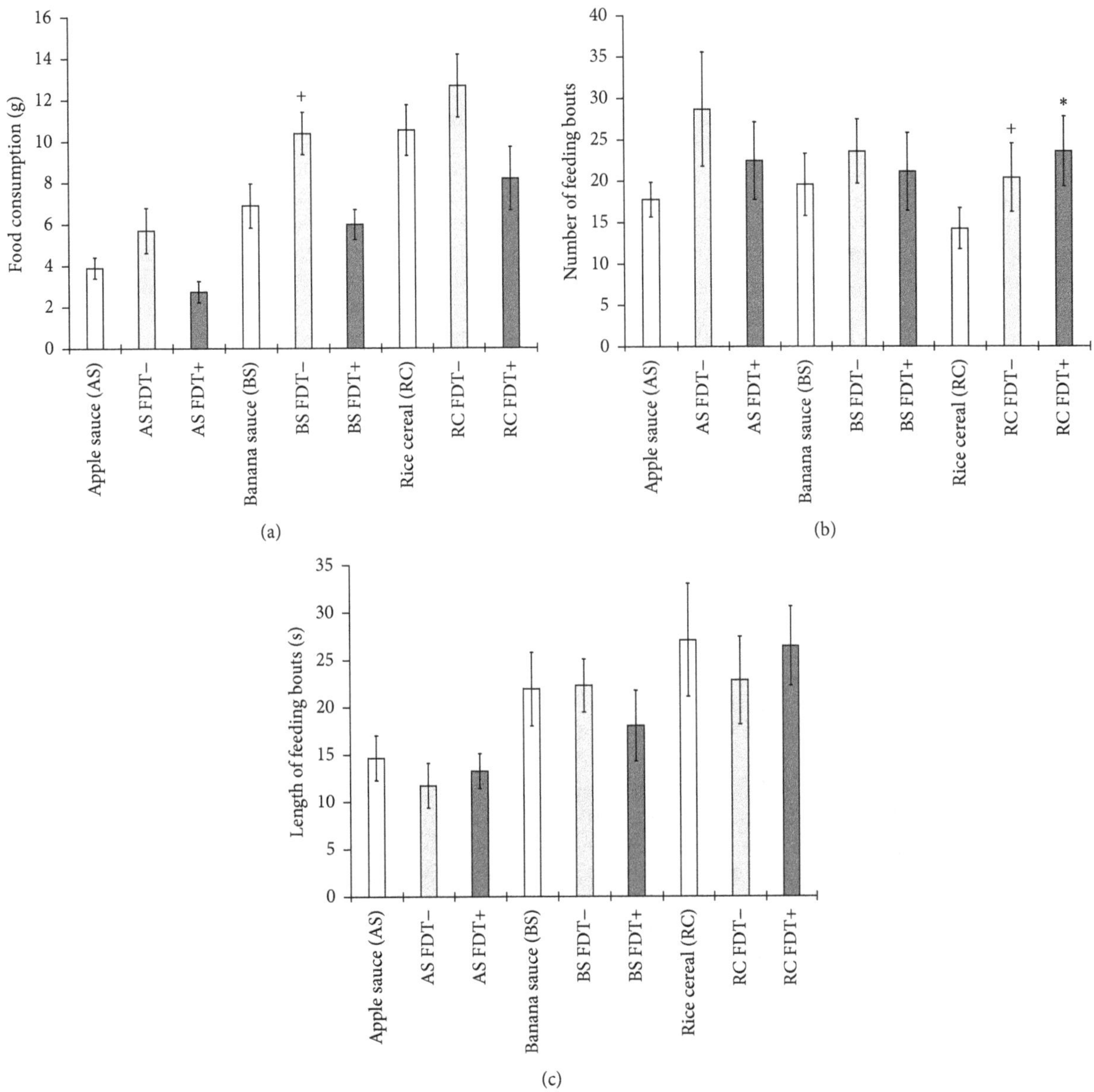

FIGURE 7: Consumption patterns of applesauce (AS), banana sauce (BS), or rice cereal (RC) alone (open bars), with the FDT− placebo (light bars) and the FDT+ (dark bars) with bars representing means with SEM error bars. Star ($p < .01$) and plus ($p < .05$) symbols represent significant increases compared with control foodstuffs (open bars). (a) Total grams consumed during the 1-h consumption test. (b) Average number of feeding bouts defined by a pause ≥ 1 second. (c) Average length of each feeding bout.

FDT+ ILIs suggests that the FDT containing the LPV/r elicits aversive orosensory signals not unlike strong bitter tastants, whereas the ILIs for the placebo FDT− (166.3 ± 8.4) and body-weight-adjusted FDT 1 : 30 (201.9 ± 21.4) did not differ from water (150.7 ± 2.3).

During long-term 23-h tests, rats were able to discern a difference between the placebo FDT− and the FDT+ containing LPV/r, demonstrating a slight reduction in licking to the FDT+ compared with control and FDT− solutions; however, this slight decrease is not indicative of a strong aversive sensation, as seen with the dramatic reduction in 42% EtOH with and without LPV/r (Figure 3(a)). As discussed below, the consumption patterns of milk with FDT+ reveal a potential negative postingestive influence on consumption. However, there was no evidence of postingestive influences on the consumption patterns of water containing FDT+. The decreases in licks during the first minute of each meal and increases in the percentage of ILIs greater than 250 ms suggest that FDT+ can be detected in water and that the orosensory perception is mildly aversive (Figure 6). Thus, masking of the FDT+ may be required for maximal patient adherence. Overall, the long-term consumption patterns support the evidence from brief-access tests that body-weight-adjusted FDT+ is detectable but not strongly aversive to rats and that placebo FDT− is treated no differently than control solutions. Therefore, it can be concluded that the aversive sensory signals are associated with the presence of LPV/r and not the formulation of the freeze-dried FDT suspension.

*4.2. Masking of FDT Containing LPV/r.* While sucrose was sufficient to mask the bitterness of high quinine concentrations, the lack of masking by sucrose of the averseness of FDT+ suggests that FDT+ may elicit negative sensory cues other than bitter taste. As shown in Figure 2(d), 750 mM (25% w/w) sucrose effectively eliminated negative taste reactivity behaviors to the strong quinine as represented by ILIs less than 500 ms. This suggests that sucrose had the ability to mask the strong quinine in a manner that eliminated the gaping and lateral tongue movement reflexes which produce longer ILIs. However, the same 750 mM sucrose had no effect on the ILIs for any of the concentrated FDT+ ratios. This suggests that the negative taste reactivity behaviors were still elicited by the FDT+ formulation even with the addition of sucrose (Figure 2(c)).

In contrast to concentrated FDT+ 1 : 1 ratio avoidance when presented in solution form, when the same single FDT+ in one mL of water ratio was mixed into 50 g of baby foodstuffs, there was no evidence of avoidance. In fact, the number of feeding bouts increased for RC when FDT+ was added to it. The presence of calories in foodstuffs and the ability of complex foodstuffs to mask nongustatory orosensory cues such as tactile sensations are two differences between solution and baby foodstuff testing paradigms that could explain the differential avoidance of FDT+. The inability of caloric content in 750 mM sucrose to mask FDT+ suggests that calories alone are not sufficient to overcome the negative hedonic value associated with concentrated FDT+. Therefore, it is likely that the baby foodstuffs were more efficient at masking negatively associated olfactory, textural, lubricious, or astringent trigeminal sensations potentially associated with FDT+.

*4.3. Interactions between Milk and FDT+.* The pattern of consumption of milk containing FDT+ during the 23-h long-term tests suggests negative postingestive influences. The reduction in licking to milk and FDT+ was due to several factors, including a decrease in the number of licking sessions (meals) and a decrease in the average licks per meal. Accompanying the decrease in licks per meal was a significant increase in meal duration rather than a decrease in meal duration, which might be expected. The increase in meal duration coupled with a decrease in licks per meal reflects a slower lick rate with more frequent and lengthy pauses during the meal and fewer licks per burst. This slower pattern of consumption is associated with negative postingestive influences such as gastric distress [28–30]. Dextran, a polymer bulking agent in the FDT, has been reported to interact with casein proteins in milk through electrostatic interaction, causing aggregation leading to destabilization of milk. It is possible that destabilized milk may have altered properties, thereby impacting the sensory response or digestion in rodents [31–33]. The decrease in chow consumption and body weight selectively during the milk with FDT+ test sessions further supports the premise that negative postingestive feedback such as gastric distress was influencing the consummatory behavior of the rats.

## 5. Conclusions

The novel delivery mechanism of LPV/r contained in freeze-dried FDTs has several innovative improvements to the standard liquid formulation, including heat stability, ease of distribution, and ready reconstitution in a small (1 mL) liquid sample of water [8]. This study suggests that the FDT–placebo formulation itself is palatable and does not influence consumption patterns when dissolved in water, milk, or baby foodstuffs. The presence of LPV/r in the FDT+ formulation is mildly aversive at body-weight-adjusted dosage and strongly aversive at concentrated dosages (1 : 3, 1 : 2, and 1 : 1 FDT+ : mL $H_2O$). Sucrose was an ineffective masking agent of the concentrated FDT+; however, baby foodstuffs did effectively mask any negative hedonic qualities of the strongest 1 : 1 FDT+ concentration. Therefore, consumption of the FDT+ with baby food may result in maximal patient adherence for antiretroviral therapy.

## Disclosure

All authors contributed to the interpretation of the data analysis and manuscript composition and revision and approved the final draft. An earlier version of this work was presented as a poster at the Thirty-Ninth Annual Meeting of the Association for Chemoreception Sciences. The findings and conclusions contained within are those of the authors and do not necessarily reflect positions or policies of the Gates Foundation.

## Conflicts of Interest

All authors declare that they have no conflicts of interest.

## Acknowledgments

David W. Pittman, Alexandra M. Brantly, Manjari Lal, and Manshun Lai conceived and developed the studies. David W. Pittman and Alexandra M. Brantly conducted the long-term access and food intake studies. David W. Pittman, Alexandra M. Brantly, Alexandra L. Drobonick, Hannah T. King, Daniel C. Mesta, and Caroline G. Richards conducted the brief-access study. Alexandra M. Brantly, Alexandra L. Drobonick, Kassie Franck, Tonya Foster, and Amber Parnell (all Wofford College) collected the food-intake data. David W. Pittman and Alexandra M. Brantly analyzed all data. Funding for this study was provided by Wofford College and PATH's Innovation Fund, which was supported by a grant from the Bill & Melinda Gates Foundation [OPP1110874].

## References

[1] The Joint United Nations Programme on HIV/AIDS (UNAIDS), AIDSinfo, UNAIDS, Geneva, Switzerland, 2016, http://aidsinfo.unaids.org/.

[2] National Institutes of Health, *Kaletra Dosage, Side Effects*, Rockville, Maryland, United States of America, 2016, https://aidsinfo.nih.gov/drugs/316/lopinavir—ritonavir/0/patient.

[3] M.-R. B-Lajoie, O. Drouin, G. Bartlett et al., "Incidence and Prevalence of Opportunistic and Other Infections and the Impact of Antiretroviral Therapy among HIV-infected Children in Low- and Middle-income Countries: A Systematic Review and Meta-analysis," *Clinical Infectious Diseases*, vol. 62, no. 12, pp. 1586–1594, 2016.

[4] V. Prasad, U. Schwerdtfeger, F. El-Awa, D. Bettcher, and V. da Costa e Silva, "Closing the door on illicit tobacco trade, opens the way to better tobacco control," *Eastern Mediterranean Health Journal*, vol. 21, no. 6, pp. 379-380, 2015.

[5] World Health Organization, *United Nations International Children's Emergency Fund,Fact sheet on lopinavir and ritonavir (Lpv/R) oral pellets*, World Health Organization, Geneva, Switzerland, 2015.

[6] V. Musiime, Q. Fillekes, A. Kekitiinwa et al., "The pharmacokinetics and acceptability of lopinavir/ritonavir minitab sprinkles, tablets, and syrups in african HIV-infected children," *Journal of Acquired Immune Deficiency Syndromes*, vol. 66, no. 2, pp. 148–154, 2014.

[7] A. F. Schlatter, A. R. Deathe, and R. C. Vreeman, "The need for pediatric formulations to treat children with HIV," *AIDS Research and Treatment*, vol. 2016, Article ID 1654938, 8 pages, 2016.

[8] M. Lal, *Saving Lives at Birth, A pediatric-friendly ARV dosage form: validation of palatability, flexibility, and accurate dosing of LPV/r*, 2015, https://savinglivesatbirth.net/summaries/2015/435.

[9] K. C. Berridge, "Measuring hedonic impact in animals and infants: Microstructure of affective taste reactivity patterns," *Neuroscience & Biobehavioral Reviews*, vol. 24, no. 2, pp. 173–198, 2000.

[10] H. J. Grill and R. Norgren, "The taste reactivity test. I. Mimetic responses to gustatory stimuli in neurologically normal rats," *Brain Research*, vol. 143, no. 2, pp. 263–279, 1978.

[11] D. H. McBurney and J. F. Gent, "On the nature of taste qualities," *Psychological Bulletin*, vol. 86, no. 1, pp. 151–167, 1979.

[12] J. A. Mennella, A. C. Spector, D. R. Reed, and S. E. Coldwell, "The bad taste of medicines: overview of basic research on bitter taste," *Clinical Therapeutics*, vol. 35, no. 8, pp. 1225–1246, 2013.

[13] R. K. Palmer, "The Pharmacology and Signaling of Bitter, Sweet, and Umami Taste Sensing," *Molecular Interventions*, vol. 7, no. 2, pp. 87–98, 2007.

[14] O. Pineño, "Enhanced consumption of an aversively conditioned taste following the presentation of a "medicine" taste," *Behavioural Processes*, vol. 84, no. 2, pp. 625–628, 2010.

[15] M. G. Bhat, R. M. Jordt, M. A. Khan, C. E. Foley, and T. A. Gilbertson, "Validation of a rat behavioral avoidance model from a drug delivery perspective," *International Journal of Pharmaceutics*, vol. 303, no. 1-2, pp. 31–36, 2005.

[16] D. W. Pittman, C. E. Labban, A. A. Anderson, and H. E. O'Connor, "Linoleic and oleic acids alter the licking responses to sweet, salt, sour, and bitter tastants in rats," *Chemical Senses*, vol. 31, no. 9, pp. 835–843, 2006.

[17] J. C. Smith, "The history of the "Davis Rig".," *Appetite*, vol. 36, no. 1, pp. 93–98, 2001.

[18] C. D. Dotson and A. C. Spector, "The relative affective potency of glycine, L-serine and sucrose as assessed by a brief-access taste test in inbred strains of mice," *Chemical Senses*, vol. 29, no. 6, pp. 489–498, 2004.

[19] J. I. Glendinning, J. Gresack, and A. C. Spector, "A high-throughput screening for identifying mice with aberrant taste and oromotor function," *Chemical Senses*, vol. 27, no. 5, pp. 461–474, 2002.

[20] D. W. Pittman, M. R. Mcginnis, L. M. Richardson, E. J. Miller, M. L. Alimohamed, and J. P. Baird, "Multiple processes underlie benzodiazepine-mediated increases in the consumption of accepted and avoided stimuli," *Chemical Senses*, vol. 37, no. 5, pp. 431–444, 2012.

[21] S. J. Cooper and S. Higgs, "Benzodiazepine effects on licking responses for sodium chloride solutions in water-deprived male rats," *Physiology & Behavior*, vol. 85, no. 3, pp. 252–258, 2005.

[22] J. D. Davis, T. M. Kung, and R. Rosenak, "Interaction between orosensory and postingestional stimulation in the control of corn oil intake by rats," *Physiology & Behavior*, vol. 57, no. 6, pp. 1081–1087, 1995.

[23] A. C. Spector, P. A. Klumpp, and J. M. Kaplan, "Analytical issues in the evaluation of food deprivation and sucrose concentration effects on the microstructure of licking behavior in the rat," *Behavioral Neuroscience*, vol. 112, no. 3, pp. 678–694, 1998.

[24] Y. Nakamura and N. Katakura, "Generation of masticatory rhythm in the brainstem," *Neuroscience Research*, vol. 23, no. 1, pp. 1–19, 1995.

[25] Y. Nakamura, N. Katakura, M. Nakajima, and J. Liu, "Rhythm generation for food-ingestive movements," *Progress in Brain Research*, vol. 143, pp. 97–103, 2004.

[26] J. B. Travers, L. A. Dinardo, and H. Karimnamazi, "Motor and premotor mechanisms of licking," *Neuroscience & Biobehavioral Reviews*, vol. 21, no. 5, pp. 631–647, 1997.

[27] J. A. W. M. Weijnen, "Licking behavior in the rat: Measurement and situational control of licking frequency," *Neuroscience & Biobehavioral Reviews*, vol. 22, no. 6, pp. 751–760, 1998.

[28] J.-P. Baird, S. J. St. John, and E. A.-N. Nguyen, "Temporal and qualitative dynamics of conditioned taste aversion processing: Combined generalization testing and licking microstructure analysis," *Behavioral Neuroscience*, vol. 119, no. 4, pp. 983–1003, 2005.

[29] M. A. Fudge, M. Kavaliers, J.-P. Baird, and K.-P. Ossenkopp, "Tamoxifen produces conditioned taste avoidance in male rats: An analysis of microstructural licking patterns and taste reactivity," *Hormones and Behavior*, vol. 56, no. 3, pp. 322–331, 2009.

[30] A. Rebecca Glatt, S. J. John, L. Lu, and J. D. Boughter, "Temporal and qualitative dynamics of conditioned taste aversions in C57BL/6J and DBA/2J mice self-administering LiCl," *Physiology & Behavior*, vol. 153, pp. 97–108, 2016.

[31] U. Pachekrepapol, D. S. Horne, and J. A. Lucey, "Interactions between acidified dispersions of milk proteins and dextran or dextran sulfate," *Journal of Dairy Science*, vol. 97, no. 9, pp. 5371–5382, 2014.

[32] U. Pachekrepapol, D. S. Horne, and J. A. Lucey, "Effect of dextran and dextran sulfate on the structural and rheological properties of model acid milk gels," *Journal of Dairy Science*, vol. 98, no. 5, pp. 2843–2852, 2015.

[33] X. Li, F. Deng, Y. Hua, A. Qiu, C. Yang, and S. Cui, "Effect of molecular weight of dextran on the phase behavior and microstructure of preheated soy protein/dextran mixtures," *Carbohydrate Polymers*, vol. 72, no. 1, pp. 160–168, 2008.

# 16

# The Impact of Perceived Stigma, Quality of Life, and Spiritual Beliefs on Suicidal Ideations among HIV-Positive Patients

**Nooshin Zarei**[1] **and Hassan Joulaei**[2]

[1]*Shiraz HIV/AIDS Research Center, Institute of Health, Shiraz University of Medical Sciences, Shiraz, Iran*
[2]*Health Policy Research Center, Institute of Health, Shiraz University of Medical Sciences, Shiraz, Iran*

Correspondence should be addressed to Hassan Joulaei; joulaei_h@yahoo.com

Academic Editor: Krishna Mohan

*Background.* Suicidal ideation is considered a major health problem associated with HIV/AIDS. Suicide rates among people living with HIV/AIDS (PLHA) are more than three times higher in the general population and that is a significant difference. This study aimed at investigating the related factors of suicidal ideations among HIV-positive patients in Southwest Iran. *Study Design.* A cross-sectional study. *Methods.* 351 adult volunteer HIV-infected patients that referred to the Voluntary Counseling and Testing (VCT) center in the south of Iran were evaluated based on convenience sampling. Data was collected utilizing a structured questionnaire from March to August 2015. *Results.* Over the six months prior to the study, 15.4% of the entire sample had been diagnosed with suicidal ideation. There was a significant correlation between the quality of life, spiritual beliefs, perceived stigma, and age with suicidal ideation. Suicidal ideation is significantly different in terms of gender and marital status. Perceived stigma and spiritual beliefs showed the highest effect on suicidal ideations, respectively. *Conclusions.* Having religious beliefs due to accelerating psychological adaptation can motivate HIV patients to survive and have also been considered effective in preventing women from suicide. Perceived stigma and quality of life are other factors that should be taken into consideration as key elements in suicide preventive programs.

## 1. Introduction

Suicidal ideation is considered a major health problem associated with HIV/AIDS [1, 2]. It is more common than suicide attempt and increases the risk of suicidal attempt and completed suicide [3]. Suicide rates among people living with HIV/AIDS (PLHA) are more than three times higher in the general population [4]. According to a systematic review study, the prevalence of suicidal ideation among patients with HIV varied from 13.6 to 31.0% until January 2015 [2]. The prevalence of suicidal ideation in the general population of Iran is 10 to 12.7% [5, 6].

Previous studies showed that younger and low educated PLHA have more suicidal ideations [7, 8]. Those with suicidal ideation reported high levels of depressive symptoms and mental problems [9–11], and this is positively linked with higher levels of internalized AIDS stigma among PLHA [12].

Consequently, hopelessness and negative evaluations lead to low engagement in treatment and health services and a tendency to ignore coping strategies to deal with such symptoms which in turn lead to an increase in social isolation and more risk of suicide [13]. The negative correlation between suicidal ideation and spiritual beliefs implied the importance of spirituality in coping with different health problems and HIV as well [14, 15]. Patients with a poorer quality of life (QoL) were more likely to experience depression and suicide risk than patients with higher QoL that is associated with daily functioning [16–18]. In addition, the consideration of suicidal ideations in HIV/AIDS is important not only because it predicts future attempted suicide, but also because it has been associated with poor quality of life and poor adherence with antiretroviral therapy [19, 20].

Although knowledge about the prevalence of suicidal attempts is important, suicidal ideation is more relevant and significant to understand. Perhaps by understanding the tendencies of people before committing suicide, some measures can be taken to prevent suicide. Few studies have been carried out on suicidal attempts and ideations among PLHA in Iran that consider effective factors such as spirituality, but perceived stigma as a key determinant factor is neglected [21, 22].

Due to the culture of the Iranians, stigmatized attitude is associated with more prominent role of guilt and knowing the patients involved in immoral behavior. Therefore, internal stigma and discrimination are higher in Iran in comparison with other countries which can lead to more suicidal ideation in HIV-positive individuals [23].

Therefore, this study was designed to investigate the impact of perceived stigma, quality of life, spiritual beliefs, and some other related factors on suicidal ideations among HIV-positive patients.

## 2. Methods

The population of this cross-sectional study consisted of all patients living with HIV/AIDS in Fars province. Although the exact number is unknown, according to the latest reports of the Deputy of Health in Shiraz University of Medical Sciences in September 2013, the total number of PLHA in Fars province of Iran was 4410; of them, 81% were male and 19% female.

People in the community are urged to undergo HIV testing in three ways; community awareness and education, venues such as Drop-In Center (DIC) to encourage sex workers, injecting drug users and other high-risk groups for voluntary testing, and the peers. In spite of implementing different programs to drive people for voluntary HIV testing, most of them were anonymous and not readily available. That is why respondents were selected from patients who were referred to the Voluntary Counseling and Testing (VCT) Center.

So, 351 adult volunteer HIV-infected patients referring to the VCT center in Fars province, Iran, were enrolled in the study. The questionnaire was used as a data collection tool and because some subjects were less educated, an expert who worked at the VCT filled out the questionnaires to communicate better with the patients in order to ensure accurate input of answers. The data was collected from March to August 2015 based on convenience sampling. Ethical approval was obtained from the Ethics Committee of the Shiraz University of Medical Sciences.

Inclusion criteria were HIV-positive patients in Fars province who referred to VCT center and mandatorily completed an informed consent form. Patients who did not possess any of these criteria were excluded from the study.

*2.1. Research Tool.* A questionnaire was designed and used as a tool for measuring and collecting the data. The questionnaire included demographic information, 7 items for perceived stigma, 21 items for measuring the quality of life, 13 items for spiritual and religious beliefs, and 4 items for measuring suicidal ideations using Likert's scale. For this scale, we asked participants if they had these ideations within six months prior to the study. Moreover, the interaction of the personnel with patients was also evaluated.

QoL was measured with the ACTG SF-21 which was originally adapted from the Medical Outcomes Study HIV Health Survey (MOS-HIV), a measure with well-established reliability and validity [24]. The ACTG SF-21 consisted of 8 domains: general health perceptions, physical functioning, role functioning, social functioning, pain, mental health, cognitive functioning, and energy/fatigue. Across all domains, higher scores indicate better quality of life. To evaluate stigma and discrimination, 12 items (four-choice question, 7 for internal and 5 for external/social stigma) were asked that was used by USAIDS in 2006 [25]. The range of total score was 12 to 48. Scores of 12–22.6, 22.6–33.26, and 33.26–44 were labeled as low, moderate, and high, respectively.

Despite a valid Persian questionnaire for measuring religious beliefs [26], we still have no valid questionnaire for measuring spiritual beliefs. To ensure the validity of the selected items, we solicited experts' views. A pilot study was carried out in order to gain the internal validity of the questionnaire and to determine the participant's full understanding of the questions or not. The range of total score of religious beliefs of the participants in 13 items using 5-point Likert scale. Each item score was varied between 0 (never) and 4 (always).

Although the scales were used in national projects, and the valid ACTG SF-21 questionnaire was translated in Persian, the items were pretested on 60 subjects of the study population after customization. The Cronbach's alpha was used to ensure the reliability of the items. The amounts of internal/perceived stigma, spiritual beliefs, and suicidal ideations were obtained, 0.743, 0.771, and 0.821, respectively, which were acceptable according to the sample volume of the pretest. In order to check on face validity, the surveyed items are sent to experts to obtain suggestions for modification. There was an attempt to select items that are based on common sense and seem right to the readers.

*2.2. Data Analysis.* The data were analyzed using SPSS software, version 21. Descriptive statistics such as mean, standard deviation, and frequency distribution tables were applied to describe the results. To compare suicidal tendencies among different genders, we used independent sample $T$-test. A binary logistic regression analysis was applied to identify the predictive variables of suicidal ideation. Bivariate relationships were examined between suicidal ideation, perceived stigma, quality of life, spiritual beliefs, age, and educational level through calculation of spearman correlation coefficients. Finally, a multiple regression model was run to assess the importance of each variable in explaining the suicidal ideations.

## 3. Results

Majority of the participants in the current study were married (40.5%) with education level (67.3%) less than high school diploma. Majority of them (56.1%) were at the low level of self-assessed socioeconomic status. In terms of the employment status, although all of the participants were in

TABLE 1: Demographic characteristics of the participants.

| Sociodemographic characteristics | N (%) | p value |
|---|---|---|
| *Age** (years) | 39.53 ± 7.5 | 0.120 |
| *HIV infection duration* (years) | 5 ± 2.61 | 0.044 |
| *Gender* | | |
| Male | 241 (68.7) | 0.007 |
| Female | 110 (31.3) | |
| *Marital status* | | |
| Single | 109 (31.1) | 0.005 |
| Married | 142 (40.5) | |
| Divorced | 74 (21.1) | |
| Widowed | 26 (7.4) | |
| *Education level* | | |
| Illiterate | 7 (2) | 0.083 |
| Less than diploma | 267 (76.1) | |
| Diploma | 60 (17.1) | |
| University degree | 17 (4.8) | |
| *Occupational status* | | |
| Employed | 102 (29.0) | 0.003 |
| Unemployed | 246 (70.1) | |
| Retired | 3 (0.9) | |
| *Socioeconomic status* | | |
| Lower class | 193 (56.1) | 0.001 |
| Lower middle class | 127 (36.9) | |
| Upper-middle class | 24 (7.0) | |
| Upper class | 0 (0.0) | |

*Mean ± SD.

the working age, most of them were unemployed (70.1%) (Table 1).

As to the routes of HIV transmission, 186 (52.9%) participants declared shared injection drug use, 92 (26.2%) had sexual contact with their infected spouse, 47 (13.4%) experienced extra-marital and unsafe contacts, and 26 (7.4%) pointed to the other routes such as tattoos.

Overall, 54 (15.4%) of the entire sample had suicidal tendencies over six months prior to the study. Males reported more suicidal tendencies ($M = 10.31$, SD = 23.99) than females ($M = 4.32$, 16.51), and the difference was statistically significant ($t = -2.712$, $p = 0.007$).

It is also important to note that spiritual beliefs among females were more ($M = 10.53$, SD = 1.24) than males ($M = 9.37$, SD = 2.01) and the difference was significant ($t = 6.63$, $p = 0.0001$). As to the quality of life scale, the data analysis showed that there was a significant difference between men and women ($t = 5.25$, $p = 0.0001$). The score of this scale was higher for females ($M = 291.97$, SD = 145.13) in comparison with males ($M = 204.29$, SD = 143.32). There was also a significant difference in duration of HIV infection between patients with suicidal ideations (5.10 ± 2.59) and without the ideations (4.25 ± 2.57) ($t = 2.18$, $p = 0.044$).

The suicidal ideation was significantly different in terms of marital status, as well ($F = 4.42$, $p = 0.005$). The score was higher for single patients ($M = 1.48$, SD = 1.009), in comparison with married ones ($M = 1.21$, SD = 0.769). In addition, the suicidal ideation was different according to different socioeconomic status ($f = 8.003$, $p = 0001$).

According to Spearman correlations, significant negative correlations between the QoL and spiritual beliefs with suicidal ideation were recorded, while the correlation between perceived stigma and suicidal ideations was positive. All the mentioned correlations were significant even after controlling for duration of HIV infection as a possible confounder (Table 2).

A significant negative correlation between all the QoL dimensions and suicidal ideation was recorded based on the correlation tests (Table 3).

The results of linear multiple regression model indicated the effect of each variable controlling for other explanatory variables. Perceived stigma and spiritual beliefs showed the highest effect on suicidal ideations, respectively ($\beta = 0.598$, $-0.155$). Determination coefficient for the model ($R^2 = 0.42$) shows that 42 percent of variance in suicidal ideations was explained by the variables examined (Table 4).

## 4. Discussion

Considering the fact that suicidal ideation is a health problem associated with HIV, this study was conducted to investigate

TABLE 2: The correlations between suicidal ideation and QoL, perceived stigma, and spiritual beliefs.

| | Suicidal ideation | QoL score | Perceived stigma | Spiritual beliefs |
|---|---|---|---|---|
| Suicidal ideation | 1.0 | | | |
| QoL score | −0.258** | 1.0 | | |
| Perceived stigma | 0.543** | −0.496** | 1.0 | |
| Spiritual beliefs | −0.265** | 0.206** | −0.133* | 1.0 |

**Correlation is significant at the 0.01 level (2-tailed). *Correlation is significant at the 0.05 level (2-tailed).

some of the related factors of such ideations. According to the results of the present study, 15.4% of PLHA had suicide ideations over the six months prior to the study, whereas in the general population this rate is between 10 and 12.7% [5, 6]. It is expected that the prevalence of lifetime suicidal ideation is more dramatic, while a person who lives with HIV virus is under intense internal pressure. This fact indicates the importance of considering the influencing factors that would reduce the incidence of suicide among PLHA.

The results showed that younger PLHA have more suicidal ideation that is consistent with previous studies [8]. In spite of the results of previous studies that showed a significant relationship between the lower level of education and suicide ideation [27], we did not find any relationship between these factors. One of the possible reasons for such difference is that the studied sample was relatively homogenous in terms of education and most of them had low literacy.

The results showed that patients with suicidal ideations had more length of time since HIV diagnosis. Previous studies found different results; although a study in Iran found no significant relationship between suicidal ideation scores and time from HIV infection diagnosis, a study in China found that most HIV-positive individuals made their first suicidal attempt/ideation immediately after their HIV diagnosis within a month [21, 28]. The possible reason for such a difference is that we had no HIV-infected patient who is in the early stages of coping with an HIV diagnosis in the current study. Therefore, we compared the patients who have been infected for at least two and a half years. The reasonable reason is living longer with HIV may increase posttraumatic stress disorder and depression symptoms [29, 30].

A significant point of consideration in this study is that males reported more suicidal ideations than females, which is not inconsistent with the previous results [27]; and there are probable reasons. Among the studied samples, most of them were married. The results revealed a significant difference in suicidal ideations between single and married patients. Factually, having a family and being in a family union increase their motivation to survive, especially because the majority of them had children and felt responsible towards them. The other reasons can be the higher quality of life, on the one hand, and more spiritual beliefs among the studied women, on the other hand. According to the previous studies, religion helps the patients to cope better with the suicidal crisis [31]. It also seems that having religious beliefs due to increased life expectancy and motivation of survival can be effective and prevents patients from committing suicide.

The significant negative correlation between suicidal ideation and spiritual beliefs implied the importance of spirituality and such beliefs which are consistent with other studies and can accelerate with psychological adaptation among PLHA [14, 32].

Suicidal ideation is negatively correlated with QoL both overall and each of the QoL subscales. Previous findings also confirm that patients with a poorer quality of life were more likely to experience suicide risk than patients who had higher QoL [16, 33].

Perceived stigma was identified as an important factor for suicidal ideations in this study as well. The results of a study that was done by Amiya et al. showed that depressive symptoms, rather than suicidal ideations, were positively linked with higher levels of internalized AIDS stigma among PLHA [12]. According to the results, both perceived stigma and spiritual beliefs were the most effective factors of suicidal ideation which should be considered more in the preventive strategies to reduce suicidal ideations.

Considering the high prevalence of perceived stigma in HIV-infected patients in the same context [34], harm reduction programs and counseling services with more emphasis on reducing internal HIV-stigma and increasing spiritual beliefs should be implemented to decrease the possible suicidal ideations and attempts among HIV patients.

## Additional Points

*Limitations.* Respondents were selected from the patients who had referred to the Voluntary Counseling and Testing (VCT) Center and benefited from the consulting services of the center. Therefore, lack of access to the patients outside VCT was a limitation of the current study.

*Suggestions for Future Studies.* The interventional studies through counseling services for HIV-infected patients should be considered in future studies to decrease perceived stigma as a key factor of suicidal ideation among the patients.

## Conflicts of Interest

The authors wish to confirm that there are no known conflicts of interest associated with this publication.

## Acknowledgments

The authors are grateful to Research Deputy of Shiraz University of Medical Sciences that financially supported this project (no. 95-01-59-12669) and also the patients.

TABLE 3: The correlations between suicidal ideation and QoL dimensions.

| | Suicidal ideations | General health | Physical functioning | Role functioning | Social functioning | Cognitive functioning | Pain | Mental health | Energy/fatigue |
|---|---|---|---|---|---|---|---|---|---|
| Suicidal ideations | 1.0 | | | | | | | | |
| General health perceptions | −0.303** | 1.0 | | | | | | | |
| Physical functioning | −0.118* | 0.467** | 1.0 | | | | | | |
| Role functioning | −0.184** | 0.542** | 0.470** | 1.0 | | | | | |
| Social functioning | −0.167** | 0.563** | 0.436** | 0.600** | 1.0** | | | | |
| Cognitive functioning | −0.228** | 0.514** | 0.514** | 0.468** | 0.530** | 1.0 | | | |
| Pain | −.140** | 0.550** | 0.512** | 0.520** | 0.512** | 0.494** | 1.0 | | |
| Mental health | −0.278** | 0.614** | 0.439** | 0.459** | 0.497** | 0.509** | 0.478** | 1.0 | |
| Energy/fatigue | −0.196** | 0.553** | 0.483** | 0.455** | 0.481** | 0.456** | 0.445** | 0.580** | **1.0** |

**Correlation is significant at the 0.01 level (2-tailed). *Correlation is significant at the 0.05 level (2-tailed).

TABLE 4: The linear multiple regression for suicidal ideations as a dependent variable.

| Variables | Std. error | Beta | $t$ | $p$ value |
|---|---|---|---|---|
| Age | .002 | −.087 | −1.841 | 0.067 |
| Social class | .027 | −.115 | −2.412 | 0.016 |
| Male | .041 | .011 | .199 | 0.842 |
| Employed | .040 | −.002 | −.034 | 0.973 |
| Single | .041 | .011 | .194 | 0.846 |
| Divorced/widowed | .038 | −.016 | −.322 | 0.747 |
| HIV infection duration | .049 | .024 | .515 | 0.607 |
| Perceived stigma | .003 | .596 | 11.662 | 0.001 |
| Quality of life | .000 | .092 | 1.604 | 0.110 |
| Religious beliefs | .009 | −.140 | −2.949 | 0.003 |

## References

[1] A. W. Carrico, "Elevated suicide rate among HIV-positive persons despite benefits of antiretroviral therapy: implications for a stress and coping model of suicide," *The American Journal of Psychiatry*, vol. 167, no. 2, pp. 117–119, 2010.

[2] G. Serafini, F. Montebovi, D. A. Lamis et al., "Associations among depression, suicidal behavior, and quality of life in patients with human immunodeficiency virus," *World Journal of Virology*, vol. 4, no. 3, pp. 303–312, 2015.

[3] G. Alexopoulos, C. F. Reynolds III, and M. L. Bruce, "Reducing suicidal ideation and depression in older primary care patients: 24-month outcomes of the PROSPECT study," *The American Journal of Psychiatry*, vol. 166, no. 8, pp. 882–890, 2009.

[4] D. W. Capron, A. Gonzalez, J. Parent, M. J. Zvolensky, and N. B. Schmidt, "Suicidality and anxiety sensitivity in adults with HIV," *AIDS Patient Care and STDs*, vol. 26, no. 5, pp. 298–303, 2012.

[5] S. K. Malakouti, M. Nojomi, J. Bolhari, M. Hakimshooshtari, M. Poshtmashhadi, and D. De Leo, "Prevalence of suicide thoughts, Plans and attempts in a community sample from Karaj, Iran," *Community Mental Health Journal*, vol. 45, no. 1, pp. 37–41, 2009.

[6] X.-L. Cao, B-.L. Zhong, Y.-T. Xiang et al., "Prevalence of suicide ideation, attempts and the associated factors among a sample of Iranian population in south part of the country: a population based study," *Iranian Journal of Psychiatry*, vol. 49, no. 4, pp. 296–308, 2015.

[7] M. K. Nock, G. Borges, E. J. Bromet et al., "Cross-national prevalence and risk factors for suicidal ideation, plans and attempts," *The British Journal of Psychiatry*, vol. 192, no. 2, pp. 98–105, 2008.

[8] M. Preau, A. D. Bouhnik, P. Peretti-Watel, Y. Obadia, and B. Spire, "Suicide attempts among people living with HIV in France," *AIDS Care*, vol. 20, no. 8, pp. 917–924, 2008.

[9] R. O. Shittu, M. K. Alabi, L. O. Odeigah et al., "Suicidal ideation among depressed people living with HIV/AIDS in Nigeria, West Africa," *Open Journal of Medical Psychology*, vol. 3, no. 3, pp. 262–270, 2014.

[10] S. T. Lawrence, J. H. Willig, H. M. Crane et al., "Routine, self-administered, touch-screen, computer-based suicidal ideation assessment linked to automated response team notification in an HIV primary care setting," *Clinical Infectious Diseases*, vol. 50, no. 8, pp. 1165–1173, 2010.

[11] P. Razavi, K. Hajifathalian, B. Saeidi et al., "Quality of life among persons with HIV/AIDS in Iran: internal reliability and validity of an international instrument and associated factors," *AIDS Research and Treatment*, vol. 2012, Article ID 849406, 6 pages, 2012.

[12] R. M. Amiya, K. C. Poudel, K. Poudel-Tandukar, B. D. Pandey, and M. Jimba, "Perceived family support, depression, and suicidal ideation among people living with HIV/AIDS: A cross-sectional study in the Kathmandu Valley, Nepal," *PLoS ONE*, vol. 9, no. 3, Article ID e90959, 2014.

[13] P. T. Yanos, D. Roe, K. Markus, and P. H. Lysaker, "Pathways between internalized stigma and outcomes related to recovery in schizophrenia spectrum disorders," *Psychiatric Services*, vol. 59, no. 12, pp. 1437–1442, 2008.

[14] J. M. Simoni, M. G. Martoneb, and J. F. Kerwinb, "Spirituality and psychological adaptation among women with HIV/AIDS: Implications for counseling," *Journal of Counseling Psychology*, vol. 49, no. 2, pp. 139–147, 2002.

[15] S. Z. Tabei, N. Zarei, and H. Joulaei, "The impact of spirituality on health," *Shiraz E Medical Journal*, vol. 17, no. 6, 2016.

[16] M. Pompili, A. Pennica, G. Serafini et al., "Depression and affective temperaments are associated with poor health-related quality of life in patients with HIV infection," *Journal of Psychiatric Practice*, vol. 19, no. 2, pp. 109–117, 2013.

[17] H. Jin, J. Hampton Atkinson, X. Yu et al., "Depression and suicidality in HIV/AIDS in China," *Journal of Affective Disorders*, vol. 94, no. 1-3, pp. 269–275, 2006.

[18] L. Schlebusch and N. Vawda, "HIV-infection as a self-reported risk factor for attempted suicide in South Africa," *African Journal of Psychiatry*, vol. 13, no. 4, pp. 280–283, 2010.

[19] E. Kinyanda, S. Hoskins, J. Nakku, S. Nawaz, and V. Patel, "The prevalence and characteristics of suicidality in HIV/AIDS as seen in an African population in Entebbe district, Uganda," *BMC Psychiatry*, vol. 12, article 63, 2012.

[20] L. Sherr, F. Lampe, M. Fisher et al., "Suicidal ideation in UK HIV clinic attenders," *AIDS*, vol. 22, no. 13, pp. 1651–1658, 2008.

[21] F. Dabaghzadeh, F. Jabbari, H. Khalili, and L. Abbasian, "Associated factors of suicidal thoughts in HIV-positive individuals," *Iranian Journal of Psychiatry*, vol. 10, no. 3, pp. 185–191, 2015.

[22] AS. Anari, R. Bidaki, H. Soltani, H. Zolala, R. Asadi, Z. Khajekarimaddini et al., "Frequency of Suicide Ideation and Attempt in HIV infected patients referred to behavioral health counseling center of Rafsanjan (RUMS) and Kerman University of medical sciences (KUMS) in 2012," *Galen Medical Journal*, vol. 4, no. 1, pp. 33–38, 2015.

[23] S. SeyedAlinaghi, K. Paydary, P. Afsar Kazerooni et al., "Evaluation of stigma index among people living with HIV/AIDS

(PLWHA) in six cities in Iran," *Thrita*, vol. 2, no. 4, pp. 69–75, 2013.

[24] A. W. Wu, R. D. Hays, S. Kelly, F. Malitz, and S. A. Bozzette, "Applications of the medical outcomes study health-related quality of life measures in HIV/AIDS," *Quality of Life Research*, vol. 6, no. 6, pp. 531–554, 1997.

[25] L. Nyblade and K. Y. MacQuarrie, *Can We Measure HIV/AIDS-related Stigma and Discrimination? Current Knowledge about Quantifying Stigma in Developing Countries*, USAIDS, 2006.

[26] M. Khodayarifard, B. Ghobari–Bonab, M. Shokoohi–Yekta et al., "Developing a Religiosity Scale for Iranian College Student," *Procedia - Social and Behavioral Sciences [Persian]*, vol. 82, pp. 432–435, 2013.

[27] M. K. Nock, T. E. Joiner Jr., K. H. Gordon, E. Lloyd-Richardson, and M. J. Prinstein, "Non-suicidal self-injury among adolescents: Diagnostic correlates and relation to suicide attempts," *Psychiatry Research*, vol. 144, no. 1, pp. 65–72, 2006.

[28] Y. Wu, H. Yang, J. Wang, H. Yao, X. Zhao, J. Chen et al., "Prevalence of suicidal ideation and associated factors among HIV-positive MSM in Anhui, China," *International Journal of STD & AIDS*, vol. 26, no. 7, pp. 496–503, 2015.

[29] S. Arseniou, A. Arvaniti, and M. Samakouri, "HIV infection and depression.," *Psychiatry and Clinical Neurosciences*, vol. 68, no. 2, pp. 96–109, 2014.

[30] M. Rzeszutek, W. Oniszczenko, M. Żebrowska, and E. Firląg-Burkacka, "HIV infection duration, social support and the level of trauma symptoms in a sample of HIV-positive polish individuals," *AIDS Care Psychological and Socio-medical Aspects of AIDS/HIV*, vol. 27, no. 3, pp. 363–369, 2015.

[31] J. Osafo, B. L. Knizek, C. S. Akotia, and H. Hjelmeland, "Influence of Religious Factors on Attitudes Towards Suicidal Behaviour in Ghana," *Journal of Religion and Health*, vol. 52, no. 2, pp. 488–504, 2013.

[32] N. A. Cooperman and J. M. Simoni, "Suicidal ideation and attempted suicide among women living with HIV/AIDS," *Journal of Behavioral Medicine*, vol. 28, no. 2, pp. 149–156, 2005.

[33] D. L. Haller and D. R. Miles, "Suicidal ideation among psychiatric patients with HIV: Psychiatric morbidity and quality of life," *AIDS and Behavior*, vol. 7, no. 2, pp. 101–108, 2003.

[34] N. Zarei, H. Joulaei, and M. Fararouei, "Perceived Stigma and Quality of Life Among Women Living with HIV/AIDS," *Women's Health Bulletin*, vol. 4, no. 1, 2016.

# 17

# Quality of Life of People Living with HIV/AIDS in the Ho Municipality, Ghana

**James Osei-Yeboah,[1] William K. B. A. Owiredu,[2,3] Gameli Kwame Norgbe,[4] Sylvester Yao Lokpo,[1] Christian Obirikorang,[2] Emmanuel Alote Allotey,[1] John Gameli Deku,[1] Emmanuel Akomanin Asiamah,[1] Nana Yaw Barimah Manaphraim,[1] Prince Senyo Kwasi Nyamadi,[1] Edward Yiadom Boakye,[1] Tibemponi Ntoni,[1] Roseline Avorkliyah,[1] Romeo Asumbasiya Aduko,[1] Seyram Tetteh Quarshie,[5] and Maxwell Jenkins Gbemu[6]**

[1] *Department of Medical Laboratory Sciences, School of Allied Health Sciences, University of Health and Allied Sciences, Ho, Ghana*
[2] *Department of Molecular Medicine, School of Medical Sciences, Kwame Nkrumah University of Science and Technology, Kumasi, Ghana*
[3] *Department of Clinical Biochemistry, Diagnostic Directorate, Komfo Anokye Teaching Hospital, Kumasi, Ghana*
[4] *School of Allied Health Sciences, University of Health and Allied Sciences, Ho, Ghana*
[5] *Health Information Unit, Ho Municipal Hospital, Ghana Health Service, Ho, Volta Region, Ghana*
[6] *Laboratory Department, Volta Regional Hospital, Ghana Health Service, Ho, Volta Region, Ghana*

Correspondence should be addressed to James Osei-Yeboah; joyeboah@uhas.edu.gh

Academic Editor: Robert R. Redfield

Quality of life (QoL) is an important component in the evaluation of the wellbeing of people living with HIV/AIDS (PLHIV). This study was aimed at evaluating the QoL of PLHIV attending the antiretroviral clinics in the Ho municipality. A cross-sectional study was conducted from January 2017 to April 2017 involving 158 purposively selected HIV-positive patients who were attending the antiretroviral clinics both in the Volta Regional Hospital and Ho Municipal Hospital. An Interviewer administered standard questionnaire (WHOQOL-HIV Bref) was used to collect information on sociodemography, medical history, and the quality of life (QoL) of the respondents. Among these 158 HIV-positive respondents, 126 (79.75) and 14 (8.86) presented with excellent and good overall QoL, respectively, whilst 18 (11.39) had their life negatively affected by HIV/AIDS. Religious/personal beliefs (19.62%) were the most affected QoL component, followed by the physical (15.82%) and level of independence (15.19%) domains. Patients' occupation, perception of health, sexual activity, and state of the disease were associated with poor overall QoL. In general, being an HIV-infected man, symptomatic patient, not being sexually active, or being ART naïve was also associated with poorer QoL in several HIV/AIDS QoL domains.

## 1. Introduction

The Human Immunodeficiency virus (HIV) infection and its associated pandemic of Acquired Immune Deficiency Syndrome (AIDS) have burdened the population with serious public health and socioeconomic challenges over the years [1]. The disease does not only affect the patients' physical condition, but also affects their sociocultural relations, mental health, and financial aspects of life [2, 3].

The introduction of antiretroviral treatment (ART) has drastically changed the course of the disease from a rapidly progressive catastrophic illness to a chronic disease with reduction in mortality rate, opportunistic infections, and length of hospitalisation [4, 5]. However the increase in the access to biomedical interventions such as ART for people living with HIV/AIDS (PLHIV), in the developing world, has not been adequately matched with the requisite psychosocial treatments to help improve the effectiveness of biomedical interventions [3]. Optimizing care for PLHIV requires an understanding of the factors that contribute to physical health, psychological wellbeing, social relationships, and quality of life [5].

Quality of life has been considered synonymous with health status, functional status, psychological wellbeing, happiness with life, satisfaction of needs, and assessment of one's own life [6]. Assessment of quality of life has become an important outcome measure in the management of HIV/AIDS and reflects improvement or otherwise of the health experience and satisfaction with care among patients living with HIV/AIDS [7, 8].

In Ghana, the Volta region with an HIV prevalence of 2.7% higher than the national prevalence of 2.4% is one of the top HIV regions according to the 2016 national sentinel survey report [9]. According to Folasire et al. [10], QoL assessment helps in making judgments about areas of need and the planning of interventions in the management of PLHIV. A review of the Ghanaian literature shows no available data on QoL of PLHIV in the regional jurisdiction of Volta, the site of the current study. To address this knowledge gap, this study was aimed at assessing the QoL of PLHIV, in the Ho municipality in the Volta region of Ghana, using the World Health Organization instrument for quality of life, the brief version (WHOQoL-Bref).

## 2. Methods

*2.1. Study Design and Study Site.* A hospital-based cross-sectional study was conducted from January 2017 to April 2017 involving one hundred and fifty-eight (158) purposively selected HIV-positive patients, who were attending the Antiretroviral Clinics at the Volta Regional Hospital (VRH) and the Ho Municipal Hospital. The study participants were selected from a pool of patients 18 to 70 years old, who live in the Ho municipality.

*2.2. Sample Size Determination.* Using the average monthly attendance of HIV/AIDS patients of sixty-five (65) for two previous months (November 2016 and December 2016), a total study population of 260 was generated for the four-month study duration. Using the Raosoft online sample size calculator (http://www.raosoft.com/samplesize.html), the recommended minimum sample of 156 participants was calculated at 95% confidence level, 5% margin of error, and a response distribution of 50%.

*2.3. Instrument for Data.* A questionnaire, consisting of sociodemographic, medical, and the WHOQOL-HIV Bref instrument was administered at the time of the interview to assess each study participant.

The questionnaire consisted of 31 items in six (6) domains (physical health, psychological health, level of independence, social relationships, environment, and religious/personal beliefs, as well as one item each for overall quality of life and general health perception). The physical health domain measured pain and discomfort, energy and fatigue, and sleep and rest. The psychological domain measured positive feelings, thinking, learning, memory and concentration, self-esteem, bodily image and appearance, and negative feelings. The level of independence domain measured mobility, activities of daily living, dependence on medications or treatments, and work capacity. The social relationships domain measured personal relationships, social support, and sexual activity. The environmental domain measured physical safety and security, home environment, financial resources, health and social care: accessibility and quality, opportunities for acquiring new information and skills, participation in and opportunities for recreation and leisure activities, and physical environment (pollution, noise, traffic, climate, and transport). The religious/personal beliefs domain measured forgiveness and blame, concerns about the future, and death and dying [11]. Each item contained a 5-point Likert-type scale that best represented their opinion, based on their life over the previous 4 weeks. On the scale, one (1) indicated low and negative perceptions, whilst five (5) indicated high and positive perceptions, which denoted better QoL. Negatively worded items were reverse scored, and all scores were checked for appropriate range (between (1) and (5)).

*2.4. Data Analysis.* The percentage scores were calculated as the sum of individual scores obtained in a domain divided by the total attainable score in that domain multiplied by 100. Thus the percentage scores range from a minimum of 25 to a maximum of 100 [12]. Quality of life scores were categorized into three (3) sections; with scores ≥ 80 denoting excellent QoL, 60 to 79 denoting a good QoL, and <60 representing poor QoL [13]. Statistical analysis was performed using the Statistical Package for Social Science (SPSS) software package, version 21.0. Data were presented using frequency and percentages, median and corresponding interquartile range in parenthesis for descriptive variables, and testing between proportions were carried out using Fisher Exact and chi square test where appropriate, whilst Independent Sample Mann–Whitney $U$ test was used to compare two medians. At all times, $p < 0.05$ was considered as statistically significant.

*2.5. Ethical Consideration.* Informed consent was obtained from all participants after the study procedure was clearly explained to them in a language they understand (either English or Ewe). Approval for the study was obtained from the facilities at both the Volta Regional Hospital (VRH), Ho, and the Ho Municipal Hospital. Ethical Clearance for the study was granted by the Ethical Review Committee of the School of Allied Health Sciences of the University of Health and Allied Sciences, Ho *(UHAS-SAHS-ERSC:026A/2017).* No patient was denied the appropriate care for declining to participate in the study.

## 3. Results

The study population consisted of 158 patients, 88 (55.70%) from the Volta Regional Hospital and 70 (44.30%) from the Ho Municipal Hospital. The male population represented 42 (26.58%) and the female 116 (73.42%) of patients from the two facilities. Majority of the participants 104 (65.82%) had primary school education and 62 (39.24%) were married as at

TABLE 1: Sociodemographic characteristics of people living with HIV/AIDS in Ho municipality.

| Parameter | Frequency | Percentage |
|---|---|---|
| Total | 158 | 100 |
| Facility | | |
| Regional Hospital | 88 | 55.70 |
| Municipal Hospital | 70 | 44.30 |
| Gender | | |
| Male | 42 | 26.58 |
| Female | 116 | 73.42 |
| Educational background | | |
| No education | 14 | 8.86 |
| Primary | 104 | 65.82 |
| Secondary | 30 | 18.99 |
| Tertiary | 10 | 6.33 |
| Marital status | | |
| Single | 85 | 53.80 |
| Cohabitation | 11 | 6.96 |
| Married | 62 | 39.24 |
| Occupation status | | |
| Formal | 16 | 10.13 |
| Informal | 125 | 79.11 |
| Not employed | 17 | 10.76 |
| Stage of disease | | |
| Asymptomatic | 126 | 79.75 |
| Symptomatic | 32 | 20.25 |
| Antiretroviral therapy | | |
| ART | 101 | 63.92 |
| ART naïve | 57 | 36.08 |

Data is presented as frequency with corresponding percentage.

the time of data collection. One hundred twenty-five (79.11%) participants were employed in the informal sector and 10.76% of participants had no gainful employment. Majority of the participants were in the asymptomatic stage of the disease 126 (79.75%) and a total of 101 (63.92%) patients were on ART (See Table 1).

The overall quality of life median percentage score and interquartile range among the study respondents were 71.29 and 9.31, respectively. The psychological domain recorded the lowest median percentage score (68.00) and highest component score was observed in the social relationship domain (75.00). Though not statistically significant, the median scores of the overall QoL, the physical and social relationship, and spiritual/religion/personal beliefs domains were higher for the females compared to their male counterparts (See Table 2).

Among the study population, 126 (79.75) were graded as presenting with an excellent overall QoL, 14 (8.86) presented with good overall QoL, and 18 (11.39) had their life negatively affected by the disease. On the question of health satisfaction of PLHIV, 123 (77.85%) appraised their health as excellent, 11 (6.96%) assessed their health as good, and 24 (15.19%) appraised their health as poor. Religious/personal beliefs domain which looks at the patients' inclination to forgiveness and blame and concerns about the future, death, and dying recorded the poorest score 31 (19.62%), followed by physical component (pain and discomfort, sleep and rest, mobility, activities of daily living, and work capacity), 25 (15.82%), and level of independence 24 (15.19%) (See Table 3).

As seen from Table 4, the respondents' facility of care, gender, educational background, marital status, and antiretroviral therapy had no significant association with the quality of life. Participants who were not gainfully employed presented with the highest affected quality of life. Patients who perceived themselves as having poor health significantly presented with a lower quality of life 18 (20.45) compared to their counterparts who perceived themselves as healthy 0 (0.00%). Significantly poorer QoL was observed among patients who were sexually inactive 15 (18.52) and symptomatic HIV/AIDS patients 8 (25.00) (See Table 4).

A significant gender variation of psychological quality of life among the study population was observed. The male population presented with a poorer psychological QoL (23.81%) than their female counterparts (9.48%). Non-sexually active HIV/AIDS patients had a significantly poorer quality of life (19.75%) compared to sexually active patients (6.49%) for the psychological domain. Patients seeking care at the Ho Municipal Hospital had better quality of life compared to those at the Volta Regional Hospital the psychological quality of life domain and general health perceptions. Symptomatic HIV/AIDS patients had a poorer quality of life (31.25% and 21.88%) as compared to the asymptomatic patients (11.11% and 14.29%) for general health perceptions and physical quality of life domains, respectively. However asymptomatic HIV/AIDS patients had a poorer score (22.22%), compared to the symptomatic patients (9.38%), under the spiritual/religion/personal beliefs. Patients who were not on ART had a significantly poorer quality of life (29.82%) as against patients on ART (13.86%) for spirituality/religiosity/personal beliefs QoL domain (See Table 5).

## 4. Discussion

Quality of life (QoL) refers to the degree of excellence in a person's life at any given period that contributes to satisfaction and happiness of the person and benefits society [14]. The current study aimed to assess the quality of life of people living with HIV/AIDS in the Ho Municipality of Ghana. The demographic profile of the participants showed that majority (73.42%) of the study participants were females. Gender vulnerability to HIV infection is tilted towards females in the Ghanaian and African society [1, 15]. Furthermore, most of the respondents (74.68%) had not attained secondary education at the time of the study. This finding compares with the demographic characteristics of the HIV/AIDS population in the work of S. I. Bello, and I. K. Bello [1] in Nigeria where formal education levels were low among PLHIV.

In the current study, the overall median percentage score of QoL was 71.29, which is lower than reported by Acharya [16] and Giri et al. [17] (80.00) among Nepalese PLHIV, but higher than reported by Oliveira et al. [18], (62.5) among Brazilian PLHIV. Other works in the literature in the African

TABLE 2: Quality of life score and component quality of life scores stratified by gender.

| Parameter | Total (158) | Female (116) | Male (42) | $p$ value |
|---|---|---|---|---|
| Overall QoL | 71.29 (9.31) | 71.63 (8.23) | 69.42 (10.15) | 0.167 |
| Physical | 70.00 (25.00) | 75.00 (25.00) | 70.00 (20.00) | 0.292 |
| Psychological | 68.00 (12.00) | 68.00 (12.00) | 68.00 (13.00) | 0.071 |
| Level of independence | 70.00 (15.00) | 70.00 (15.00) | 70.00 (16.25) | 0.080 |
| Social relationships | 75.00 (15.00) | 75.00 (15.00) | 70.00 (20.00) | 0.239 |
| Environment | 72.50 (12.50) | 72.50 (12.50) | 72.50 (12.50) | 0.777 |
| Spiritual/religion/personal beliefs | 70.00 (25.00) | 70.00 (25.00) | 67.50 (21.25) | 0.635 |

Data is presented as median (interquartile range). $p$ is significant at 0.05.

TABLE 3: Components of the quality of life of people living with HIV/AIDS in the Ho municipality.

| Parameter | Excellent | Good | Poor |
|---|---|---|---|
| Overall QoL | 126 (79.75) | 14 (8.86) | 18 (11.39) |
| Health satisfaction | 123 (77.85) | 11 (6.96) | 24 (15.19) |
| Physical | 56 (35.44) | 77 (48.73) | 25 (15.82) |
| Psychological | 33 (20.89) | 104 (65.82) | 21 (13.29) |
| Level of independence | 40 (25.32) | 94 (59.49) | 24 (15.19) |
| Social relationships | 51 (32.28) | 89 (56.33) | 18 (11.39) |
| Environment | 26 (16.45) | 123 (77.85) | 9 (5.70) |
| Spiritual/religion/personal beliefs | 62 (39.24) | 65 (41.14) | 31 (19.62) |

Data is presented as frequency with corresponding percentage in parenthesis.

TABLE 4: Variables associated with the overall Quality of Life of People Living with HIV and AIDS in the Ho municipality.

| Parameter | Excellent | Good | Poor | $p$ value |
|---|---|---|---|---|
| Facility | | | | |
| Regional Hospital | 68 (77.27) | 7 (7.96) | 13 (14.77) | 0.3121 |
| Municipal Hospital | 58 (82.86) | 7 (10.00) | 5 (7.14) | |
| Gender | | | | |
| Male | 31 (73.81) | 5 (11.90) | 6 (14.29) | 0.5295 |
| Female | 95 (81.90) | 9 (7.76) | 12 (10.34) | |
| Educational Background | | | | |
| None | 9 (64.29) | 4 (28.57) | 1 (7.14) | 0.2201 |
| Basic | 84 (80.77) | 8 (7.69) | 12 (11.54) | |
| Secondary | 24 (80.00) | 2 (6.67) | 4 (13.33) | |
| Tertiary | 9 (90.00) | 0 (0.00) | 1 (10.00) | |
| Marital status | | | | |
| Single | 69 (81.18) | 7 (8.23) | 9 (10.59) | 0.9547 |
| Cohabitation | 8 (72.73) | 1 (9.09) | 2 (18.18) | |
| Married | 49 (79.03) | 6 (9.68) | 7 (11.29) | |
| Occupational status | | | | |
| Formal | 13 (81.25) | 1 (6.25) | 2 (12.50) | 0.0017 |
| Informal | 104 (83.20) | 12 (9.60) | 9 (7.20) | |
| Not employed | 9 (52.94) | 1 (5.88) | 7 (41.18) | |
| Antiretroviral Therapy | | | | |
| ART | 82 (81.19) | 10 (9.90) | 9 (8.91) | 0.3813 |
| ART Naive | 44 (77.19) | 4 (7.02) | 9 (15.79) | |
| Perception of Health | | | | |
| Ill health | 62 (70.45) | 8 (9.09) | 18 (20.45) | 0.0003 |
| Healthy | 64 (91.43) | 6 (8.57) | 0 (0.00) | |
| Sexual activity | | | | |
| Active | 66 (85.71) | 8 (10.39) | 3 (3.90) | 0.0144 |
| Nonactive | 60 (74.07) | 6 (7.41) | 15 (18.52) | |
| Disease state | | | | |
| Symptomatic | 22 (68.75) | 2 (6.25) | 8 (25.00) | 0.0242 |
| Asymptomatic | 104 (82.54) | 12 (9.52) | 10 (7.94) | |

Data is presented as frequency with corresponding percentage in parenthesis. $p$ is significant at 0.005.

TABLE 5: Associated variable with the component of quality of life of people living with HIV/AIDS in the Ho municipality.

| QoL Domain | Parameter | Excellent | Good | Poor | *p* value |
|---|---|---|---|---|---|
| Psychological quality of life | | | | | |
| Gender | Male | 5 (11.90) | 27 (64.29) | 10 (23.81) | 0.0303 |
| | Female | 28 (24.14) | 77 (66.38) | 11 (9.48) | |
| Sexual activity | Active | 18 (23.38) | 54 (70.13) | 5 (6.49) | 0.0476 |
| | Non Active | 15 (18.52) | 50 (61.73) | 16 (19.75) | |
| Facility | Regional | 11 (12.50) | 63 (71.59) | 14 (15.91) | 0.0128 |
| | Municipal | 22 (31.43) | 41 (58.57) | 7 (10.00) | |
| Spiritual/religion/personal beliefs | | | | | |
| Disease state | Symptomatic | 21 (65.63) | 8 (25.00) | 3 (9.38) | 0.0027 |
| | Asymptomatic | 41 (32.54) | 57 (45.24) | 28 (22.22) | |
| Therapy | ART | 44 (43.56) | 43 (42.57) | 14 (13.86) | 0.0449 |
| | Naive | 18 (31.58) | 22 (38.60) | 17 (29.82) | |
| General health perceptions | | | | | |
| Disease state | Symptomatic | 20 (62.50) | 2 (6.25) | 10 (31.25) | 0.0178 |
| | Asymptomatic | 103 (81.75) | 9 (7.14) | 14 (11.11) | |
| Facility | Regional | 65 (73.86) | 4 (4.55) | 19 (21.59) | 0.0244 |
| | Municipal | 58 (82.86) | 7 (10.00) | 5 (7.14) | |
| Physical quality of life | | | | | |
| Disease state | Symptomatic | 5 (15.63) | 20 (62.50) | 7 (21.88) | 0.0312 |
| | Asymptomatic | 51 (40.48) | 57 (45.24) | 18 (14.29) | |

Data is presented as frequency with corresponding percentage in parenthesis. *p* is significant at 0.05.

setting presented their QoL scores in means, therefore making direct comparison of scores with the current study not plausible [1, 6, 10]. With the exception of the psychological domain in the Brazilian study [18], all the component QoL percentage median scores recorded in this study were found to be higher than that recorded by the previous cited works.

The social and environment domains which are a reflection of the physical environment, poor living conditions, and how PLHIV are affected by societal discrimination and stigmatization, as well as HIV/AIDS' influence on patients' sexual desire, personal relationships, and family life, could be said to be better in Ho municipality than in other jurisdictions [1, 6, 16–18]. This may be due to effective social support network and reduced exposure to discrimination and stigmatization [10].

In this study population, HIV/AIDS negatively affected the quality of life of 11.39%, with the most affected domain being the spiritual/religious/personal belief domains (19.62%). The least affected domain was the environmental domain (5.70%), which measured physical safety and security, home environment, financial resources, health and social care, accessibility and quality, opportunities for acquiring new information and skills, participation in and opportunities for recreation and leisure activities, and physical environment [19].

Though not statistically significant, the study observed that, with the exception of one, all the patients who had attained tertiary level education at the time of the study presented with excellent quality of life (Table 4). According to Liping et al. [20] who also reported a similar finding in an earlier work, the reason may be that people with higher educational attainment have a more enlightened attitude towards the disease with the increasing public awareness of HIV. Patients who are more educated can better understand the disease state and the instructions given on drug usage, which invariably enhances their QoL [1].

The symptomatic patients significantly presented with a lower overall quality of life, lower physical QoL, and lower general perception of health but had better spirituality/religiosity/personal beliefs and this agrees with the findings of Folasire et al. [10] in a study conducted in Nigeria. Accounting for high QoL score in the spirituality/religiosity/personal beliefs domain among PLHIV in Northern Ethiopia, Tesfay et al. [21] posited that people tend to be spiritual and religious when confronted with issues that are beyond them; they engage in spiritual and religious reflections, treasuring the gifts in their lives, accepting and surrendering to the approach of their death. This state of heightened spirituality reflects on the high score on the spirituality/religiosity/personal beliefs domain.

According to Shan et al. [22], among medical history variables, HIV-infected persons with worse health conditions are inclined to have worse QoL. One of the most acknowledged clinical variables associated with QoL of PLHIV is the breakdown of immunity which is the main cause of symptoms in HIV and is associated with lower QoL [20, 22].

Contrary to the findings of Manhas [19] who attributed the lower quality of life among women living with HIV/AIDS in India to their male counterpart as a reflection of a patriarchal society where gender inequality leads to higher discrimination, stigmatization, and abuse of a female living with HIV/AIDS, in the current study the male participants presented with a poorer psychological quality of life (Table 5). On the other hand Folasire et al. [10] did not find any significant difference in QoL scores between males and females living with HIV/AIDS in Nigeria.

As mentioned by other reports, QoL is associated with employment and income status [3, 22, 23]; this study found that patients who were not gainfully employed presented with a significantly lower QoL, (41.18%), which was more than five times when compared with those who were employed in the informal sector and more than thrice those employed in the formal sector ($p = 0.0017$) (Table 4).

Patients' self-appraisal of their health significantly predicted their quality of life, with lower QoL recorded among those who perceived themselves as ill. The significantly better quality of life in the psychological and health perception among patients attending ART clinic at the Municipal hospital compared to those obtaining care from the regional hospital may require further studies to establish the causal relationship. However, some studies have alluded to the impact of health professionals on the wellbeing of patients presenting with chronic diseases such as PLHIV through comprehensive and consistent counseling of patients on antiretroviral drugs and education on their disease state [1].

## 5. Conclusion

In general, being an HIV-infected man, symptomatic patient, not being sexually active, or being ART naïve was linked to poorer QoL in several HIV/AIDS QoL domains. Furthermore, where PLHIV's receive care also affects their QoL.

Our findings suggest that patient-reported measures of health status and related concepts may help provide a feasible, reliable, and valid method to assess the impact of HIV/AIDS and future management interventions to improve patient outcomes.

## Conflicts of Interest

The authors have declared that no conflicts of interest exist.

## Authors' Contributions

This work was carried out with collaboration between all authors.

## Acknowledgments

The authors acknowledge the help they received from the ARV clinics and laboratory scientists at the Volta Regional Hospital and Ho Municipal Hospital in conducting this study.

## References

[1] S. I. Bello and I. K. Bello, "Quality of life of HIV/AIDS patients in a secondary health care facility," *Proceedings (Baylor University Medical Center)*, vol. 26, no. 2, pp. 116–119, 2013.

[2] D. Tate, R. H. Paul, T. P. Flanigan et al., "The impact of apathy and depression on quality of life in patients infected with HIV," *AIDS Patient Care and STDs*, vol. 17, no. 3, pp. 115–120, 2003.

[3] T. Abrefa-Gyan, L. J. Cornelius, and J. Okundaye, "Sociodemographic factors, social support, quality of life, and HIV/AIDS in Ghana," *Journal of Evidence-Informed Social Work*, vol. 13, no. 2, pp. 206–216, 2016.

[4] M. Préau, C. Leport, D. Salmon-Ceron et al., "Health-related quality of life and patient-provider relationships in HIV-infected patients during the first three years after starting PI-containing antiretroviral treatment," *AIDS Care Psychological and Socio-medical Aspects of AIDS/HIV*, vol. 16, no. 5, pp. 649–661, 2004.

[5] A. Enimil, N. Nugent, C. Amoah et al., "Quality of life among Ghanaian adolescents living with perinatally acquired HIV: a mixed methods study," *AIDS Care Psychological and Socio-medical Aspects of AIDS/HIV*, vol. 28, no. 4, pp. 460–464, 2016.

[6] A. Fatiregun, K. Mofolorunsho, and K. Osagbemi, "Quality of life of people living with HIV/AIDS In Kogi State, Nigeria," *Benin Journal of Postgraduate Medicine*, vol. 11, no. 1, 2009.

[7] K. H. Basavaraj, M. A. Navya, and R. Rashmi, "Quality of life in HIV/AIDS," *Indian Journal of Sexually Transmitted Diseases and AIDS*, vol. 31, no. 2, pp. 75–80, 2010.

[8] H. Jia, C. R. Uphold, S. Wu, K. Reid, K. Findley, and P. W. Duncan, "Health-related quality of life among men with HIV infection: effects of social support, coping, and depression," *AIDS Patient Care and STDs*, vol. 18, no. 10, pp. 594–603, 2004.

[9] NACP, *2016 HIV Sentinel Survey Report*, National AIDS Control Programme, Accra, Ghana, 2017.

[10] O. F. Folasire, A. E. Irabor, and A. M. Folasire, "Quality of life of people living with HIV and AIDS attending the antiretroviral clinic, University College Hospital, Nigeria," *African Journal of Primary Health Care and Family Medicine*, vol. 4, no. 1, article 294, 8 pages, 2012.

[11] S. M. Skevington, "Advancing cross-cultural research on quality of life: observations drawn from the WHOQOL development," *Quality of Life Research*, vol. 11, no. 2, pp. 135–144, 2002.

[12] B. Pedroso, G. L. Gutierrez, E. Duarte, L. A. Pilatti, and C. T. Picinin, "Quality of life assessment in people living with HIV/AIDS: clarifying the WHOQOL-HIV and WHOQOL-HIV-Bref instruments," in *Global View of HIV Infection*, InTech, 2011.

[13] A. A. Rubaish, "The usefulness of global student rating items under end program evaluation surveys in quality improvements: an institutional experience in higher education, Saudi Arabia," *iBusiness*, vol. 3, pp. 353–358, 2011.

[14] O. O. Oguntibeju, "Quality of life of people living with HIV and AIDS and antiretroviral therapy," *HIV/AIDS—Research and Palliative Care*, vol. 4, pp. 117–124, 2012.

[15] F. Starace, L. Cafaro, N. Abrescia et al., "Quality of life assessment in HIV-positive persons: application and validation of the WHOQOL-HIV, Italian version," *AIDS Care Psychological and Socio-medical Aspects of AIDS/HIV*, vol. 14, no. 3, pp. 405–415, 2002.

[16] D. Acharya, "Assessment of quality of life of people living with HIV and AIDS receiving anti-retroviral therapy in Kathmandu Valley," *Journal of Institute of Medicine*, vol. 37, no. 1, pp. 9–13, 2014.

[17] S. Giri, M. Neupane, S. Pant et al., "Quality of life among people living with acquired immune deficiency syndrome receiving anti-retroviral therapy: A study from Nepal," *HIV/AIDS—Research and Palliative Care*, vol. 5, pp. 277–282, 2013.

[18] F. B. M. Oliveira, M. E. B. Moura, T. M. E. De Araújo, and E. M. L. R. Andrade, "Quality of life and associated factors in people

living with HIV/AIDS," *Acta Paulista de Enfermagem*, vol. 28, no. 6, pp. 510–516, 2015.

[19] C. Manhas, "Self-esteem and quality of life of people living with HIV/AIDS," *Journal of Health Psychology*, vol. 19, no. 11, pp. 1471–1479, 2014.

[20] M. Liping, X. Peng, L. Haijiang, J. Lahong, and L. Fan, "Quality of life of people living with HIV/AIDS: a Cross-sectional study in zhejiang province, China," *PLoS ONE*, vol. 10, no. 8, Article ID e0135705, 2015.

[21] A. Tesfay, A. Gebremariam, M. Gerbaba, and H. Abrha, "Gender differences in health related quality of life among people living with HIV on highly active antiretroviral therapy in mekelle town, northern ethiopia," *BioMed Research International*, vol. 2015, Article ID 516369, pp. 1–9, 2015.

[22] D. Shan, Z. Ge, S. Ming et al., "Quality of life and related factors among HIV-positive spouses from serodiscordant couples under antiretroviral therapy in Henan Province, China," *PLoS ONE*, vol. 6, no. 6, Article ID e21839, 2011.

[23] R. L. Hipolito and D. C. de Oliveira, "Quality of Life of people living with HIV/AIDS: a cross-sectional study," *Brazilian Journal of Nursing*, vol. 15, pp. 575–578, 2016.

18

# A Critical Review of the Evidence Concerning the HIV Latency Reversing Effect of Disulfiram, the Possible Explanations for Its Inability to Reduce the Size of the Latent Reservoir In Vivo, and the Caveats Associated with Its Use in Practice

**Harry D. J. Knights**

*Brasenose College, University of Oxford, Oxford, UK*

Correspondence should be addressed to Harry D. J. Knights; harry.knights16@imperial.ac.uk

Academic Editor: Guido Poli

Combination antiretroviral therapy (cART) effectively suppresses the replication of human immunodeficiency virus type 1 (HIV-1), improves immune function, and decreases the morbidity of acquired immune deficiency syndrome (AIDS). However, it is unable to eradicate the virus because it does not eliminate latently infected cells. The latent reservoir poses the major barrier to an HIV-1 cure. The "shock and kill" strategy aims to reactivate the virus and destroy latently infected cells. Many latency reversing agents (LRAs) reactivate HIV in vitro, but the absence of damaging side-effects and efficacy in vivo make disulfiram particularly promising. However, in clinical trials to date, disulfiram treatment has not resulted in a reduction in the size of the latent reservoir. In this article I will therefore discuss the evidence for the latency reversing effect of disulfiram, the possible explanations for its inability to reduce the size of the latent reservoir in vivo, and the caveats associated with its use in practice. These considerations will help to inform judgements about the prospect of an HIV cure from disulfiram based treatments.

## 1. Introduction

Combination antiretroviral therapy (cART) for people infected with human immunodeficiency virus type 1 (HIV-1) effectively suppresses viral replication to below the limit of detection [1]. This successfully improves immune function and substantially decreases the morbidity and mortality of acquired immune deficiency syndrome (AIDS) [1]. However, it fails to eliminate the virus because a latent form of HIV persists [2, 3].

The latent reservoir consists of between $10^5$ and $10^6$ long-lived resting memory $CD4^+$ T cells (Tm) harbouring an integrated, replication competent HIV genome [2–4]. Provided the host cell stays quiescent, the provirus remains transcriptionally silent [5]. This means that latently infected cells do not express viral antigen and therefore cannot be targeted by the immune system [3, 5]. However, following cellular activation, the provirus is transcribed and virus is produced, reestablishing active infection [2, 3]. The latent reservoir is extremely stable; it has been estimated to have a half-life of 44 months in HIV patients receiving cART, requiring 73.4 years to be completely destroyed [6]. This might be explained by the vertical transmission of infectious proviruses during the clonal expansion of Tm cells [7]. The recently discovered long-lived latently infected stem cell-like Tm cells (Tscm) [8] may also be involved. However, the significance of this rare population of cells remains unclear.

The stability of the latent reservoir means that HIV patients have to maintain cART for life. This is expensive, requires lifelong compliance, has undesirable side-effects, and creates stigma, providing the rational for the development of an HIV cure. Two types of cure are recognised: sterilising and functional. A sterilising cure would completely eradicate the virus (including latent virus), while a functional cure would result in long-term host-mediated control of viral replication and consequently lasting remission of symptoms in the absence of cART, with replication competent virus remaining within the body.

The "shock and kill" [9] strategy has recently gained a lot of attention. This aims to reactivate the latent virus, reducing the size of the latent reservoir through direct viral cytopathic killing and immune-mediated destruction while cellular reinfection is blocked with cART [9]. Although this has traditionally been considered a sterilising cure strategy, recent studies on the natural hosts of Simian immunodeficiency viruses (SIVs) suggest that reduced central memory $CD4^+$ T cell (Tcm) infection, in the absence of viral eradication, might be responsible for their functional cure [10, 11]. It is therefore tempting to speculate that incomplete shock and kill strategies might reduce the size of the Tm pool enough for continued antiretroviral treatment to establish a functional cure in humans. Therefore, precisely what type of cure shock and kill is aiming to achieve is open to debate.

Early shock and kill attempts revolved around the use of immune activators: anti-CD3 immunoglobulin, IL-2, and TNF$\alpha$ [12, 13]. However, they entailed a high risk of global T cell activation and systemic induction of proinflammatory cytokines [12, 13]. Therefore, latency reversing agents (LRAs) that activate HIV from latency without global T cell activation were needed. Since the turn of the century, an array of different compounds have shown promise in vitro [14–16]. Two of these, the histone deacetylase inhibitors (HDACI) [17–19] and disulfiram [20, 21], have recently shown success in vivo. However, there have been indications in the literature of widespread and damaging HDACI side-effects [22], including disruption of the antiviral immune system [23], raising concerns about the feasibility of prolonged administration. Accordingly, in this article I will focus on disulfiram, although other LRAs will be discussed where appropriate.

*1.1. Disulfiram.* The latency reversal capabilities of disulfiram and its metabolites were first uncovered in 2011 by Xing et al. [15]. They established latency in $CD4^+$ lymphoblasts by infecting them with HIV and then allowing them to return to a resting state. Elegantly, since they used recombinant HIV expressing GFP, they were able to assess reactivation by flow cytometry. Using this technique, they screened the John Hopkins Drug Library and found eight hits; one of them, disulfiram, had been used to safely treat alcoholism for decades under the trade-name "Antabuse" [24]. Crucially, disulfiram treatment did not increase cell size (an indicator of activity), the production of proinflammatory cytokines, or the expression of activation markers. Therefore, the latency reversal effect of disulfiram appeared to be HIV specific and not due to global T cell activation. The proposed mechanism is outlined in Figure 1.

The in vitro effect, however, did not translate into an effect on patient cells. In 2014, Bullen et al. examined the latency reversal effect of disulfiram on resting $CD4^+$ T cells freshly isolated from HIV patients on cART [26]. Unexpectedly, they found that disulfiram did not induce viral outgrowth and virus release or cause increases in intracellular HIV mRNA. This suggested, in contrast to studies on in vitro models, that disulfiram does not reactivate latency in patient cells. The reasons for this discrepancy are unclear. One explanation is that current in vitro models for HIV latency do not fully recapitulate the mechanisms governing HIV latency in patient cells. Disappointingly, therefore, this study suggested

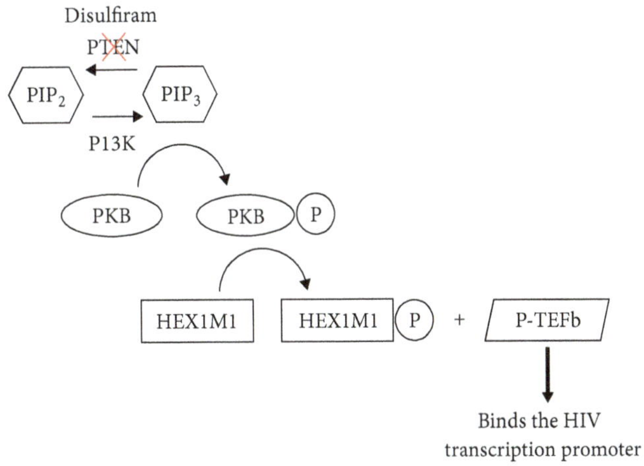


FIGURE 1: The mechanism of disulfiram activation of HIV transcription. Disulfiram activates the PKB/Akt signalling pathway by depleting PTEN (see Doyon et al. [25]).

that disulfiram would be unlikely to drive eradication of the latent reservoir in vivo.

At first, this was consistent with evidence from clinical trials. In 2014, Spivak et al. [20] administered 500 mg of disulfiram daily for two weeks to HIV patients on stable cART. While cART is extremely effective at suppressing viral replication, patients on cART still develop a residual viraemia [27–29]. This is caused by the release of virus from latently infected cells following activation [28]. Therefore, the authors were able to determine latency reactivation in vivo by measuring plasma HIV RNA. In the original analysis, they found no significant change to plasma HIV RNA during disulfiram administration. However, in a post hoc analysis, a transient increase was detected in patients sampled immediately after dosing and patients with higher plasma disulfiram concentrations. These findings inspired a subsequent phase 2 dose-escalation study [21]. Patients received 500, 1000, or 2000 mg of disulfiram daily for three days. A dose-related increase in cell-associated unspliced HIV RNA was observed during and after dosing. It remains unclear why Bullen et al. were unable to detect the same increase in intracellular HIV RNA ex vivo on patient cells. It is possible the immune system is having a synergistic effect on latency reactivation in vivo [26]. Collectively, these landmark clinical studies suggest that disulfiram provides a window of effective latency reactivation in vivo. This provides the first evidence of successful latency reversal in HIV infected individuals by a safe, well-tolerated drug and well-established drug.

## 2. Discussion

There are a number of problems with the use of disulfiram to eradicate the latent reservoir that need to be discussed.

*2.1. The Persistence of the Latent Reservoir.* Inconsistent with the shock and kill hypothesis, none of the disulfiram studies reported a decrease in the frequency of latently infected cells.

Understanding why this is the case will be essential for the development of effective shock and kill cure strategies.

Disulfiram might simply not be potent enough to achieve the magnitude of latency reversal required to cause virus-mediated cell lysis. If correct, it might be necessary to use disulfiram in combination with other mechanistically distinct LRAs to enhance the reactivating effect [30]. This might be compounded by the high frequency of viral escape mutations in patients on cART [31] and the impaired cytotoxic T cell (CTL) cytolytic capacity associated with chronic HIV infections [32], both predicted to inhibit the immune-mediated destruction of reactivated cells.

Interestingly, this is consistent with a study by Shan et al. showing that in vitro latency reversal using an HDACI, suberoylanilide hydroxamic acid (SAHA), did not result in the death of infected Tm cells despite viral cytopathic effects and the presence of autologous CTLs [33]. Instead, the efficient killing of infected cells required antigen-specific stimulation of patient CTLs prior to latency reactivation. It therefore appears that a balance between overstimulation, leading to global T cell activation, and understimulation, leading to the survival of reactivated cells, needs to be achieved. This has led to the general consensus that prestimulation of the antiviral immune response might be necessary for the successful "kill" of reactivated cells. Further studies will be required to confirm whether this applies to disulfiram in vivo.

*2.2. The Presence of Other Viral Reservoirs.* Many studies have examined the effect of disulfiram on latently infected Tm cells. However, less have investigated the effect of disulfiram on other cells. Many different cell types including macrophages [34], dendritic cells [35], and haematopoietic progenitor cells (HPCs) [36] are susceptible to HIV in vitro. Moreover, macrophages [34], microglia [37, 38], astrocytes [37–39], and HPCs [36] from HIV patients have been shown to contain HIV DNA. These findings have led to the proposition that latently infected Tm cells might not be the only viral reservoir in vivo. Whether or not this is the case is still far from certain. While other cell types can be infected in vivo and contain integrated HIV genomes, whether they persist for years in the setting of cART and can be reactivated to produce infectious virus is a contentious issue [40] (for a review, see Kandathil et al. 2016 [41]). Therefore, from a clinical perspective, it is unclear whether they are capable of reseeding infection.

Crucially, however, if non-Tm reservoirs do develop, they will be important to eradication efforts and will likely become more so once the Tm reservoir has been eliminated. Specifically, if disulfiram cannot target these reservoirs, cART could never be stopped for fear of viral rebound "restocking" the cleared reservoirs.

*2.3. The Possibility of a CNS Reservoir.* Recently, the possibility of a CNS reservoir has been the centre of attention [40]. This is because the CNS has a unique set of characteristics that could greatly affect the outcome of LRA use:

(1) The potential to develop HIV-associated neurocognitive disorders (HANDs) [42].

(2) Restricted LRA penetration [43] which may limit the "shock."

(3) Altered immune surveillance [44] which may compromise the "kill."

(4) Restricted cART penetration [45] which may allow continued viral replication, counteracting the clearance of the latent reservoir.

(5) Phylogenetically distinct HIV clades within the CNS which may respond differently to the LRA [46].

(6) Latently infected cells within the CNS (microglia and possibly astrocytes) are long-lived [47].

The development of HANDs is of particular importance. Owing to the success of cART, the life expectancy of HIV patients has increased dramatically over the last 20 years [48]. As a result, secondary HIV pathologies (such as HANDs) are becoming more frequent [40]. The pathophysiology underlying the development of HANDs is not known. However, one possibility is that they are caused by a long-lived infected CNS cell population that is releasing virus within the brains of suppressed patients. If this is the case, shock and kill strategies will need to target these cells. Conveniently, disulfiram easily crosses the blood-brain barrier because of its small size [49]. This means it is anatomically able to target any latently infected cells residing within the CNS. However, Gray et al. found it did not induce viral transcription in monocyte-derived macrophages, a cellular model for brain perivascular macrophages and microglia, or primary foetal astrocytes [50]. This result is disappointing: if reproducible in vivo, disulfiram may not improve the cognitive decline of HIV patients. Specific techniques for targeting CNS latency may therefore be needed in conjunction with disulfiram treatment.

However, the degree to which their cellular model represents latently infected CNS cells in vivo needs careful consideration. In particular, they validate their model by confirming the cell replication kinetics are equivalent to cultured microglia; this, however, is just one cell characteristic. They also used a lentiviral vector whose long-terminal repeat (LTR) was derived from the X4-tropic laboratory strain of HIV-1, NL4-3. The authors hypothesised that LTRs derived from CNS-tropic strains of HIV might respond differently to disulfiram. However, this is now known not to be the case. In a later study, the same group showed disulfiram did not activate transcription in human foetal astrocytic cells transfected with HIV containing LTRs from the CNS compartment of HIV patients [51]. Nevertheless, these findings need to be confirmed in animal models and then in vivo on HIV patients before any conclusions can be drawn about the efficacy of disulfiram on latently infected CNS cells.

On the other hand, if it transpires that disulfiram cannot target latently infected CNS cells, it is possible that this may not affect its therapeutic potential. Specifically, whether HANDs are caused by the release of virus from long-lived latently infected CNS cells remains unknown. Instead, it is possible that HANDs are a consequence of untreated viral infection prior to the initiation of cART or during periods of interrupted treatment. Moreover, only around 10% of HIV patients have detectable levels of HIV RNA in their cerebrospinal fluid (CSF) [52]. This might suggest that the presence of latently infected cells within the CNS is an uncommon occurrence. As a result, the precise implications of disulfiram being unable to reverse latency in CNS cells remain unclear.

Furthermore, it must also be considered that successful shock and kill within the CNS has the potential to cause cognitive decline itself through the destruction of infected glial cells and subsequent neuroinflammation. This would be a particular concern for patients with a larger number of latently infected cells within the CNS (perhaps because of late cART initiation or a long infection period). It might, therefore, be better to leave such patients on strict cART regimes. On the other hand, there may be situations where mild or transient neuronal dysfunction is an acceptable "price" for HIV eradication, similar to the "chemo brain" some patients experience following systemic cancer chemotherapy [53]. Either way, if LRAs like disulfiram were to be used clinically, neurocognitive monitoring would be essential to ensure any neurocognitive decline is detected in time for treatment to be stopped.

There is also the challenge of achieving adequate CNS penetration of antiretroviral agents to ensure the clearing of the CNS viral reservoir is not masked by continued CNS viral replication and propagation. The antiretroviral drug CNS penetration-effectiveness (CPE) rank [54] provides a useful guide and can be augmented by novel nanoformulation delivery techniques [55]. However, CNS penetration is potentially double-edged; in vitro studies suggest some antiretrovirals, particularly the NRTI abacavir and the NNRTI nevirapine, can be neurotoxic [56]. Therefore, while CNS cART infiltration will be essential for successful shock and kill, this problem should be approached with caution for fear of worsening any HANDs and impairing CNS function.

*2.4. Measuring the Size of the Viral Reservoir.* Parallel to the problem of eliminating the latent reservoir is the challenge of measuring the size of the latent pool to determine when the virus has been eradicated. This highlights another key problem facing efforts to eradicate HIV using disulfiram: techniques for measuring reservoir size are inaccurate and complicated. An in-depth analysis of the pros and cons of the different techniques used is beyond the scope of this article (for a review, see Bruner et al. [57]). However, in brief, there are two types: quantitative viral outgrowth assays (Q-VOA) and polymerase chain reaction- (PCR-) based methods.

The Q-VOA uses phytohemagglutinin to globally activate Tm cells ex vivo and reinstate HIV production. The virus is then expanded and quantified by ELISA for the HIV p24 antigen. While this approach has long been the "gold standard," a recent study identified intact proviruses from p24 negative samples [58], suggesting that the Q-VOA underestimates the size of the in vivo reservoirs. This is believed to be because reactivation is stochastic, such that each provirus has a finite probability of being induced following activation [59]. Furthermore, the Q-VOA is labour intensive and expensive, has a 1–3 week culture time, and requires large blood volumes. Accordingly, it remains unsuitable for large scale clinical trials.

Alternatively, the PCR methods directly measure the frequency of cells containing HIV genomes [60]. Here, PCR is performed on blood Tm cell DNA and the infected cell frequency is calculated by comparison to a standard curve constructed using known copy numbers of proviral DNA. Although PCR methods are simple and require small blood volumes, they quantify large numbers of dysfunctional, replication incompetent viral genomes [61]. In fact, PCR methods typically yield infected cell frequencies 2-3 logs higher than the Q-VOA [61]. Generally, therefore, the Q-VOA provides an underestimate and PCR an overestimate, of the true size of the latent pool. Using this information, it would be useful to create an equation to more precisely calculate true reservoir size from the Q-VOA and PCR estimates. This could be done in vitro by controlling latent reservoir size, measuring it with the Q-VOA and PCR methods, and then comparing the values.

Furthermore, nonspecificity means it is very difficult for PCR methods to detect small changes in the number of intact proviruses capable of reseeding infection. This is problematic because very few latently infected cells contain an intact provirus [62], and therefore successful shock and kill will only result in a small absolute reduction in the number of intact proviruses. Therefore, it is possible that the disulfiram studies underestimated the latency reversing effect on replication competent provirus.

To this end, perhaps the best technique to date has been the *tat/rev* induced limiting dilution assay (TILDA) [63]. This measures the frequency of cells containing inducible multiply spliced *tat/rev* RNA. This is usually absent from latent cells and is only induced upon reactivation [64]. Conversely, many defective genomes have deletions encompassing the tat and rev genes [58]. As a result, the latent cell frequency measured by TILDA lies somewhere between the Q-VOA and PCR estimates, indicative of greater accuracy. There are also no RNA extraction or virus amplification steps, meaning it takes just two days, and it offers similar advantages to PCR with regard to simplicity and small blood volume requirement. This makes TILDA a potentially useful assay for large scale clinical trials. However, again there are limitations: it relies on the amplification of a highly variable HIV genome region, suggesting that the required primers may not recognise all viral quasispecies.

Furthermore, as previously discussed, other latent cell types exist within tissues. This would not be a hindrance if the size of blood and tissue reservoirs was tightly correlated, but there is conflicting and limited evidence for this [65]. It might therefore be necessary to combine these quantification methods with tissue sampling techniques. This has been done previously [66]. However, biopsies pose their own limitations: they are invasive and cannot be taken from all tissues, especially the CNS. For the CNS, it may be possible to estimate the number of latently infected cells from the CSF viral load. However, further studies will be needed to confirm whether CSF viral load is dependent on the frequency of latently infected cells that may be residing within the CNS.

As can be seen, all techniques for quantifying the reservoir have their own advantages and disadvantages. This poses a serious problem for HIV eradication efforts. Without a high-throughput, sensitive, and well-validated assay it will remain difficult for researchers to move forward with clinical trials, accurately evaluate the efficacy of LRAs like disulfiram, and ever confirm that a sterilising cure has been achieved.

## 3. Conclusions

Overall, there is strong evidence that disulfiram effectively and specifically reverses HIV latency in cellular models. While this failed to translate into an effect on patient cells, subsequent clinical trials identified an effect in vivo. However, so far, this has failed to result in a reduction in the size of the latent reservoir in HIV patients. Possible explanations for this include insufficient potency and failed immune clearance. Therefore, it is likely that combining disulfiram with other mechanistically distinct LRAs and the use of preimmune stimulation will help overcome these challenges. Furthermore, future studies will be needed to assess whether non-Tm reservoirs are able to reseed the infection after prolonged cART. If they are, safe shock and kill techniques for nonblood reservoirs will need to be explored. Finally, more refined techniques for measuring the size of the latent reservoir safely in different tissues need to be developed. Therefore, while disulfiram shows promise as an HIV cure strategy, further studies are needed to solve the problems highlighted in this article before any conclusions about its clinical efficacy can be drawn.

## Conflicts of Interest

The author has no conflicts of interest.

## Acknowledgments

The author acknowledges Professor William James for his assistance.

## References

[1] F. J. Palella Jr., K. M. Delaney, A. C. Moorman et al., "Declining morbidity and mortality among patients with advanced human immunodeficiency virus infection. HIV outpatient study investigators," *The New England Journal of Medicine*, vol. 338, no. 13, pp. 853–860, 1998.

[2] D. Finzi, M. Hermankova, T. Pierson et al., "Identification of a reservoir for HIV-1 in patients on highly active antiretroviral therapy," *Science*, vol. 278, no. 5341, pp. 1295–1300, 1997.

[3] J. K. Wong, M. Hezareh, H. F. Günthard et al., "Recovery of replication-competent HIV despite prolonged suppression of plasma viremia," *Science*, vol. 278, no. 5341, pp. 1291–1295, 1997.

[4] T.-W. Chun, L. Carruth, D. Finzi et al., "Quantification of latent tissue reservoirs and total body viral load in HIV-1 infection," *Nature*, vol. 387, no. 6629, pp. 183–188, 1997.

[5] M. Hermankova, J. D. Siliciano, Y. Zhou et al., "Analysis of human immunodeficiency virus type 1 gene expression in latently infected resting $CD4^+$ T lymphocytes in vivo," *Journal of Virology*, vol. 77, no. 13, pp. 7383–7392, 2003.

[6] J. D. Siliciano, J. Kajdas, D. Finzi et al., "Long-term follow-up studies confirm the stability of the latent reservoir for HIV-1 in resting CD4+ T cells," *Nature Medicine*, vol. 9, no. 6, pp. 727–728, 2003.

[7] F. R. Simonetti, M. D. Sobolewski, E. Fyne et al., "Clonally expanded $CD4^+$ T cells can produce infectious HIV-1 in vivo," *Proceedings of the National Academy of Sciences of the United States of America*, vol. 113, no. 7, pp. 1883–1888, 2016.

[8] M. J. Buzon, H. Sun, C. Li et al., "HIV-1 persistence in $CD4^+$ T cells with stem cell-like properties," *Nature Medicine*, vol. 20, no. 2, pp. 139–142, 2014.

[9] G. Lehrman, I. B. Hogue, S. Palmer et al., "Depletion of latent HIV-1 infection in vivo: a proof-of-concept study," *The Lancet*, vol. 366, no. 9485, pp. 549–555, 2005.

[10] C. M. Beaumier, L. D. Harris, S. Goldstein et al., "CD4 downregulation by memory CD4+ T cells in vivo renders African green monkeys resistant to progressive SIVagm infection," *Nature Medicine*, vol. 15, no. 8, pp. 879–885, 2009.

[11] M. Paiardini, B. Cervasi, E. Reyes-Aviles et al., "Low levels of SIV infection in sooty mangabey central memory $CD4^+$ T cells are associated with limited CCR5 expression," *Nature Medicine*, vol. 17, no. 7, pp. 830–836, 2011.

[12] T.-W. Chun, D. Engel, S. B. Mizell et al., "Effect of interleukin-2 on the pool of latently infected, resting CD4+ T cells in HIV-1-infected patients receiving highly active anti-retroviral therapy," *Nature Medicine*, vol. 5, no. 6, pp. 651–655, 1999.

[13] J. M. Prins, S. Jurriaans, R. M. E. Van Praag et al., "Immunoactivation with anti-CD3 and recombinant human IL-2 in HIV-1-infected patients on potent antiretroviral therapy," *AIDS*, vol. 13, no. 17, pp. 2405–2410, 1999.

[14] X. Contreras, M. Schweneker, C.-S. Chen et al., "Suberoylanilide hydroxamic acid reactivates HIV from latently infected cells," *The Journal of Biological Chemistry*, vol. 284, no. 11, pp. 6782–6789, 2009.

[15] S. Xing, C. K. Bullen, N. S. Shroff et al., "Disulfiram reactivates latent HIV-1 in a Bcl-2-transduced primary $CD4^+$ T cell model without inducing global T cell activation," *Journal of Virology*, vol. 85, no. 12, pp. 6060–6064, 2011.

[16] L. Ylisastigui, N. M. Archin, G. Lehrman, R. J. Bosch, and D. M. Margolis, "Coaxing HIV-1 from resting CD4 T cells: histone deacetylase inhibition allows latent viral expression," *AIDS*, vol. 18, no. 8, pp. 1101–1108, 2004.

[17] N. M. Archin, A. L. Liberty, A. D. Kashuba et al., "Administration of vorinostat disrupts HIV-1 latency in patients on antiretroviral therapy," *Nature*, vol. 487, no. 7408, pp. 482–485, 2012.

[18] J. H. Elliott, F. Wightman, A. Solomon et al., "Activation of HIV transcription with short-course vorinostat in HIV-infected patients on suppressive antiretroviral therapy," *PLoS Pathogens*, vol. 10, no. 11, Article ID e1004473, 2014.

[19] T. A. Rasmussen, M. Tolstrup, C. R. Brinkmann et al., "Panobinostat, a histone deacetylase inhibitor, for latent-virus reactivation in HIV-infected patients on suppressive antiretroviral therapy: a phase 1/2, single group, clinical trial," *The Lancet HIV*, vol. 1, no. 1, pp. e13–e21, 2014.

[20] A. M. Spivak, A. Andrade, E. Eisele et al., "A pilot study assessing the safety and latency-reversing activity of disulfiram in HIV-1-infected adults on antiretroviral therapy," *Clinical Infectious Diseases*, vol. 58, no. 6, pp. 883–890, 2014.

[21] J. H. Elliott, J. H. McMahon, C. C. Chang et al., "Short-term administration of disulfiram for reversal of latent HIV infection: a phase 2 dose-escalation study," *The Lancet HIV*, vol. 2, no. 12, pp. e520–e529, 2015.

[22] S. Subramanian, S. E. Bates, J. J. Wright, I. Espinoza-Delgado, and R. L. Piekarz, "Clinical toxicities of histone deacetylase inhibitors," *Pharmaceuticals*, vol. 3, no. 9, pp. 2751–2767, 2010.

[23] R. B. Jones, R. O'Connor, S. Mueller et al., "Histone deacetylase inhibitors impair the elimination of HIV-infected cells by cytotoxic T-lymphocytes," *PLoS Pathogens*, vol. 10, no. 8, Article ID e1004287, 2014.

[24] R. G. Bell and H. W. Smith, "Preliminary report on clinical trials of antabuse," *Canadian Medical Association Journal*, vol. 60, no. 3, pp. 286–288, 1949.

[25] G. Doyon, J. Zerbato, J. W. Mellors, and N. Sluis-Cremer, "Disulfiram reactivates latent HIV-1 expression through depletion of the phosphatase and tensin homolog," *AIDS*, vol. 27, no. 2, pp. F7–F11, 2013.

[26] C. K. Bullen, G. M. Laird, C. M. Durand, J. D. Siliciano, and R. F. Siliciano, "New ex vivo approaches distinguish effective and ineffective single agents for reversing HIV-1 latency in vivo," *Nature Medicine*, vol. 20, no. 4, pp. 425–429, 2014.

[27] G. Dornadula, H. Zhang, B. VanUitert et al., "Residual HIV-1 RNA in blood plasma of patients taking suppressive highly active antiretroviral therapy," *The Journal of the American Medical Association*, vol. 282, no. 17, pp. 1627–1632, 1999.

[28] F. Maldarelli, S. Palmer, M. S. King et al., "ART suppresses plasma HIV-1 RNA to a stable set point predicted by pretherapy viremia," *PLoS Pathogens*, vol. 3, no. 4, p. e46, 2007.

[29] S. Palmer, F. Maldarelli, A. Wiegand et al., "Low-level viremia persists for at least 7 years in patients on suppressive antiretroviral therapy," *Proceedings of the National Academy of Sciences of the United States of America*, vol. 105, no. 10, pp. 3879–3884, 2008.

[30] G. M. Laird, C. K. Bullen, D. I. S. Rosenbloom et al., "Ex vivo analysis identifies effective HIV-1 latency-reversing drug combinations," *The Journal of Clinical Investigation*, vol. 125, no. 5, pp. 1901–1912, 2015.

[31] K. Deng, M. Pertea, A. Rongvaux et al., "Broad CTL response is required to clear latent HIV-1 due to dominance of escape mutations," *Nature*, vol. 517, no. 7534, pp. 381–385, 2015.

[32] A. Sáez-Cirión, C. Lacabaratz, O. Lambotte et al., "HIV controllers exhibit potent CD8 T cell capacity to suppress HIV infection ex vivo and peculiar cytotoxic T lymphocyte activation phenotype," *Proceedings of the National Academy of Sciences of the United States of America*, vol. 104, no. 16, pp. 6776–6781, 2007.

[33] L. Shan, K. Deng, N. S. Shroff et al., "Stimulation of HIV-1-specific cytolytic T lymphocytes facilitates elimination of latent viral reservoir after virus reactivation," *Immunity*, vol. 36, no. 3, pp. 491–501, 2012.

[34] S. Gartner, P. Markovits, D. M. Markovitz, M. H. Kaplan, R. C. Gallo, and M. Popovic, "The role of mononuclear phagocytes in HTLV-III/LAV infection," *Science*, vol. 233, no. 4760, pp. 215–219, 1986.

[35] S. Popov, A.-L. Chenine, A. Gruber, P.-L. Li, and R. M. Ruprecht, "Long-term productive human immunodeficiency virus infection of CD1a-sorted myeloid dendritic cells," *Journal of Virology*, vol. 79, no. 1, pp. 602–608, 2005.

[36] C. C. Carter, A. Onafuwa-Nuga, L. A. McNamara et al., "HIV-1 infects multipotent progenitor cells causing cell death and establishing latent cellular reservoirs," *Nature Medicine*, vol. 16, no. 4, pp. 446–451, 2010.

[37] M. J. Churchill, P. R. Gorry, D. Cowley et al., "Use of laser capture microdissection to detect integrated HIV-1 DNA in macrophages and astrocytes from autopsy brain tissues," *Journal of NeuroVirology*, vol. 12, no. 2, pp. 146–152, 2006.

[38] K. A. Thompson, C. L. Cherry, J. E. Bell, and C. A. McLean, "Brain cell reservoirs of latent virus in presymptomatic HIV-infected individuals," *American Journal of Pathology*, vol. 179, no. 4, pp. 1623–1629, 2011.

[39] C. A. Wiley, R. D. Schrier, J. A. Nelson, P. W. Lampert, and M. B. Oldstone, "Cellular localization of human immunodeficiency virus infection within the brains of acquired immune deficiency syndrome patients," *Proceedings of the National Academy of Sciences of the United States of America*, vol. 83, no. 18, pp. 7089–7093, 1986.

[40] B. J. Brew, K. Robertson, E. J. Wright et al., "HIV eradication symposium: will the brain be left behind?" *Journal of NeuroVirology*, vol. 21, no. 3, pp. 322–334, 2015.

[41] A. J. Kandathil, S. Sugawara, and A. Balagopal, "Are T cells the only HIV-1 reservoir?" *Retrovirology*, vol. 13, no. 1, p. 86, 2016.

[42] R. K. Heaton, D. B. Clifford, D. R. Franklin et al., "HIV-associated neurocognitive disorders persist in the era of potent antiretroviral therapy: CHARTER Study," *Neurology*, vol. 75, no. 23, pp. 2087–2096, 2010.

[43] M. J. Churchill, D. J. Cowley, S. L. Wesselingh, P. R. Gorry, and L. R. Gray, "HIV-1 transcriptional regulation in the central nervous system and implications for HIV cure research," *Journal of NeuroVirology*, vol. 21, no. 3, pp. 290–300, 2015.

[44] M. J. Carson, J. M. Doose, B. Melchior, C. D. Schmid, and C. C. Ploix, "CNS immune privilege: hiding in plain sight," *Immunological Reviews*, vol. 213, no. 1, pp. 48–65, 2006.

[45] S. Letendre, J. Marquie-Beck, E. Capparelli et al., "Validation of the CNS penetration-effectiveness rank for quantifying antiretroviral penetration into the central nervous system," *Archives of Neurology*, vol. 65, no. 1, pp. 65–70, 2008.

[46] M. Ait-Khaled, J. E. McLaughlin, M. A. Johnson, and V. C. Emery, "Distinct HIV-1 long terminal repeat quasispecies present in nervous tissues compared to that in lung, blood and lymphoid tissues of an AIDS patient," *AIDS*, vol. 9, no. 7, pp. 675–683, 1995.

[47] S. Kramer-Hämmerle, I. Rothenaigner, H. Wolff, J. E. Bell, and R. Brack-Werner, "Cells of the central nervous system as targets and reservoirs of the human immunodeficiency virus," *Virus Research*, vol. 111, no. 2, pp. 194–213, 2005.

[48] H. Samji, A. Cescon, R. S. Hogg et al., "Closing the gap: increases in life expectancy among treated HIV-positive individuals in the United States and Canada," *PLoS ONE*, vol. 8, no. 12, Article ID e81355, 2013.

[49] D. I. Eneanya, J. R. Bianchine, D. O. Duran, and B. D. Andresen, "The actions of metabolic fate of disulfiram," *Annual Review of Pharmacology and Toxicology*, vol. 21, pp. 575–596, 1981.

[50] L. R. Gray, H. On, E. Roberts et al., "Toxicity and in vitro activity of HIV-1 latency-reversing agents in primary CNS cells," *Journal of NeuroVirology*, vol. 22, no. 4, pp. 455–463, 2016.

[51] L. R. Gray, D. Cowley, C. Welsh et al., "CNS-specific regulatory elements in brain-derived HIV-1 strains affect responses to latency-reversing agents with implications for cure strategies," *Molecular Psychiatry*, vol. 21, no. 4, pp. 574–584, 2016.

[52] A. Edén, D. Fuchs, L. Hagberg et al., "HIV-1 viral escape in cerebrospinal fluid of subjects on suppressive antiretroviral treatment," *Journal of Infectious Diseases*, vol. 202, no. 12, pp. 1819–1825, 2010.

[53] C. B. Brezden, K.-A. Phillips, M. Abdolell, T. Bunston, and I. F. Tannock, "Cognitive function in breast cancer patients

receiving adjuvant chemotherapy," *Journal of Clinical Oncology*, vol. 18, no. 14, pp. 2695–2701, 2000.

[54] S. Letendre, "Central nervous system complications in HIV disease: HIV-associated neurocognitive disorder," *Topics in Antiviral Medicine*, vol. 19, no. 4, pp. 137–142, 2011.

[55] H. Dou, C. B. Grotepas, J. M. McMillan et al., "Macrophage delivery of nanoformulated antiretroviral drug to the brain in a murine model of NeuroAIDS," *Journal of Immunology*, vol. 183, no. 1, pp. 661–669, 2009.

[56] K. Robertson, J. Liner, and R. B. Meeker, "Antiretroviral neurotoxicity," *Journal of NeuroVirology*, vol. 18, no. 5, pp. 388–399, 2012.

[57] K. M. Bruner, N. N. Hosmane, and R. F. Siliciano, "Towards an HIV-1 cure: measuring the latent reservoir," *Trends in Microbiology*, vol. 23, no. 4, pp. 192–203, 2015.

[58] Y.-C. Ho, L. Shan, N. N. Hosmane et al., "Replication-competent noninduced proviruses in the latent reservoir increase barrier to HIV-1 cure," *Cell*, vol. 155, no. 3, pp. X540–551, 2013.

[59] A. D. Weinberger and L. S. Weinberger, "Stochastic fate selection in HIV-infected patients," *Cell*, vol. 155, no. 3, pp. 497–499, 2013.

[60] C. Vandergeeten, R. Fromentin, E. Merlini et al., "Cross-clade ultrasensitive PCR-based assays to measure HIV persistence in large-cohort studies," *Journal of Virology*, vol. 88, no. 21, pp. 12385–12396, 2014.

[61] S. Eriksson, E. H. Graf, V. Dahl et al., "Comparative analysis of measures of viral reservoirs in HIV-1 eradication studies," *PLoS Pathogens*, vol. 9, no. 2, Article ID e1003174, 2013.

[62] K. M. Bruner, A. J. Murray, R. A. Pollack et al., "Defective proviruses rapidly accumulate during acute HIV-1 infection," *Nature Medicine*, vol. 22, no. 9, pp. 1043–1049, 2016.

[63] F. A. Procopio, R. Fromentin, D. A. Kulpa et al., "A novel assay to measure the magnitude of the inducible viral reservoir in HIV-infected individuals," *EBioMedicine*, vol. 2, no. 8, pp. 874–883, 2015.

[64] S. R. Lewin, M. Vesanen, L. Kostrikis et al., "Use of real-time PCR and molecular beacons to detect virus replication in human immunodeficiency virus type 1-infected individuals on prolonged effective antiretroviral therapy," *Journal of Virology*, vol. 73, no. 7, pp. 6099–6103, 1999.

[65] G. Pantaleo, C. Graziosi, J. F. Demarest et al., "HIV infection is active and progressive in lymphoid tissue during the clinically latent stage of disease," *Nature*, vol. 362, no. 6418, pp. 355–358, 1993.

[66] R. D. Hockett, J. M. Kilby, C. A. Derdeyn et al., "Constant mean viral copy number per infected cell in tissues regardless of high, low, or undetectable plasma HIV RNA," *Journal of Experimental Medicine*, vol. 189, no. 10, pp. 1545–1554, 1999.

# 19

# Antiretroviral Treatment Adherence: Knowledge and Experiences among Adolescents and Young Adults in Soweto, South Africa

**Stefanie Hornschuh, Janan Janine Dietrich, Celokuhle Tshabalala, and Fatima Laher**

*Perinatal HIV Research Unit, Chris Hani Baragwanath Academic Hospital, Faculty of Health Sciences, University of the Witwatersrand, Gauteng 1864, South Africa*

Correspondence should be addressed to Stefanie Hornschuh; hornschuhs@phru.co.za

Academic Editor: Stefan Baral

Human immunodeficiency virus (HIV) management of adolescents and young adults (AYAs) is particularly pertinent to sub-Saharan Africa, where the pediatric HIV burden is marked. Antiretroviral treatment (ART) adherence is a major challenge for AYAs. This qualitative study explored knowledge and experiences of adherence amongst AYAs attending treatment at the Perinatal HIV Research Unit (PHRU), Soweto, South Africa. Four focus group discussions (FGDs) and eight in-depth interviews (IDIs) were conducted with HIV-infected 15–25-year-old ART recipients. Transcripts were coded thematically. Participants ($n$ = 26) were aged median 18.5 years, 59.1% female and 69.2% virally suppressed <400 cp/ml. Three main themes emerged during FGDs and IDIs: (i) correct knowledge about how to be adherent, benefits, and nonadherence consequences, (ii) social, personal, and medication-related barriers to adherence, and (iii) reminder, concealment, and motivational strategies to optimize adherence. Interventions to improve AYA adherence could focus on practical strategies, including status disclosure and medication concealment.

## 1. Introduction

The highest global burden of HIV is in South Africa, where prevalence was 12.2% (6.4 million people) in 2012 [1]. Amongst AYAs aged 15 to 24 years, prevalence was 7.1% [1]. About two-thirds of infected AYAs in South Africa acquired the virus through vertical transmission [2]. Before South Africa implemented prevention of mother-to-child transmission interventions, an estimated 60.000 perinatal HIV infections occurred per annum [3]; since then, improved ART access has reduced this number drastically. In 2013 alone, there were still 16.000 new infections in the 0–14-year-old age group in South Africa [4]. With ART advances, these children can and do survive into adolescence and adulthood [5, 6].

ART use results in substantial reductions in HIV-related morbidity and mortality [7, 8]. However, for ART to be effective, sustained viral suppression must be achieved through near-perfect pill adherence [9–11]. Lifelong adherence to daily pills is a known challenge for patients [12]. Nonadherence may result in drug resistance, treatment failure, and subsequent reduced treatment options [13, 14].

A recent study conducted in Zimbabwe between 2004 and 2010 to examine whether adolescents treated for HIV achieved similar treatment outcomes to adults found that HIV-infected adolescents are at higher risk for treatment failure than their adult counterparts [15]. Therefore, knowledge about adherence is critical, and there is a body of publications about adherence barriers and facilitators in the southern African context, especially quantitative research amongst adult patients [16]. Amongst adult patients in the region, various barriers to ART adherence have been identified: fear of HIV status disclosure, HIV-related stigma, alcohol use and drug abuse, forgetfulness, complicated ART regimens, pill burden, side effects, transportation costs, and financial constraints [17, 18]. In one study in South Africa, Peltzer et al. [19] found that determinants for adult nonadherence to ART included poor environment, experiences of HIV-related discrimination, and use of herbal medicine. Determinants of ART adherence included low depression scores, good adherence information, behavioural skills, and social support [19].

It is possible that many of the adherence barriers and facilitators for adults also apply to AYAs, but the latter's higher risk treatment failure does seem to suggest that additional concerns may need to be considered if we are to understand AYA adherence. AYAs in general are particularly vulnerable to adherence problems as they experience unique obstacles owing to the changes during adolescence, including psychological, cognitive, and social development [20, 21]. Even so, there are fewer publications focusing on AYA adherence in Africa. One qualitative study with 23 AYAs in Kenya found that adherence was affected by the need for secrecy to avoid inadvertent disclosure and stigmatisation, pill burden, medication fatigue, lack of planning when travelling, and using adherence as leverage in conflicts [22]. Our study qualitatively explored the experiences of HIV-infected AYAs with regard to ARV adherence.

## 2. Methods

We conducted a qualitative study through FGDs, IDIs, and a demographics questionnaire.

*2.1. Setting.* The study was conducted from March to August 2012 at the PHRU, located at the Chris Hani Baragwanath Academic Hospital in Soweto, South Africa. Soweto is a group of urban townships southwest of Johannesburg, with an estimated population of over one million people [23]. PHRU offers HIV testing, prevention, and treatment for infants, children, adolescents, and adults. At PHRU, HIV-infected AYAs were treated at either its pediatric or adult HIV clinic.

*2.2. Participants.* Eligibility criteria were age between 15 and 25 years at the time of study, HIV infection by self-report to study staff, receipt of ART at either the PHRU adult or pediatric treatment clinic, and ability to provide voluntary written informed consent and, if applicable, assent.

*2.3. Data Collection Procedures.* Potential participants were identified via the PHRU clinic database matching study age and treatment criteria. Potential participants, and their parents for those below 18 years of age, were briefly told about the study telephonically by a study representative and invited to a private room at the PHRU to receive information in full. All participants who provided voluntary written informed consent, and if applicable assent, were assisted by a female interviewer to complete a brief questionnaire about sociodemographic information. The questionnaire structure has been described previously and collected information about HIV transmission mode, HIV status disclosure, and socioeconomic status [24].

Four FGDs were first conducted to identify major themes. Once these were completed, AYAs who had not participated in the FGDs were invited to the IDIs, which attempted to elicit, in an environment without the interference of peer influence, more detailed information on the main themes which had been identified. All interviews were organized in the same location nearby to but removed from the clinic to create similar conditions.

*2.3.1. Focus Group Discussions.* The semistructured FGD interview guide questions elicited the level of knowledge and participant perceptions about adherence and adherence barriers and facilitators.

FGD questions about ART adherence were as follows:

(1) Tell me everything you know about ART adherence.

(2) Who explained to you how to be adherent?

(3) Everyone who takes medication every day has days when they feel like they don't want to take medication. Who can tell us what happens to them on those days?

(4) Can you think of reasons why young people can't take their medication as they are supposed to do?

IDI questions about ART adherence were as follows:

(1) FGD questions listed above were also asked in IDIs.

(2) In your opinion, why is it important for someone who is HIV positive to take his/her medication properly?

(3) Did you ever face problems with your medication (e.g., side effects, switch of medication)? What were your experiences?

The interview guide was piloted with a convenience sample of three voluntary AYA patients from the pediatric HIV clinic who gave their opinions regarding the questions and their understanding so that the guide could be refined.

With the finalized interview guide, four FGDs were conducted, each consisting of three to six participants. The FGDs were stratified by clinic and gender: (1) female patients from the pediatric clinic, (2) female patients from the adult clinic, (3) male patients from the pediatric clinic, and (4) a mixed group of male and female patients from the adult clinic. FGDs were between 45 and 90 minutes' long and were audio-recorded. Interviews were facilitated by two young local multilingual female interviewers who were experienced in AYA qualitative research and trained on HIV and treatment issues for AYA. Questions were open-ended and probed where necessary to ensure robust data generation. The FGDs were conducted in a mix of English, Zulu, and Sotho [local languages in South Africa], with the facilitators being fluent in all three languages. Audio-recorded transcripts were transcribed and translated into English.

*2.3.2. In-Depth Interviews.* Eight IDIs were conducted, each around 60 minutes long and audio-recorded. IDI participants were not the same as the FGD participants. Interviews were facilitated by one of the two female interviewers who had conducted the FGDs. The question guide asked the same questions that had been in the FGDs to confirm whether responses that had been given in a peer-context would be different from those given without peer influence, and extra questions probed the level of understanding about the importance of adherence and the experiences of adverse effects of medications (see FGD and IDI questions about antiretroviral therapy adherence in Section 2.3.1). Audio-recorded transcripts were transcribed and translated into English.

*2.3.3. Biological Marker of Adherence.* Because ART adherence is a behaviour that can be linked with a biological marker, we collated the most recent HIV-1 viral load of the participants from the clinic records. However, viral load data was unknown to the interviewers at the time of the interviews with the participants so as to prevent influencing the course of the discussion.

*2.4. Ethical and Community Approval.* Ethical approval was obtained from the University of the Witwatersrand Human Research Ethics Committee. The Soweto adolescent community advisory board found that the study was relevant and appropriate. Study participant confidentiality was maintained by use of study numbers (not names) during the study proceedings and on the study documents. Participants, and parents/legal guardians if applicable, were given a reimbursement of R50 (~USD4) for transport costs.

*2.5. Data Analysis.* Quantitative data gained from the sociodemographic questionnaire were entered into Microsoft Office Excel to ensure accuracy across the data. Descriptive statistics and frequencies were calculated using Statistical Package for Social Sciences (SPSS) version 22.0. The most recent HIV-1 viral load was used to determine participants overall adherence; participants that were virally suppressed <400 cp/ml versus those that were not virally suppressed >400 cp/ml.

The FGD and IDI transcripts were hand-coded by the primary author using thematic analysis. First, the primary author entered a process of data immersion by reading and rereading transcripts. Thereafter, the primary investigator developed a code-book with the second author. Codes were developed based on the interview guide and addressed the following aspects: correct knowledge about how to be adherent; correct knowledge about adherence benefits and nonadherence consequences; social, personal, and medication-related barriers to adherence; and reminder, concealment, and motivational strategies to optimize adherence. Codes were then grouped into categories to develop subthemes. Relevant quotations selected from the transcripts were used to support the identified themes.

## 3. Results

*3.1. Participant Characteristics.* Overall, 186 ART patients between the ages of 15 and 25 years were identified; 123 had documented telephone numbers in the clinic databases or patient records and 26 participated in the study. The response rate for study participation was 22.4% (17/76) for females and 19.1% (9/47) for males. A total of 18 participants participated in the FGDs, 13 females (72.2%) and 5 males (22.8%). IDIs were conducted with 8 participants, equally divided by gender as 4 females and 4 males.

Table 1 shows participant characteristics. The median age of participants was 18.5 years [interquartile range (IQR) 17.0–21.5 years]. Seventeen (65.4%) participants indicated that they had acquired HIV through vertical transmission. The majority ($n$ = 17, 65.4%) were receiving ART at the pediatric clinic facility. The HIV status of all participants was known to at least one household member, most commonly their siblings ($n$ = 14, 53.8%), biological mother ($n$ = 12, 46.2%), and grandparents ($n$ = 12, 46.2%). Sixteen (61.5%) participants were classified as food insecure. The most recent viral load laboratory results showed that 18/26 (69.2%) participants were virally suppressed (<400 cp/ml) at the time of participation.

Three main themes emerged during FGDs and IDIs: (i) AYAs have correct knowledge about how to be adherent, benefits of adherence, and the consequences of nonadherence, (ii) despite correct theoretical knowledge about adherence, real life barriers existed that could result in suboptimal adherence, and (iii) there were facilitators and strategies to optimize adherence (Figure 1).

Table 1: Characteristics of adolescents and young adults who participated in FGDs and IDIs ($n$ = 26).

| Characteristics | |
|---|---|
| Median age, years (IQR) | 18.5 (17.0–21.5) |
| Gender, $n$ (%) | |
| Female | 17 (59.1) |
| Male | 9 (40.9) |
| Self-reported mode of HIV acquisition | |
| Vertical transmission | 17 (65.4) |
| Heterosexual transmission | 4 (15.4) |
| Unknown | 5 (19.2) |
| Treatment clinic attendance, $n$ (%) | |
| Adult clinic | 9 (34.6) |
| Pediatric clinic | 17 (65.4) |
| People to whom HIV status is disclosed*, $n$ (%) | |
| Biological mother | 12 (46.2) |
| Biological father | 2 (7.7) |
| Sibling/s | 14 (53.8) |
| Grandparent/s | 12 (46.2) |
| Cousin/s | 4 (15.4) |
| Partner/s | 4 (15.4) |
| Friend/s | 3 (11.8) |
| Teacher/s | 1 (3.8) |
| Other | 8 (30.8) |
| Food security, $n$ (%) | |
| Insecure | 16 (61.5) |
| Marginally secure | 5 (19.2) |
| Secure | 5 (19.2) |
| Biological marker of ART adherence | |
| Virologically suppressed < 400 cp/ml, $n$ (%) | 18 (69.2) |
| Female** | 12/17 (70.6) |
| Male | 6/9 (66.7) |

*Multiple responses allowed.
**One missing value for most recent viral load.

*3.2. Correct Knowledge about How to Be Adherent, Benefits, and Consequences of Nonadherence.* Most participants

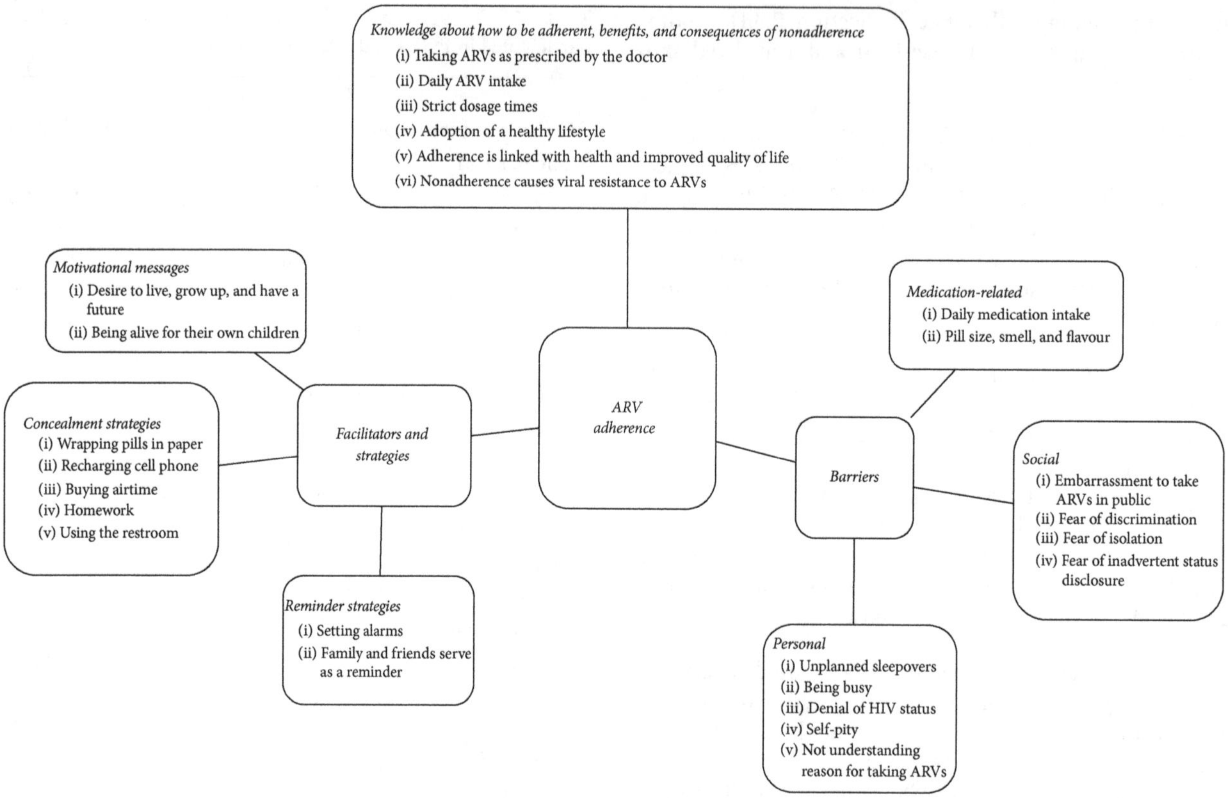


FIGURE 1: Summary of themes and subthemes emerging from FGDs and IDIs.

provided accurate basic knowledge about how to take their antiretrovirals (ARVs) properly. Most FGD participants agreed that the medication schedule should be followed as prescribed. FGD and IDI participants emphasized that taking medication every day without missing days and that following strict dosing times were important parts of adherence. However, though correct information about dosing was known to participants, the rationale for the dosing schedule was not always known. A 25-year-old female FGD participant said "If they [the doctors] say 3 times a day and you take 2, they have their reasons why you have to take it 3 times a day." Two participants agreed that a time period of twelve hours should lapse between the first and the second doses. Two participants emphasized that adopting a healthy lifestyle was also part of adherence to treatment: "You should start making decisions about [your] life, like for instance eating healthy food and living a healthy lifestyle" (17-year-old female FGD participant).

Many said they had started treatment in childhood. Explanations about how and why treatment should be taken were often introduced by the clinic staff, but three IDI participants said a family member had taught them. One 22-year-old female IDI participant, infected through vertical transmission, said that "both the doctor and my aunt explained perfectly well to me and the importance of me taking it [ARVs]."

Participants stated their perceptions about the benefits of ARV adherence. Three participants agreed that outcomes of strict adherence to ARVs would be prolonged life and improvement of quality of life. An 18-year-old male IDI participant stated that strict adherence would decrease the risk of HIV transmission.

Even though participants had difficulties in explaining the biological rationale of why ARVs had to be taken as prescribed, they were aware that there were consequences of nonadherence. They showed awareness that nonadherence could cause viral resistance to ARVs. For instance, a 19-year-old female FGD participant stated "If they [HIV patients] won't be taking their medication they'll end up getting different kind of viruses and that will influence them…" Another participant stated "They [doctors] told me that if I miss a dose the virus will grow and end up showing itself" (17-year-old male FGD participant).

Others perceived suboptimal ARV adherence to decrease overall health and quality of life, as expressed by one 21-year-old male IDI participant: "It is important [being adherent to ARVs] because as you are seeing me today as strong as I am, it is because of those pills and if you don't take them you go back to getting sick." A female FGD participant, aged 24 years, talked of the outcome of her experience being nonadherent to her ARVs as such "You'll pick up sickness, be in hospital in and out…."

*3.3. Barriers to Suboptimal Adherence.* At first, participants were uncomfortable admitting that they missed doses. Those that said they had been nonadherent declared to have done so unintentionally. Participants became more comfortable describing possible reasons for suboptimal adherence when the interviewer asked them to talk about "others" and not themselves necessarily. In this context of referring to others, participants easily volunteered personal, social, and medication-related reasons for suboptimal adherence and eased into talking about their own barriers to adherence.

*3.3.1. Personal Barriers.* Some participants said that when they became forgetful about their medication reminder system, their adherence would suffer. One 18-year-old female FGD participant said "Sometimes I cannot carry a pill reminder with me to school because the last time I did that it got lost at school and it cost me to buy another one." Five other participants admitted that they forgot taking their medication during an unplanned sleepover or simply forgot to take a dose while being in a rush or being busy. A 16-year-old male IDI participant described such a situation during a school trip: "I was not at home and I was on a school trip...I forgot them [ARVs], because I was too excited about the trip."

Another personal barrier to adherence was a level of denial and anger about childhood HIV persisting into adolescence and young adulthood despite treatment adherence in childhood. A 21-year-old female FGD participant, infected through vertical transmission, talked about how she used nonadherence to test out her disbelief that she would still have HIV after a whole childhood of taking treatment. "I am a very suicidal person...there are times where I would just give up...you are taking treatment...I'm still getting sick...I am still losing weight...but growing up realizing that this [ARVs] is something I [have] been drinking since I was a child – no man let me just live it like that [without ARVs]. Well I have been testing. I cannot say I have not been missing my doses – I have missed doses; I've defaulted a lot of times... I wanted to see what [was] going to happen to me and you find two to three months you are healthy and the next month you are out and you starting to get sick then you ask yourself why am I still sick with the very same sickness that I have been taking treatment for. Like, there [are] so many questions...".

The need for assimilation and not wanting to feel different was another personal reason named for neglecting doses. A female FGD participant aged 17-years, infected through vertical transmission, expressed "... If there is a family gathering...and they are not taking them and I have to take them, I feel different and think why I should drink them."

There was also mention of nonadherence as a means of dealing with conflict situations, with the intention to do self-harm: "Me and my granny were not in good terms...I would do that [not taking ARVs] just to make a revenge because I would think she doesn't love me and it's better if I kill myself and not taking the pills" (18-year-old male IDI participant).

*3.3.2. Social Barriers.* Social reasons for suboptimal adherence were heavily clustered around the idea of stigma. AYAs felt that taking medication in front of friends and family members would cause them to become embarrassed about having HIV, and furthermore they feared they would be discriminated against. Therefore, they generally took medication in secret so they could avoid inadvertent HIV status disclosure.

However, beyond stigma, there was also the idea that adherence could interfere with perceived normative AYA social behaviour. Drinking alcohol at parties was perceived as normative social behaviour, and it was perceived that ART and alcohol should not be taken together. One 24-year-old female FGD participant said "You are at a party and you are thinking about your medication so you thinking of going home fast. And what [is] bad is that you [are] not supposed to mix the medication with alcohol. So those are the challenges that we are facing as young people."

*3.3.3. Medication-Related Barriers.* Many participants expressed feeling tired or bored of taking their ARVs daily. A 24-year-old female FGD participant said "This thing of them [clinic staff] telling us to drink them [ARVs] every day and every day... it [is] just too much work. At least if other pills they make them to be syrups instead of pills." Others reported being tired of the big size, smell, and taste of the pills. A 16-year-old male FGD participant explained that "the pills need a flavour and ...taste...sometimes I feel like I don't want to take them anymore and...some of them are just so big."

*3.4. Facilitators and Strategies for Optimal Adherence.* Participants described several strategies that they acquired to support optimal adherence to ARVs including reminder, concealment strategies, and motivational messages.

*3.4.1. Reminder Strategies.* Participants mentioned different reminder methods including alarms, medication charts, family members, and friends. Four participants reported that they set daily alarms that reminded them to take their ARVs in time. However, for one female participant, setting alarms was risky, as she thought it could reveal her HIV status inadvertently to others. The best option for her was to disclose to a trusted person who would be able to remind her to take her daily ARVs.

Some participants stated they used their closest family and friends, who knew their status, as an additional reminder to take medication. A female FGD participant aged 16 years explained that "for me, drinking the medication in front of other people is not a problem. When me and my mother are visiting, my mother will tell me straight that I go and take my medication. Even if they ask me what the medication is for I'll tell them straight...and they keep quiet."

*3.4.2. Concealment Strategies.* In contrast, some participants were uncomfortable disclosing their HIV status to family members or friends, particularly when there was not enough trust. They acquired concealment strategies to take their ARVs in order to avoid inadvertent HIV status disclosure, discrimination, and isolation. Some participants reported wrapping their pills in paper or tissue to hide them from other people. A 25-year-old female participant said "The pills are always in my jean pockets or my breast inside the tissue. If I do not have water I opt for a chewing gum or some sweets. I put them one by one so that they won't ask any questions." Others invented reasons to be able to take their ARVs secretly, such as needing to get away to recharge cell phones, buy airtime for cell phones, do homework, or go to the restroom.

*3.4.3. Motivational Messages.* Many participants developed motivational messages with the desire to live, to grow up, to have a future and career. Those motivational messages kept them focused on being adherent to their ARVs despite the side effects that some of them experienced. For instance, one male IDI participant aged 20 years said "...I didn't want to become a statistics being another number...I wanted to live and continue my life and that's the reason why I am here, so I might as well live it." Two others confessed that their main motivation for taking their ARVs properly is their child: "Now I have a reason why I should take my treatment, I have a child now, so I have to look up, that you know that not only for me, I am not living for myself now, this I [have] somebody to look out for..." (21-year-old FGD female participant).

The majority of participants stated that they accepted their HIV status and were driven to be adherent by the desire to gain a long and healthy future life: "Why should I be ashamed of my life, this is how I have to live my life, take my pills, because without them I could get AIDS and AIDS kills...If I get ashamed of them [ARVs] it means I am ashamed of myself" (16-year-old male FGD participant).

## 4. Discussion

This qualitative study is one of the few studies to explore the knowledge in regard to adherence barriers and facilitators and experiences of ART adherence with AYAs who were mostly perinatally infected and from a developing setting.

As expected, AYAs in our study shared many adherence challenges previously identified in quantitative research amongst adult patients: fear of HIV status disclosure, HIV-related stigma, alcohol use, forgetfulness, and depression [17–19]. However, not all challenges were mutual. Our AYAs did not emphasize ART side effects as a challenge, even though studies in adults have found this. And unlike adults [19], AYAs did not speak of financial constraints. This is understandable because, even though most come from impoverished circumstances, AYAs may not hold financial responsibility in the household. A study in the South African private sector, which serves better-resourced patients who are able to pay for care, found 43.6%–55.8% viral suppression at 24 months on treatment in 10–30-year-olds, and correspondingly poor adherence [25]. In contrast, almost seventy percent of our study participants had suppressed viral loads, admittedly a biased sample because their willingness to participate in the study may reflect better adherence behaviours, but it is similar to AYAs in other resource-limited settings [26]. Taken together, it demonstrates that AYAs can overcome poor environments to maintain excellent treatment outcomes. The self-motivating strategies for adherence described by AYAs in our study show their resilience in trying to achieve this.

Our study identified unique adherence challenges that AYAs face, which are different from adults; some of these may be unique to AYAs who were infected at a young age. For example, we described a perinatally infected AYA who doubted persistence of the virus after a childhood of ART adherence and used nonadherence as a method to establish the ongoing pathogenicity of the disease.

Another issue for the subset of AYAs who were infected at a very young age is status disclosure and how that could affect adherence. In our study, AYAs, even perinatally infected ones, demonstrated correct basic knowledge about medication adherence and its benefits as well as consequences of nonadherence. Indeed, many have been in care since childhood and credit their knowledge source to their healthcare providers. This is encouraging because it implies that, for the perinatally infected AYAs in this study, healthcare providers have generally been able to transfer knowledge from parents and caregivers to the patients as they grow into adolescence. Clinical care that includes counselling, a supportive environment, a relationship of trust with the provider, and open discussion of patient concerns can help patients develop adequate adherence strategies [27–29]. This kind of optimal care is facilitated when vertically infected children are made aware of their HIV diagnosis in a timely manner [30]. Many children in developing countries are not told about their HIV diagnosis [31–33]. In a recent study conducted among pediatric ART children aged 4 to 17 years in Gauteng, South Africa, only 34% were disclosed about their HIV status [32]. Indeed, it is plausible that some of the one-fifth of adolescents in our study who stated that they do not know their infection route are perinatal infections who have not been disclosed to, placing them at risk of not understanding the importance of adherence, and dropping out of adherence, as they become adults. The disclosure process and the timing of disclosure as well as the relationship with the healthcare provider and their parents play an important role in regard to ARV medication management for AYA patients and are an area that requires further research [33, 34]. Learning about HIV status in a timely and appropriate manner has benefits in achieving long-term disease management and improvement of ARV adherence [18, 30].

Other challenges for AYA stem from how ART interrelates with the normative increased socialisation of adolescence. AYA described adherence challenges in relation to taking alcohol with medication. But mostly, they feared that public pill taking would inadvertently disclose their status, embarrass them, and stigmatise them at sleepovers, parties, family functions, and hanging out with friends. As with adults, this was a prominent reason for skipping doses in our study and supported by findings from another study conducted in Chicago, United States, among adolescents and young adults [28]. Although the majority claimed that at least one household member knew their status, few to very close friends were aware of their status, and this confirms assertions that the fear of stigma remains high even in high HIV prevalence settings [22, 35].

*Limitations.* Because of the poor participation and the fairly high proportion of virally suppressed participants in our sample, we do not know to what extent these findings would be valid for participants who have very poor adherence and are lost to follow-up. A possible reason for the poor participation could be fear of implied HIV status disclosure in a peer group setting.

The presence of other peers during FGDs could have affected participants' responses, but we conducted IDIs with different individuals to ensure that data was not only received from a peer-influenced environment. Although there was evidence of social desirability bias, we attempted to limit it by encouraging participants to talk about nonadherence in others when they did not want to admit to it initially in themselves. This gave way to personal anecdotes of times they had experienced nonadherence.

## 5. Conclusion

Despite having good knowledge about ART, AYAs may face circumstances which can derail optimal adherence. AYAs may present with specific adherence problems, such as denial about HIV persistence after a childhood of treatment and the issues that HIV/AIDS poses to them during a phase of development in which social assimilation gains prominence in their lives. AYAs may find it difficult to open up about these circumstances as they struggle internally to resolve them. It may be useful for the healthcare practitioner facing a poorly adherent AYA patient to learn from the strategy we employed in our interviews: inviting AYAs to share general, not necessarily personal, barriers to adherence. Regardless, in a world where HIV discrimination remains a reality, secretiveness may be a practical and palatable strategy which a healthcare worker can suggest to AYAs to help maintain adherence while public disclosure is unthinkable for the individual. Parallel interventions may be motivational messaging focusing on the known long-term health, longevity, and prevention benefits of achieving viral suppression through adherence and practical strategies for status disclosure where appropriate.

## Competing Interests

The authors declare that they have no competing interests.

## Acknowledgments

The authors thank Dineo Tsotetsi for translations and transcriptions, Matamela Makongoza for conducting the interviews, Dr. Lerato Mohapi and Dr. Avy Violari for facilitating clinic access, and the AYA participants and their parents for their study participation and sharing their time and insights with the authors. This research was supported by the University of the Witwatersrand through a grant awarded to Dr. Laher.

## References

[1] O. Shisana, T. Rehle, L. C. Simbayi et al., *South African National HIV Prevalence, Incidence, Behaviour and Communication Survey 2012*, HSRC Press, Cape Town, South Africa, 2014.

[2] M. D. Nglazi, K. Kranzer, P. Holele et al., "Treatment outcomes in HIV-infected adolescents attending a community-based antiretroviral therapy clinic in South Africa," *BMC Infectious Diseases*, vol. 12, no. 1, article 21, 2012.

[3] P. Chigwedere, G. R. Seage III, S. Gruskin, T.-H. Lee, and M. Essex, "Estimating the lost benefits of antiretroviral drug use in South Africa," *Journal of Acquired Immune Deficiency Syndromes*, vol. 49, no. 4, pp. 410–415, 2008.

[4] UNAIDS, *Global Report: UNAIDS Report on the Global AIDS Epidemic*, UNAIDS, Geneva, Switzerland, 2013.

[5] N. Dowshen and L. D'Angelo, "Health care transition for youth living with HIV/AIDS," *Pediatrics*, vol. 128, no. 4, pp. 762–771, 2011.

[6] P. Macpherson, C. Munthali, J. Ferguson et al., "Service delivery interventions to improve adolescents' linkage, retention and adherence to antiretroviral therapy and HIV care," *Tropical Medicine and International Health*, vol. 20, no. 8, pp. 1015–1032, 2015.

[7] F. J. Palella Jr., K. M. Delaney, A. C. Moorman et al., "Declining morbidity and mortality among patients with advanced human immunodeficiency virus infection," *New England Journal of Medicine*, vol. 338, no. 13, pp. 853–860, 1998.

[8] K. K. Venkatesh, M. N. Lurie, and K. H. Mayer, "How HIV treatment could result in effective prevention," *Future Virology*, vol. 5, no. 4, pp. 405–415, 2010.

[9] D. L. Paterson, S. Swindells, J. Mohr et al., "Adherence to protease inhibitor therapy and outcomes in patients with HIV infection," *Annals of Internal Medicine*, vol. 133, no. 1, pp. 21–30, 2000.

[10] E. Wood, J. S. G. Montaner, B. Yip et al., "Adherence and plasma HIV RNA responses to highly active antiretroviral therapy among HIV-1 infected injection drug users," *CMAJ*, vol. 169, no. 7, pp. 656–661, 2003.

[11] P. G. Yeni, S. M. Hammer, M. S. Hirsch et al., "Treatment for adult HIV infection: 2004 recommendations of the international AIDS society-USA panel," *The Journal of the American Medical Association*, vol. 292, no. 2, pp. 251–265, 2004.

[12] A. Adefolalu and Z. Nkosi, "The complex nature of adherence in the management of HIV/AIDS as a chronic medical condition," *Diseases*, vol. 1, no. 1, pp. 18–35, 2013.

[13] Department of Health, *National Consolidated Guidelines for the Prevention of Mother-to-Child Transmission of HIV (PMTCT) and the Management of HIV in Children, Adolescents and Adults*, Department of Health, Pretoria, South Africa, 2014.

[14] P. L. Williams, D. Storm, G. Montepiedra et al., "Predictors of adherence to antiretroviral medications in children and adolescents with HIV infection," *Pediatrics*, vol. 118, no. 6, pp. e1745–e1757, 2006.

[15] A. Shroufi, H. Gunguwo, M. Dixon et al., "HIV-infected adolescents in southern Africa can achieve good treatment outcomes: Results From A Retrospective Cohort Study," *AIDS*, vol. 27, no. 12, pp. 1971–1978, 2013.

[16] S. L. Reisner, M. J. Mimiaga, M. Skeer, B. Perkovich, C. V. Johnson, and S. A. Safren, "A review of HIV antiretroviral adherence and intervention studies among HIV-infected youth," *Topics in HIV Medicine*, vol. 17, no. 1, pp. 14–25, 2009.

[17] E. J. Mills, J. B. Nachega, I. Buchan et al., "Adherence to antiretroviral therapy in sub-Saharan Africa and North America. A meta-analysis," *The Journal of the American Medical Association*, vol. 296, no. 6, pp. 679–690, 2006.

[18] A. A. Reda and S. Biadgilign, "Determinants of adherence to antiretroviral therapy among HIV-infected patients in Africa," *AIDS Research and Treatment*, vol. 2012, Article ID 574656, 8 pages, 2012.

[19] K. Peltzer, N. Friend-Du Preez, S. Ramlagan, and J. Anderson, "Antiretroviral treatment adherence among HIV patients in KwaZulu-Natal, South Africa," *BMC Public Health*, vol. 10, article 111, 10 pages, 2010.

[20] S. L. Becker, C. M. Dezii, B. Burtcel, H. Kawabata, and S. Hodder, "Young HIV-infected adults are at greater risk for medication nonadherence," *Medscape General Medicine*, vol. 4, no. 3, p. 21, 2002.

[21] D. A. Murphy, M. Sarr, S. J. Durako et al., "Barriers to HAART adherence among human immunodeficiency virus-infected adolescents," *Archives of Pediatrics & Adolescent Medicine*, vol. 157, pp. 249–255, 2003.

[22] C. J. Kunapareddy, W. Nyandiko, T. Inui, S. Ayaya, D. G. Marrero, and R. Vreeman, "A qualitative assessment of barriers to antiretroviral therapy adherence among adolescents in western kenya," *Journal of HIV/AIDS and Social Services*, vol. 13, no. 4, pp. 383–401, 2014.

[23] City of Johannesburg, "The making of Soweto," 2012, http://www.joburg.org.za/index.php?option=com_content&view=article&id=920&catid=88&Itemid=159.

[24] S. Hornschuh, F. Laher, M. Makongoza, C. Tshabalala, L. D. J. Kuijper, and J. Dietrich, "Experiences of HIV-positive adolescents and young adults in care in Soweto, South Africa," *Journal of HIV/AIDS and Social Services*, vol. 13, no. 4, pp. 420–435, 2014.

[25] J. B. Nachega, M. Hislop, H. Nguyen et al., "Antiretroviral therapy adherence, virologic and immunologic outcomes in adolescents compared with adults in Southern Africa," *Journal of Acquired Immune Deficiency Syndromes*, vol. 51, no. 1, pp. 65–71, 2009.

[26] C. Obirikorang, P. K. Selleh, J. K. Abledu, and C. O. Fofie, "Predictors of adherence to antiretroviral therapy among HIV/AIDS patients in the upper west region of Ghana," *ISRN AIDS*, vol. 2013, Article ID 873939, 7 pages, 2013.

[27] C. Campbell, K. Scott, C. Madanhire, C. Nyamukapa, and S. Gregson, "A 'good hospital': nurse and patient perceptions of good clinical care for HIV-positive people on antiretroviral treatment in rural Zimbabwe—a mixed-methods qualitative study," *International Journal of Nursing Studies*, vol. 48, no. 2, pp. 175–183, 2011.

[28] D. Rao, T. C. Kekwaletswe, S. Hosek, J. Martinez, and F. Rodriguez, "Stigma and social barriers to medication adherence with urban youth living with HIV," *AIDS Care - Psychological and Socio-Medical Aspects of AIDS/HIV*, vol. 19, no. 1, pp. 28–33, 2007.

[29] K. J. Roberts, "Physician-patient relationships, patient satisfaction, and antiretroviral medication adherence among HIV-infected adults attending a public health clinic," *AIDS Patient Care and STDs*, vol. 16, no. 1, pp. 43–50, 2002.

[30] W. Bikaako-Kajura, E. Luyirika, D. W. Purcell et al., "Disclosure of HIV status and adherence to daily drug regimens among HIV-infected children in Uganda," *AIDS and Behavior*, vol. 10, 2006.

[31] S. Kallem, L. Renner, M. Ghebremichael, and E. Paintsil, "Prevalence and pattern of disclosure of HIV status in HIV-infected children in Ghana," *AIDS and Behavior*, vol. 15, no. 6, pp. 1121–1127, 2011.

[32] S. Madiba, J. Mahloko, and K. Mokwena, "Prevalence and factors associated with disclosure of HIV diagnosis to infected children receiving antiretroviral treatment in public health care facilities in Gauteng, South Africa," *Journal of Clinical Research in HIV Aids and Prevention*, vol. 1, no. 1, pp. 35–45, 2013.

[33] R. C. Vreeman, M. L. Scanlon, A. Mwangi et al., "A cross-sectional study of disclosure of HIV status to children and adolescents in Western Kenya," *PLoS ONE*, vol. 9, no. 1, Article ID e86616, 10 pages, 2014.

[34] M. D. Morobadi and L. M. Webber, "Growing up with HIV in Southern Africa-HIV-infected children and adolescents," *Journal of Human Virology & Retrovirology*, vol. 1, no. 1, 2014.

[35] P. R. Mutwa, J. I. Van Nuil, B. Asiimwe-Kateera et al., "Living situation affects adherence to combination antiretroviral therapy in HIV-infected adolescents in rwanda: a qualitative study," *PLoS ONE*, vol. 8, no. 4, Article ID e60073, 2013.

# 20

# Disclosure of Parental HIV Status to Children: Experiences of Adults Receiving Antiretroviral Treatment at an Urban Clinic in Kampala, Uganda

**Charles Peter Osingada,[1] Monica Okuga,[2] Rose Chalo Nabirye,[1] Nelson Kaulukusi Sewankambo,[3] and Damalie Nakanjako[3]**

[1]*Makerere University College of Health Sciences, School of Health Sciences, Department of Nursing, P.O. Box 7072, Kampala, Uganda*
[2]*Makerere University School of Public Health, Department of Health Policy Planning and Management, P.O. Box 7072, Kampala, Uganda*
[3]*Department of Internal Medicine, School of Medicine, Makerere College of Health Sciences, P.O. Box 7072, Kampala, Uganda*

Correspondence should be addressed to Charles Peter Osingada; ocpeter@chs.mak.ac.ug

Academic Editor: David Katzenstein

Limited data are available on the experiences of parental HIV disclosure to children in Uganda. We conducted a qualitative study comprising sixteen in-depth interviews and four focus group discussions with parents receiving highly active antiretroviral therapy. Analysis was done using Atlas.ti qualitative research software. Back-and-forth triangulation was done between transcripts of the in-depth interviews and focus group discussions, and themes and subthemes were developed. Barriers to parents' disclosure included perceptions that children are too young to understand what HIV infection means and fears of secondary disclosure by the children. Immediate outcomes of disclosure included children getting scared and crying, although such instances often gave way to more enduring positive experiences for the parents, such as support in adherence to medical care, help in household chores, and a decrease in financial demands from the children. Country-specific interventions are needed to improve the process of parental HIV disclosure to children and this should encompass preparation on how to deal with the immediate psychological challenges associated with the parent's disclosure.

## 1. Introduction

HIV and AIDS continue to be a major public health challenge worldwide more so in sub-Saharan Africa where HIV-related illness is a leading cause of morbidity and mortality. Global estimates indicated that, by the end of 2014, 36.9 million people were living with HIV infection, and of these 25.8 million were in sub-Saharan Africa [1]. Even though there has been a global decline in new HIV infections and associated deaths, the number of clients enrolled for antiretroviral therapy has steadily grown to reach at least 15.8 million [1]. According to a national survey of 2011, about 7.3% of individuals aged 15–49 years are infected with HIV [2]; the number of new infections reportedly dropped from 128068 in 2009 to about 99000 in 2014, while the estimated number of annual HIV-related deaths declined from 52799 in 2009 to 32890 in 2015 [3]. A decrease in HIV-related deaths [4] coupled with an increase in the number of people accessing antiretroviral treatment has given birth to the phenomenon of social normalization of HIV and AIDS [5] which according to Roy and colleagues depends on both disclosure of HIV status to a person's social networks and willingness and ability of the network to support the emotional and material needs of the person living with HIV [6]. In work conducted in Uganda and Tanzania, high adherence resulted from social and material support from an individual's social networks [7].

HIV status disclosure has been the subject of numerous studies on the African continent, particularly in view of increasing incidence of HIV transmission to sexual partners in several countries [8–13]. Also, following publication of the World Health Organization (WHO) guidelines on HIV counselling for children up to 12 years of age [14], there has been renewed interest in encouraging parents and caregivers to disclose their HIV status to children. A parent's disclosure of their HIV-positive status can occur at different levels. It can be limited to sharing of health information between the parent and child which then happens to result in the child knowing the parent's serostatus. Disclosure can also be planned by the parent and shared either directly or indirectly: it can take the form of full disclosure when the terms HIV and AIDS are used in sharing the health information, resulting in the child knowing the parent's HIV-positive status; or it can take the form of partial disclosure when the specific terms HIV or AIDS are not used by the parent, yet the parent's actions or conversation results in the child becoming aware of the parent's HIV-positive status.

Available literature indicates that HIV-positive individuals struggle with what, when, and how to disclose their HIV-positive status [15–17]. Nondisclosure has been justified by parents based on the premise of protecting children from the negative social and psychological consequences caused by disclosure [16, 18–20]. Nevertheless, nondisclosure has been associated with negative consequences for both the parent and child [21, 22]. In many developing countries, there is a growing demand for culturally appropriate interventions intended to increase parents' readiness to disclose their HIV status to their children [15]. Interventions to encourage parental HIV disclosure to children have been tested in the United States [21, 23] and China [24]. However, in sub-Saharan Africa, with the exception of South Africa [25–27], such interventions are uncommon. Moreover, the implementation of these kinds of interventions should be grounded on a good understanding of the local context regarding potential parental HIV disclosure. In Uganda, limited data are available on the barriers, approaches, motivators, and consequences of parental disclosure of HIV status to children. This scarcity of information provided the impetus for this study.

## 2. Methods

*2.1. Study Design and Setting.* A cross-sectional, descriptive, qualitative study was conducted among HIV-positive clients in care and treatment at the Infectious Diseases Institute at Makerere University's College of Health Sciences, Kampala, Uganda. The Infectious Diseases Institute is a Ugandan not-for-profit organization, established in 2002, whose mission is to strengthen HIV-related care, training, and research in Africa. By 2014 the Infectious Diseases Institute was providing care and treatment services to over 110000 people living with HIV in urban and rural settings in Uganda, which amounts to about 13% of the national effort [18].

*2.2. Participant Recruitment and Data Collection.* The study participants comprised adult parents who were HIV-positive, who either had or had not disclosed their HIV serostatus to their child/children, and who had a biological child aged at least 5 years or older. The age-5 lower limit was chosen based on a recommendation by the World Health Organization [14] that children of school age should be told of a caregiver's HIV-positive status. No upper limit cut-off for a child's age was stated because in African settings parents tend to perceive children as a child irrespective of their child's age. The sample was purposively determined to include both clients who had disclosed their HIV status and those who had not. Potential participants were identified by the research assistants at the clinic; to avoid disrupting the smooth running of the clinic, willing clients were given appointments to return later for an in-depth interview (IDI) and/or focus group discussion (FGD). The selection involved a process of screening all potential participants during the time when they were waiting for review of their individual treatment. Each client who met the inclusion criteria was then given an appointment for when to return for the purposes of participating in the study. Sampling was also guided by the principle of data saturation—that is, data collection was terminated when no new information appeared to be elicited from the IDIs and FGDs.

Data were first collected from participants who returned for an IDI. Each parent was taken through the process of consent, and those who provided written informed consent were then individually interviewed by one of four trained research assistants. Each interview lasted between thirty and forty-five minutes and all the interviews were conducted in Luganda (the local language of central Uganda). To ensure privacy and confidentiality, each interview was conducted in a quiet room usually used for counselling clinic clients. Each of the participants in the study, in either an IDI or FGD, was paid the equivalent of US $10 to compensate for travel and time. A total of 16 IDIs were carried out with HIV-positive parents who had or had not disclosed their status to their child/children. Of these, nine parents had disclosed their HIV status (i.e., shared health information with a child, resulting in the child knowing the parent's HIV-positive status) and seven had not. In addition, four FGDs, each with 8 or 9 participants, were carried out: two groups with men and two groups with women. We chose to conduct separate FGDs for men and women for cultural reasons, as in the Ugandan context anecdotal evidence suggests that women tend to express their opinions less freely in the presence of men. We conducted one FGD for men and one for women who had disclosed their HIV status, and likewise there was one group for men and another for women who had not disclosed their HIV status. A total of 35 clients participated in the four FGDs. The IDIs and FGDs were conducted using guides developed by the investigators after reviewing the literature on parental HIV disclosure. Different guides were developed for research with parents who had disclosed their HIV status and with those who had not. All the guides were translated into Luganda by an expert from Makerere University's Department of Linguistics, English-Language Studies and Communication. The translated guides were pretested among HIV-positive parents attending the Old Mulago HID and AIDS Clinic in the general outpatient department, which was not part of the study site so as to avoid bias that would result from patients who participated in the pretest being included in the study. Adjustments were made to the flow of questions and probes before the data collection began.

*2.3. Data Management.* Audio-recordings of the IDIs and FGDs were transcribed and translated and then analysed by an expert with a social science background, using Atlas.ti qualitative data management software. The transcripts were assigned a name that did not contain any personal identifying information, to maintain anonymity. A code book was developed after reading through a random sample of five transcripts (2 FGDs and 3 IDIs) to ascertain the emerging themes. The transcripts were then entered into Atlas.ti. Next, the codebook from the emerging issues that had been transformed into different codes was entered into Atlas.ti. Each of the transcripts was then thoroughly read and any portion of text identified that related to a particular code was highlighted and attached to the respective code. Query reports for each of the codes were produced containing short summaries of texts. Each of these short summaries was read several times and analysed manually using manifest content analysis to identify emerging patterns. Back-and-forth triangulation was done between transcripts of the FGDs and IDIs before a decision was made to group those sources together under the themes and subthemes. These themes reflected underlying meanings in the text. In presenting the results here, we quote extractions from the texts, representing the themes, to support our findings.

## 3. Results

*3.1. Sociodemographics of the Participants.* A total of 51 parents on ART participated in the study. Sixteen clients participated in IDIs: 7 males and 9 females; their ages ranged from 28 to 59 years. Thirty-five individuals participated in FGDs: 19 males and 16 females; their ages ranged from 24 to 67 years. Religious affiliations and disclosure status of each participant are shown in Table 1.

*3.2. Parents' Experiences regarding HIV Disclosure.* Experiences concerning parental HIV disclosure fell into four categories: barriers/hindrances, motivators, approaches, and consequences. Themes that emerged from the data in each category are summarised in Table 2.

*3.3. Barriers to Parental HIV Disclosure.* Table 1 summarises four themes that emerged from the data relating to barriers or hindrances to parents' disclosure: viewing disclosure as a burden, perceived immaturity of the children, strength of the relationship between the parent and child, and anticipated unfavourable level of support from the child.

*3.3.1. Viewing Disclosure as an Unnecessary Burden.* Some parents who had not disclosed their HIV status viewed sharing their serostatus as an unnecessary burden that was not worth the risk of going through it. They feared that their child/children might ask about their own HIV status, that they would probably tell the other partner/parent about their HIV test result, and that this would exert pressure on the parent to explain how the disease came into the family. One male participant in a FGD said the following:

> *Those children can put pressure on me...first of all, I have not taken them for testing, so I do not know whether they are [HIV] negative or positive. I have also feared to do this; I may take them to test and one or two are found [HIV] positive, and the woman will ask "how did it come?" And we might get misunderstandings in the home, so I kept quiet and I have peace...as you know we have responsibilities in some organizations and even in the central government, so it gave me peace for keeping my secret. (participant in men's FGD)*

*3.3.2. Children Perceived as Too Young to Understand.* Some parents chose not to disclose their HIV status because they perceived their child as too young to understand the meaning and consequences of HIV infection, and some also believed a child would not be able to keep the parent's HIV status confidential. One woman explained the following:

> *I take drugs with my husband, and [the children] donot see it, we keep it in the bedroom. Even if they go there they have not yet known it, they have never seen it anywhere. They will only see the tin, they will not know whether it is for headache or stomach pains. I will tell them when they grow up, but now they are very young, even if you tell them they will not take it seriously. (IDI with female)*

*3.3.3. Poor Relationship between Parent and Child.* Parents, but particularly fathers, often chose not to disclose their HIV status to their child because they felt the relationship between them was not good enough to facilitate disclosure. Some parents reported lacking the personal confidence to disclose their HIV status, and in other instances they felt their child was not interested in their health. Other reasons included parents viewing their adult children as being interested only in sharing the parent's property and less so in personal concerns. There were also cases where the children were regarded as being close to only one parent, which made the other uncomfortable about disclosure. This is demonstrated in explanations provided by two men:

> *Only that the other three I do not always get information about them, that is why I do not tell them some things; if I want I just pay their fees and they go to school, but they do not know some information about me...they are all spoiled and they now think like her [their mother]; they do not expect me to tell them anything good, they only respect what their mother tells them. So I have left them like that. (IDI with male)*

> *"Another thing, I have many children and they are not from the same mother; so I think that if I tell, this one will think that maybe it is this mother who did this [brought the infection into the family], but there is not much problem. (IDI with male)*

TABLE 1: Sociodemographic characteristics of study participants.

| Number | Gender | Age | Focus group discussion (FGD)/in-depth interview (IDI) | Region | Disclosure status |
|---|---|---|---|---|---|
| 1 | Female | 32 | FGD | Protestant | Not disclosed |
| 2 | Female | 41 | FGD | Protestant | Not disclosed |
| 3 | Female | 26 | FGD | Muslim | Not disclosed |
| 4 | Female | 49 | FGD | Protestant | Not disclosed |
| 5 | Female | 29 | FGD | Catholic | Not disclosed |
| 6 | Female | 24 | FGD | Protestant | Not disclosed |
| 7 | Male | 54 | FGD | Protestant | Disclosed |
| 8 | Female | 67 | FGD | Protestant | Disclosed |
| 9 | Female | 26 | FGD | Catholic | Disclosed |
| 10 | Female | 46 | FGD | Protestant | Disclosed |
| 11 | Female | 45 | FGD | Protestant | Disclosed |
| 12 | Female | 60 | FGD | Protestant | Disclosed |
| 13 | Female | 41 | FGD | Protestant | Disclosed |
| 14 | Female | 38 | FGD | Catholic | Disclosed |
| 15 | Male | 42 | FGD | Protestant | Disclosed |
| 16 | Male | 54 | FGD | Catholic | Disclosed |
| 17 | Male | 51 | FGD | Catholic | Disclosed |
| 18 | Male | 37 | FGD | Protestant | Disclosed |
| 19 | Male | 40 | FGD | Muslim | Disclosed |
| 20 | Male | 58 | FGD | Muslim | Disclosed |
| 21 | Male | 39 | FGD | Protestant | Not disclosed |
| 22 | Male | 39 | FGD | Catholic | Disclosed |
| 23 | Male | 31 | FGD | Protestant | Not disclosed |
| 24 | Male | 61 | FGD | Protestant | Not disclosed |
| 25 | Male | 42 | FGD | Catholic | Not disclosed |
| 26 | Male | 40 | FGD | Protestant | Not disclosed |
| 27 | Male | 50 | FGD | Protestant | Not disclosed |
| 28 | Male | 45 | FGD | Protestant | Not disclosed |
| 29 | Male | 40 | FGD | Protestant | Not disclosed |
| 30 | Female | 30 | FGD | Catholic | Not disclosed |
| 31 | Male | 46 | FGD | Protestant | Disclosed |
| 32 | Male | 52 | FGD | Protestant | Not disclosed |
| 33 | Male | 58 | FGD | Protestant | Disclosed |
| 34 | Female | 45 | FGD | Pentecostal | Disclosed |
| 35 | Female | 33 | FGD | Catholic | Not disclosed |
| 36 | Male | 37 | IDI | Protestant | Disclosed |
| 37 | Female | 50 | IDI | Protestant | Disclosed |
| 38 | Female | 45 | IDI | Muslim | Not disclosed |
| 39 | Male | 28 | IDI | Catholic | Not disclosed |
| 40 | Female | 44 | IDI | Muslim | Not disclosed |
| 41 | Female | 45 | IDI | Pentecostal | Disclosed |
| 42 | Male | 46 | IDI | Catholic | Disclosed |
| 43 | Male | 59 | IDI | Protestant | Not disclosed |
| 44 | Female | 56 | IDI | Pentecostal | Disclosed |
| 45 | Female | 44 | IDI | Protestant | Not disclosed |
| 46 | Female | 48 | IDI | Muslim | Not disclosed |
| 47 | Male | 33 | IDI | Protestant | Disclosed |
| 48 | Female | 35 | IDI | Catholic | Disclosed |
| 49 | Male | 43 | IDI | Muslim | Not disclosed |
| 50 | Male | 49 | IDI | Protestant | Disclosed |
| 51 | Female | 48 | IDI | Catholic | Disclosed |

TABLE 2: Barriers/hindrances to disclosure as presented by parents who did not disclose HIV serostatus to their children.

| Themes | Subthemes |
|---|---|
| Viewing disclosure as a risk or burden | (i) Parent being in poor health and therefore concerned more about their health than disclosure.<br>(ii) Parents perceived the children as already knowing their (parent's) HIV status.<br>(iii) Parents feared that the children may ask them about their own (child's) HIV status.<br>(iv) Parents feared their children's assumption that they (parents) are about to die.<br>(v) Parents preferring to have "peace of mind" and hence avoid disclosure to children. |
| Immaturity of children | (i) Children were viewed by the parent as being unable to understand the meaning and consequences of being HIV-positive.<br>(ii) Parents observed that the child might not keep the parent's HIV-positive status confidential. |
| Relationship between parent and child | (i) Relationship between parent and the children was viewed as not good enough to facilitate disclosure.<br>(ii) Parents reported not being personally confident enough to disclose their HIV status.<br>(iii) Children did not seem interested and passionate enough about the health of their parents.<br>(iv) Parents viewed their children as being interested only in sharing the parent's property.<br>(v) Children being closer to one of the parents, making the other uncomfortable to disclose their HIV status under such circumstances. |
| Anticipated support from children | (i) Parent viewed children as not being able to support them emotionally or practically.<br>(ii) Parent still felt in good health and saw no need to be supported by the children. |

*3.3.4. Anticipated Unfavourable Level of Support from a Child.* Some parents felt self-reliant because they were in otherwise good health and able to support themselves and thus did not feel the need or benefit of disclosure to their children. One man explained the following:

> *I do not have any serious problem. . .until when I reach my last day, so that gives me confidence that I do not need my children to know. . .so I saw that if I am capable I do not need to disclose. . .what I did, I got a house boy who helps me in everything. . .. I can be able to do everything on my own; I do not need any support, and whenever I need help I just run here. (participant in men's FGD)*

*3.4. Motivation of Disclosure.* A parent's motivation to disclose their HIV status was captured in four themes (Table 3). Overall, men were more likely to be motivated to disclose their HIV status to their child so as to clarify doubts about their HIV-positive status, whereas females were more likely to disclose their HIV status as a result of seeing it as an obligation to their child.

*3.4.1. Parental Obligation of Disclosure.* Some parents had disclosed their HIV status clearly because they felt it was their obligation and responsibility to their children. One mother remarked the following:

> *What forced me to disclose to them, when I produced children, I never produced a boy, I produced four children and they are all girls. One of them died and I remained with three, so it pained me a lot that if I do not tell these children. . .they are like my sisters, so I said these children should grow knowing my status, they do not have any brother in life, I am now their sister, so let me tell them. (IDI with female)*

*3.4.2. Clarification of Doubts about the Parent's HIV Status.* Some parents explained that their disclosure had arisen after they noticed suspicion among their children, who might have noticed "suspicious medicines" in the home or that the parent was attending monthly hospital appointments:

> *One time I was there and I thought I would die and these children would not know how I died or what killed me; and as you know when you die you cannot fail to get someone among ten people who will feel sorry, so I first told the boy; and I told him that I am very sick, and this disease is so serious that it does not cure, and he told me there is no disease that cannot cure; I told him that don't joke for me, I am sick, then I asked him that "have you ever seen people suffering from HIV/AIDS?" (IDI with male)*

*3.4.3. Need to Protect the Child.* Other parents had disclosed their HIV status out of a desire to protect adolescent children who were likely to engage in higher-risk sexual behaviours. One mother said the following:

> *So now she was grown, with breasts growing big, she started putting on short skirts, and that is when I called her and told her that I have HIV and it is the reason I take drugs every morning and evening. She got surprised and said that at school we learn that HIV is not cured. . .and I advised her not to go in for boys, and good enough at church they sign papers that they will not have sex until marriage, and for her she honours*

TABLE 3: Motivators to disclosure, as presented by parents who disclosed their HIV status to their children.

| Theme | Subthemes |
|---|---|
| Obligation of disclosure | (i) Parent wanting to clarify their HIV-positive status to the children.<br>(ii) Desire to prepare the children so that death of the parent would not come as a shock.<br>(iii) Parents' desire to confirm what the children had earlier suspected that the parent might be HIV-positive. |
| Clarification or "clearing the air" about the parent's HIV status | (i) Desire to clarify the "suspicious medicines" (antiretroviral drugs) that the children had already seen the parent taking.<br>(ii) Clarifying to the children about monthly hospital appointments. |
| Need to protect children | (i) Parents chose to disclose their HIV status as a way of warning them that higher-risk sexual behaviour could lead to contracting HIV.<br>(ii) Desire to show children that HIV can "kill" or is "very painful" or that it is not pleasant to take medicines every day. |
| Improved health | (i) Parents disclosed their HIV status after noticing an improvement in their health. |

*that commitment so much, and she always says "Mammy, I cannot sleep with boys, not until I put on a white gown like you did." (mother of teenager, in FGD)*

One father stated it this way:

*My children are big, and they were seeing me taking my medicine, and they are also growing; so you have to show them that love is good but it also has tears; you have to show children that HIV kills and it is very painful and it is not fun to take medicine every day. (father of teenager, in FGD)*

*3.4.4. Disclosure Based on Parent's Feeling of Improved Health.* Several parents had been motivated to disclose their HIV status based on noticing an improvement in their health and thus felt their disclosure would less likely scare the child based on this timing:

*And my daughter was worried and asking herself what I was suffering from, because I used to fall sick all the time during that time, but I could not tell her. I only used to tell her that they are still investigating, but they had already told me that I was HIV-positive. When I was admitted and I was badly off [very sick], I decided not to disclose at that moment, [instead] I told them when I came back from the hospital. (IDI with female)*

*3.5. Parents' Approaches to Disclosure.* The process of parental disclosure elicited two main themes (Table 4): as a result of circumstances and preplanning by the parent as either direct or indirect disclosure.

*3.5.1. Circumstantial Disclosure.* Some parents started the process of disclosing their HIV-positive status to their children following circumstantial prompts, such as when a child asked about the parent's HIV status or wanted to know their own status, or following death of a family member. One participant said the following:

*The child was also born [HIV] positive, so the child was started on septrin [cotrimoxazole] and when the child grew up she asked her mother that "but mummy, for how long will I take this medicine?" So the mum responded that "We shall take it until God will decide for us." Then the child asked me that "Daddy, I always see mummy taking medicine and she also gives me medicine, what is it for?" For me, I am open, so I told her A-B-C-D [and I] disclosed. (participant in men's FGD)*

*3.5.2. Planned Conversation.* For some parents the process of disclosure was planned well in advance and it entailed gathering all the children together for making a direct disclosure in a family meeting:

*So I called them together at the same time in the same room and I told them that take care, "you protect yourselves, you are young and you are girls. I, your mother, I had not told you but I am HIV-positive, if you did not know." (IDI with female)*

*3.5.3. Leaving Medicines in the Open.* Some parents initiated the process of disclosure by deliberately leaving their antiretroviral medicines out for children to see, without ever verbally disclosing their HIV-positive status. For example,

*I did not tell them abruptly, like you are there and you want to counsel your children and you tell them that I am like this, I have gone to the hospital and they tested my blood and I was found HIV-positive. But I used to leave my drugs (medicine) on the table for them to see and know for themselves. (IDI with female)*

*3.6. Positive Outcomes of Disclosure.* Positive outcomes of the parents' disclosure (Table 5) included themes wherein a child showed concern about the parent's health, parents received support from the children, children improved their behaviour, and the parent felt psychological relief after disclosure.

*3.6.1. Children Showing Concern about a Parent's Health.* In some cases, once a parent had disclosed their HIV-positive

TABLE 4: Some processes of disclosure, as presented by the patients that had disclosed their HIV status to their children.

| Themes | Subthemes |
|---|---|
| Being prompted by events | (i) When the children asked about the parent's HIV status.<br>(ii) When the children wanted to know their own HIV status. |
| Gathering children | (i) Parents planning well in advance and gathering the children together for the disclosure. |
| Offering clues | (i) Leaving the antiretroviral medicines for the children to see, without telling them that the parent is HIV-positive. |

TABLE 5: Consequences of disclosure, as presented by parents that had disclosed their HIV status.

| Themes | Subthemes |
|---|---|
| *(a) Positive consequences* | |
| Support and concern about health of the parent | (i) Reminding parents when the time for taking their drugs approached.<br>(ii) Reminding their parents about the next hospital appointment.<br>(iii) Financial assistance or helping with household chores. |
| Improved behaviour of children | (i) Change in the behaviour of the child to avoid stressing the parent. |
| *(b) Negative consequences (mainly short term)* | |
| Emotional breakdown | (i) Children responding to disclosure by crying.<br>(ii) The parent themselves crying after disclosure.<br>(iii) Stress for both parent and child. |
| Children getting scared | (i) Children responding by getting very scared. |

status, a child started reminding them to take their medicines and to keep hospital appointments. One father said the following:

> *And when time comes they tell me that "Father, your medicine?" And sometimes I take like a week when I am away from home, but they will ask you that "Daddy, how many days will you spend there?" I tell them that may be one week, and they will pack medicines for two weeks, and they will tell you that "I have put for two weeks because you might reach there and anything can happen." (IDI with male)*

*3.6.2. Parents Receiving Emotional or Practical Support from Children after Disclosure.* Some children had responded to their parent's disclosure by offering emotional, material, financial, or even food support to the parent. Their support also included help with household chores:

> *Since the children got to know about my status they provided a lot of care because they know their mum is sick; they do most of the work at home, especially the boy does not want me to go and fetch water and he fetches it himself. . .so that is it. . .they help me a lot because they do all the work. (IDI with female)*

*3.6.3. Improved Behaviour of Children.* There were cases when children were described as making excessive financial demands before the parent had disclosed their HIV status, yet after disclosure the parent reported a positive change in a child's behaviour and this lessened the parent's stress. One woman said the following:

> *So they understood and they felt concerned, and they started to give me support and they reduced on the demands they were putting on me; those who used to ask money for special hire to take them to school started taking a taxi to go to school. (IDI with female)*

*3.6.4. Parents' Psychological Relief.* Some parents reported a sense of relief after disclosure to their children. One mother said the following:

> *Those other ones were also hurt, but one of the children was more hurt, she showed that it was too much for her.... In fact I did not feel okay after telling them, but after some days I felt I had offloaded a very big luggage from my head, because it had haunted me always and I always wanted to tell them, but there was no way I would tell them because I thought it would hurt them. (IDI with female)*

*3.7. Negative Consequences of Disclosure.* Two themes commonly emerged in both the FGDs and IDIs concerning negative consequences from a parent's disclosure: emotional breakdown of either the child or parent and children getting scared by the information.

*3.7.1. Emotional Breakdown.* For most of the parents an immediate negative outcome of disclosure had been children and, in some cases, even the parent crying afterwards as, for instance, the following:

> *Then I asked him that "have you even heard about HIV?" He told me, HIV? Daddy, HIV kills, they tell us at school that HIV kills," and he told me HIV is AIDS, he was trying to explain. Then I told him that I take that medicine because I was tested and found that I was HIV-positive, the HIV that kills, but I take that medicine so that I can prolong my life. Then he broke down into tears, he cried; so I told him that "This is the reason I did not want to tell you when you are still young, but that is it." (IDI with father of teenage boy)*

> *They tried to cry a bit saying, "our daddy died and our mother's life is also in suspense," but I consoled them and told them that "Let us leave everything in God's hands; you pray for me, support me, so that I can take my medicines, because the moment I miss taking it, it is bad." (IDI with female)*

*3.7.2. Children Getting Scared.* In other cases when parents had disclosed their HIV status, the children became very scared and stressed, and this also worried the parents themselves:

> *These children [6 and 12 years] were already in school, and they could teach them about HIV at school, but they were in great fear that every day mummy has been having HIV, which means she is going to die. They were stressed, and as a parent you would see that what you have told them did them bad, they were so much affected. (IDI with female)*

> *My children [ages 6 and 12 years] realized it themselves and I never sat them down, they had already seen their dad suffering, and the elder boy asked me that "Mummy, in which health facility do you seek care?" And I told him that they had directed me to the infectious diseases clinic...the young one got scared and I told him to be firm. (participant in women's FGD)*

## 4. Discussion

As supported by our findings, parents' HIV status disclosure to children is still a challenging issue characterised by numerous obstacles, varied approaches, and mixed outcomes. We found it interesting that parents who perceived themselves as self-reliant and in otherwise good health did not consider it essential to disclose their HIV-positive status to their children. In addition, however, we observed many of the usual other hurdles to disclosure, as previously described in the literature, such as parents' perceptions that children are too young to understand the health information and that they will be subsequently unable to keep it secret [16, 18, 28–30], fear of having to explain how a parent became infected [31], and perceptions of a poor relationship between the parent and child [29].

In this study, parents' motivation for disclosure sometimes clearly related to their improved health status following an episode of severe illness. To our knowledge, this finding has not been reported by other studies in Uganda. Parents had also often disclosed their HIV status out of a sense of responsibility and obligation to their children. Similar findings have been reported by studies conducted in the United States [32] and China [33]. Importantly, this finding provides an opportunity for healthcare professionals to build on parents' inner strength and desire to protect, beyond just making the simple recommendation that parents should disclose their HIV status to their children. Thus, future interventions could aim to bolster parents' propensity to discharge their perceived responsibility in this regard. Moreover, parents who are provided with basic information and skills about disclosure are likely to be encouraged and better equipped to disclose their HIV status to their children, and this can include the benefits of improved family communication and cohesion [34, 35].

Some parents in this study cited the need to protect adolescent children from engaging in higher-risk sexual behaviour as a strong consideration for their disclosure. This finding supports the results of studies conducted in China [33], Burkina Faso [29], and the United States [35]. One implication is that the promotion of HIV status disclosure, particularly in the context of family, may pay significant dividends in regard to HIV prevention. This is so because parents who discuss with children measures to prevent HIV infection are more likely to be trusted and believed than other adults because of their experience and position in the family. This supports the need for approaches that enhance parental self-efficacy in HIV disclosure. Whereas in this study disclosure was often portrayed as a protective action, the literature is rife with examples where nondisclosure has been justified by parents based on the same premise of protecting children from the negative social and psychological consequences caused by disclosure [16, 18–20]. Nevertheless, while nondisclosure is sometimes intended to protect children, it has been associated with negative consequences for both the parent and child [21, 22]. Additional research, especially in resource limited countries with a high burden of HIV, is merited to demonstrate whether the benefits of parental disclosure far outweigh the negative outcomes.

In this study, the process of disclosure for some parents was hastened by circumstances, such as children asking parents how long they (child/children) were going to be on a medication. For other parents, disclosure was a preplanned process that involved gathering their children together for a family discussion which culminated in the parent sharing his or her HIV-positive status. Similarly, Dematteo and colleagues (2002) reported that disclosure was sometimes planned in the context of gathering for a special meal or favourite family activity. The same authors stated that disclosures had also occurred in the context of a family argument or after a parent had been drinking. The experiences of parents in this study and others reveal that there is a dearth of practical and generalizable approaches to help parents in making decisions regarding the process of disclosure. Future work in this area, especially in Uganda and similar African contexts, should focus on developing contextually appropriate interventions to encourage parents' HIV status disclosure to children.

In this study, the outcomes of parental HIV disclosure were mixed, as has been similarly demonstrated in other studies. Positive outcomes noted by parents after disclosure included children reminding the parent about taking their medication, packing medicines for the parent when they had to travel, helping more with household chores, and improving their behaviour, including reducing the financial demands the child put on the parent; comparable findings were reported by Kennedy et al. (2010) and Tiendrebeogo et al. [29]. Conversely, negative consequences of disclosure tended to be the immediate emotional burden, as many of the parents reported that a child had reacted by crying or getting scared. Perhaps it is primarily for fear of these emotional reactions that many parents avoid disclosure to children [36]. Yet, despite the negative consequences associated with parental HIV disclosure, it is suggested that parents' nondisclosure to children might actually lead to increased psychosocial vulnerability [22].

## 5. Study Limitations

The findings of this qualitative study cannot be generalized to all HIV-positive parents in Uganda. Furthermore, when interviews are used as a method of data collection, there is a tendency of participants to distort their responses to present a favourable opinion, which leads to response bias. This was minimized by emphasizing honesty throughout the data-collection period. Finally, it would have been interesting to document the consequences of parental HIV disclosure from the perspectives children, but this was outside the scope of this study. Despite these limitations, the study presents important findings that can help shape the direction of interventions to promote parental HIV disclosure in Uganda. Approaches to facilitate parental HIV disclosure in Uganda and other highly affected resource limited settings are especially needed following the recently released World Health Organization policy guidelines requiring all individuals who test HIV-positive to commence ART [37]. These policy guidelines have resulted in development of country-specific "test and treat" guidelines thus transforming HIV into a chronic infection.

## 6. Conclusions

Parental HIV disclosure remains a complex phenomenon hampered by psychological barriers and uncertain family dynamics. In situations where disclosure occurs, the outcomes may be mixed for both the parent and child. However, HIV-treatment programmes in sub-Saharan Africa require culturally suitable interventions that facilitate the process of disclosure. Particularly, interventions are needed to better prepare parents and children to deal especially with the immediate psychological problems associated with parental HIV status disclosure. In the meantime we recommend that parents and children should receive counselling before and after disclosure to deal with psychological challenges associated with disclosure.

## Ethical Approval

Ethical approval for the study was obtained from Makerere University College of Health Sciences, School of Medicine Research Ethics Committee, under Reference REC REF no. 2013-137 and from the Uganda National Council for Science and Technology (UNCST) under Reference no. SS 3321. Approval for the study was also obtained from University of Washington Human Subjects Review Committee under Reference no. 46827-J.

## Consent

Written informed consent was obtained from each participant before data collection.

## Disclosure

This study's contents are solely the responsibility of the authors and do not necessarily represent the official views of the supporting offices.

## Conflicts of Interest

The authors declare that they have no conflicts of interest.

## Authors' Contributions

Charles Peter Osingada, Monica Okuga, Rose Chalo Nabirye, Nelson Kaulukusi Sewankambo, and Damalie Nakanjako were responsible for the study conception and design. Charles Peter Osingada and Monica Okuga were responsible for the data collection and analysis. Charles Peter Osingada and Monica Okuga were responsible for data interpretation and drafting of the manuscript. Charles Peter Osingada, Monica Okuga, Rose Chalo Nabirye, Nelson Kaulukusi Sewankambo, and Damalie Nakanjako made critical revisions to the paper for important intellectual content. All authors read and approved the final manuscript.

## Acknowledgments

The authors acknowledge all the research assistants who participated in data collection and all the clients at the Infectious Diseases Institute (IDI) who participated in the study. Their profound gratitude goes to the administration at IDI for all the support extended to them during the conduct of the study. This research was supported by the Afya Bora Consortium (Health Resources & Service Administration U91HA06801B) and University of Washington Centre for AIDS Research (CFAR), a NIH funded program (P30 AI027757) which is supported by the following NIH Institutes and Centres (NIAID, NCI, NIMH, NIDA, NICHD, NHLBI, and NIA). Additional funding for this work was received from NURTURE program through Grant no. D43TW010132 supported by Office of the Director, National Institutes of Health (OD), National Institute of Dental & Craniofacial Research (NIDCR), National Institute of Neurological Disorders and Stroke (NINDS), National Heart, Lung, and Blood Institute (NHLBI), Fogarty International Center (FIC), and National Institute on Minority Health and Health Disparities (NIMHD).

## References

[1] Joint United Nations Programme on HIV/AIDS, "UNAIDS Fact sheet," 2015.

[2] Uganda Ministry of Health, "Uganda AIDS Indicator Survey," 2011.

[3] Uganda Aids Information Center, "Renewed commitment to the HIV/AIDS Fight," http://aicug.org/?q=node/1, 2016.

[4] J. Rubaihayo, N. M. Tumwesigye, J. Konde-Lule et al., "Trends and predictors of mortality among HIV positive patients in the era of highly active antiretroviral therapy in Uganda," *Infectious Disease Reports*, vol. 7, no. 3, pp. 66–73, 2015.

[5] A. Hardon and E. Moyer, "Anthropology of AIDS: Modes of Engagement," *Medical Anthropology: Cross Cultural Studies in Health and Illness*, vol. 33, no. 4, pp. 255–262, 2014.

[6] M. Roy, N. Czaicki, C. Holmes et al., "Understanding Sustained Retention in HIV/AIDS Care and Treatment: a Synthetic Review," *Current HIV/AIDS Reports*, vol. 13, no. 3, pp. 177–185, 2016.

[7] N. C. Ware, J. Idoko, S. Kaaya et al., "Explaining adherence success in sub-Saharan Africa: an ethnographic study," *PLoS Medicine*, vol. 6, no. 1, Article ID e1000011, 2009.

[8] T. Gultie, M. Genet, and G. Sebsibie, "Disclosure of HIV-positive status to sexual partner and associated factors among ART users in Mekelle hospital," *HIV/AIDS - Research and Palliative Care*, vol. 7, pp. 209–214, 2015.

[9] O. E. Amoran, "Predictors of disclosure of sero-status to sexual partners among people living with HIV/AIDS in Ogun State, Nigeria," *Nigerian Journal of Clinical Practice*, vol. 15, no. 4, pp. 385–390, 2012.

[10] T. A. Erku, B. Megabiaw, and M. Wubshet, "Predictors of HIV status disclosure to sexual partners among people living with HIV/AIDS in Ethiopia," *Pan African Medical Journal*, vol. 13, article 87, 2012.

[11] T. M. Balogun, B. Awofala, I. C. Iredu, A. O. Ajayi, and M. Ohakwere, "Seropositive status disclosure to partners and safer sexual behaviours among people living with HIV: An issue in prevention and treatment," *Nigerian Postgraduate Medical Journal*, vol. 21, no. 4, pp. 338–342, 2014.

[12] I. Yaya, B. Saka, D. E. Landoh et al., "HIV status disclosure to sexual partners, among people living with HIV and AIDS on antiretroviral therapy at Sokodé regional hospital, Togo," *PLoS ONE*, vol. 10, no. 2, Article ID e0118157, 2015.

[13] G. T. Tshweneagae, V. M. Oss, and T. Mgutshini, "Disclosure of HIV status to sexual partners by people living with HIV," *Curationis*, vol. 38, no. 1, pp. E1–6, 2015.

[14] World Health Organization, "Guideline on HIV Disclosure Counselling for Children Up to 12 Years of Age," Geneva, 2011.

[15] S. Qiao, X. Li, and B. Stanton, "Disclosure of parental HIV infection to children: A systematic review of global literature," *AIDS and Behavior*, vol. 17, no. 1, pp. 369–389, 2013.

[16] B. Thomas, A. Nyamathi, and S. Swaminathan, "Impact of HIV/AIDS on mothers in Southern India: A qualitative study," *AIDS and Behavior*, vol. 13, no. 5, pp. 989–996, 2009.

[17] S. Ashaba, A. Kaida, J. N. Coleman et al., "Psychosocial challenges facing women living with HIV during the perinatal period in rural Uganda," *PLoS ONE*, vol. 12, no. 5, Article ID e0176256, 2017.

[18] S. L. Nam, K. Fielding, A. Avalos, T. Gaolathe, D. Dickinson, and P. W. Geissler, "Discussing matters of sexual health with children: What issues relating to disclosure of parental HIV status reveal," *AIDS Care Psychological and Socio-medical Aspects of AIDS/HIV*, vol. 21, no. 3, pp. 389–395, 2009.

[19] F. L. Palin, L. Armistead, A. Clayton et al., "Disclosure of maternal HIV-infection in South Africa: Description and relationship to child functioning," *AIDS and Behavior*, vol. 13, no. 6, pp. 1241–1252, 2009.

[20] R. Ostrom Delaney, J. M. Serovich, and J.-Y. Lim, "Reasons for and against maternal HIV disclosure to children and perceived child reaction," *AIDS Care Psychological and Socio-medical Aspects of AIDS/HIV*, vol. 20, no. 7, pp. 876–880, 2008.

[21] D. A. Murphy, L. Armistead, W. D. Marelich, D. L. Payne, and D. M. Herbeck, "Pilot trial of a disclosure intervention for HIV+ mothers: The TRACK program," *Journal of Consulting and Clinical Psychology*, vol. 79, no. 2, pp. 203–214, 2011.

[22] N. Ishikawa, P. Pridmore, R. Carr-Hill, and K. Chaimuangdee, "Breaking down the wall of silence around children affected by AIDS in Thailand to support their psychosocial health," *AIDS Care Psychological and Socio-medical Aspects of AIDS/HIV*, vol. 22, no. 3, pp. 308–313, 2010.

[23] D. A. Murphy, W. N. Steers, and M. E. Dello Stritto, "Maternal disclosure of mothers' HIV serostatus to their young children," *Journal of Family Psychology*, vol. 15, no. 3, pp. 441–450, 2001.

[24] L. Zhang, W.-T. Chen, J. P. Yang et al., "Disclosing Parental HIV Status to Children in China: Lessons Learned Through an Intervention Study," *Journal of the Association of Nurses in AIDS Care*, vol. 28, no. 1, pp. 130–141, 2017.

[25] T. J. Rochat, N. Mkwanazi, and R. Bland, "Maternal HIV disclosure to HIV-uninfected children in rural South Africa: A pilot study of a family-based intervention," *BMC Public Health*, vol. 13, no. 1, article 147, 2013.

[26] T. J. Rochat, A. X. Arteche, A. Stein, J. Mitchell, and R. M. Bland, "Maternal and child psychological outcomes of HIV disclosure to young children in rural South Africa: The Amagugu intervention," *AIDS*, vol. 29, pp. S67–S79, 2015.

[27] T. J. Rochat, A. Stein, M. Cortina-Borja, F. Tanser, and R. M. Bland, "The Amagugu intervention for disclosure of maternal HIV to uninfected primary school-aged children in South Africa: a randomised controlled trial," *The Lancet HIV*, 2017.

[28] S. Qiao, X. Li, and B. Stanton, "Practice and perception of parental HIV disclosure to children in Beijing, China," *Qualitative Health Research*, vol. 24, no. 9, pp. 1276–1286, 2014.

[29] G. Tiendrebeogo, F. Hejoaka, E. M. Belem et al., "Parental HIV disclosure in Burkina Faso: Experiences and challenges in the era of HAART," *Sahara J*, vol. 10, no. 1, pp. s46–s59, 2013.

[30] D. P. Kennedy, B. O. Cowgill, L. M. Bogart et al., "Parents' disclosure of their HIV infection to their children in the context of the family," *AIDS and Behavior*, vol. 14, no. 5, pp. 1095–1105, 2010.

[31] J. P. Yang, T. Xie, J. M. Simoni et al., "A Mixed-Methods Study Supporting a Model of Chinese Parental HIV Disclosure," *AIDS and Behavior*, vol. 20, no. 1, pp. 165–173, 2016.

[32] D. J. Pilowsky, N. Sohler, and E. Susser, "Reasons given for disclosure of maternal HIV status to children," *Journal of Urban Health*, vol. 77, no. 4, pp. 723–734, 2000.

[33] J. P. Yang, T. Xie, J. M. Simoni et al., "A mixed-methods study supporting a model of chinese parental HIV disclosure," *AIDS and Behavior*, 2015.

[34] L. S. Wiener, H. B. Battles, and N. E. Heilman, "Factors Associated with Parents' Decision to Disclose Their HIV Diagnosis to Their Children," *Child Welfare*, vol. 77, no. 2, pp. 115–135, 1998.

[35] A. H. Vallerand, E. Hough, L. Pittiglio, and D. Marvicsin, "The process of disclosing HIV serostatus between HIV-positive mothers and their HIV-negative children," *AIDS Patient Care and STDs*, vol. 19, no. 2, pp. 100–109, 2005.

[36] J. Rwemisisi, B. Wolff, A. Coutinho, H. Grosskurth, and J. Whitworth, "'What if they ask how I got it?' Dilemmas of disclosing parental HIV status and testing children for HIV in Uganda," *Health Policy and Planning*, vol. 23, no. 1, pp. 36–42, 2008.

[37] World Health Organization, "Prevent HIV, Test and Treat all," 2016.

# Early Infant Diagnosis Sample Management in Mashonaland West Province, Zimbabwe, 2017

**Hamufare Mugauri,[1] Owen Mugurungi,[2] Addmore Chadambuka,[3] Tsitsi Juru,[1] Notion Tafara Gombe,[1] Gerald Shambira,[1] and Mufuta Tshimanga[1]**

[1]*Department of Community Medicine, University of Zimbabwe, Zimbabwe*
[2]*Ministry of Health and Child Care, Zimbabwe*
[3]*Elizabeth Glaser Paediatric AIDS Foundation (EGPAF), Zimbabwe*

Correspondence should be addressed to Tsitsi Juru; tsitsijuru@gmail.com

Academic Editor: Glenda Gray

*Background.* In 2016, Mashonaland West Province had 7.4% (520) dried blood spot (DBS) samples for early infant diagnosis (EID) rejected by the Zimbabwe National Microbiology Reference Laboratory (NMRL). The samples were suboptimal, delaying treatment initiation for HIV-infected children. EID is the entry point to HIV treatment services in exposed infants. We determined reasons for DBS sample rejections and suggested solutions. *Methods.* A cause-effect analysis, modelled on Ishikawa, was used to identify factors impacting DBS sample quality. Interviewer-administered questionnaires and evaluation of sample collection process, using Standard Operating Procedure (SOP) was conducted. Rejected samples were reviewed. Epi Info™ was used to analyze findings. *Results.* Eleven (73.3%) facilities did not adhere to SOP and (86.7%) did not evaluate DBS sample quality before sending for testing. Delayed feedback (up to 4 weeks) from NMRL extended EID delay for 14 (93.3%) of the facilities. Of the 53 participants, 62% knew valid sample identification. Insufficient samples resulted in most rejections (77.9%). Lack of training (94.3%) and ineffective supervision (69.8%) were also cited. *Conclusion.* Sample rejections could have been averted through SOP adherence. Ineffective supervision, exacerbated by delayed communication of rejections, extended EID delay, disadvantaging potential ART beneficiaries. Following this study, enhanced quality control through perstage evaluations was recommended to enhance DBS sample quality.

## 1. Introduction

In 2015 alone, approximately 1.4 million mothers living with HIV gave birth and 150 000 infants became infected with HIV globally [1]. Unless these children are promptly commenced on lifelong antiretroviral treatment (ART), HIV-positive infants invariably record their highest mortality in the first three months of life. However, a serious diagnostics gap exists [1]. Only 51% of infants exposed to HIV globally are tested by the time they are six weeks old, the age recommended by the World Health Organization (WHO) [2]. Half of these never receive their results. Of those who test positive and receive their results, only half are linked to care [2].

Affordable ART and treatment of opportunistic infections are becoming increasingly available but this only benefits infants who are diagnosed early. In order to achieve the fast-track targets of ending the AIDS epidemic by 2030, new HIV infections among children must be eliminated. HIV can be transmitted from mother to child during pregnancy, childbirth, and breastfeeding, yet, with antiretroviral therapy, mother-to-child transmission rates can decrease, in likelihood, to 5% or less [3].

HIV infection can be definitively diagnosed through the use of virologic assays in most nonbreastfed HIV-exposed infants at 1 to 2 months of age and in virtually all infected infants by 4 months of age. HIV antibody tests, including newer tests, do not establish the presence of HIV infection in infants because of transplacental transfer of maternal antibodies to HIV; therefore, a virologic test should be used [4]. The samples need to be of optimal quality to ensure an accurate diagnosis. Positive virologic tests (i.e., nucleic acid tests (NAT))—a class of tests that include HIV Ribonucleic

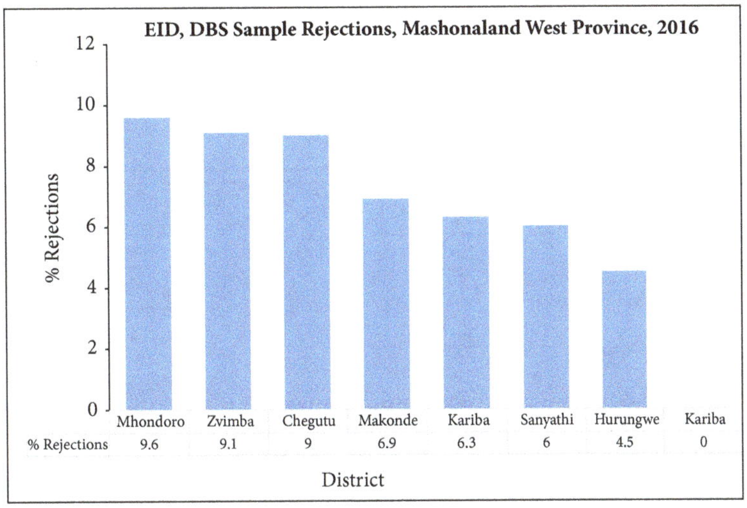


FIGURE 1: DBS rejections per district, Mashonaland West Province, Zimbabwe, 2016.

Acid (RNA) and Deoxyribonucleic Acid (DNA) polymerase chain reaction [PCR] assays, and related RNA qualitative or quantitative assays detect the HIV virus [4].

Early diagnosis of HIV allows health care providers to offer optimal care and treatment of HIV-infected children, assists in decision-making on infant feeding, and reduces illness-related stress in mothers and families. The increasing efficacy and coverage of Prevention of Mother-to-Child Transmission of HIV (PMTCT) interventions have resulted in the majority of children born to HIV-infected mothers being HIV-free [5]. Consequently, identification of infected children before the illness is possible through routine diagnostic testing of all exposed infants. WHO recommends that this be performed with virological testing at 6 weeks of age and HIV-positive infants are commenced on lifelong ART, as recommended by WHO, on provider-initiated HIV testing [6].

Among the technologies available for diagnosis of HIV in infants, PCR on DNA in blood is the most widely used and is generally considered to be the standard method. Recent studies have also demonstrated evidence that real-time PCR for HIV RNA provides a reliable and suitable alternative. HIV DNA-PCR is a qualitative test (i.e., it gives a yes/no diagnosis of HIV infection) [7]. HIV RNA detection provides additional quantitative information on virological status, and the same technology/equipment is used for monitoring the response to treatment and possible therapeutic failure [8].

Both DNA and RNA technologies are complex and expensive, requiring dedicated equipment, space, and trained technicians. However, increased automation greatly reduces the technical challenge. Some DNA and RNA (PCR) technologies support the use of DBS samples, which have considerable advantages in settings where sample-taking, transportation, and storage are problematic [9].

In Zimbabwe, ART services are increasingly being offered at primary health care facilities. Because of rapid disease progression in infants, early identification of infected infants is recognized [10]. In 2007, Zimbabwe introduced virological testing which detects a component of the HIV deoxyribonucleic acid (DNA) through the use of a polymerase chain reaction (DNA-PCR) from 6 weeks of age in HIV-exposed infants [11]. The tests are conducted at the National Microbiology Reference Laboratory (NMRL) in Harare and of late at Mpilo Central Hospital and Mutare Provincial Hospital [12].

Samples for the DNA-PCR are collected from the infants in the form of a dried blood spot (DBS) which is then sent to the National Microbiology Reference Laboratory (NMRL) via district or provincial laboratories. The sample is accompanied by a laboratory request form which captures patient identification variables (request number, province, district, health facility, mother's name, infant's name, sex, and date of birth). It also captures the date the sample was taken, mode of delivery, PMTCT prophylaxis, and infant's feeding practice, reasons for the DNA-PCR test, entry point for the test, and finally the result of the test [12].

A decline in the quality of dried blood spot (DBS) specimens for early infant diagnosis (EID) of HIV was observed in 2016. A total of 2020 (3.5%) samples were rejected by the National Microbiology Reference Laboratory (NMRL). Mashonaland West Province recorded the highest rejections countrywide at 520 (7.35%) surpassing the national rejections proportion twofold. Discrepancies in per-districts rejections were also enumerated, as shown in Figure 1 .

The rejections were for varied reasons, chiefly insufficient samples, contamination, and mismatch between sample and form, which indicate divergence from minimal quality standards as stipulated by the Standard Operating Procedure (SOP) for collection, storage, and transportation of DBS samples [13].

Rejection of samples leads to delay in providing critical lifelong antiretroviral therapy to deserving children and is contributory to the prevailing 43% paediatric ART initiations, against 74% for adults in Zimbabwe [12]. The rise in the rejection rates, above the World Health Organization (WHO) maximum threshold of 2%, presents an urgent need to

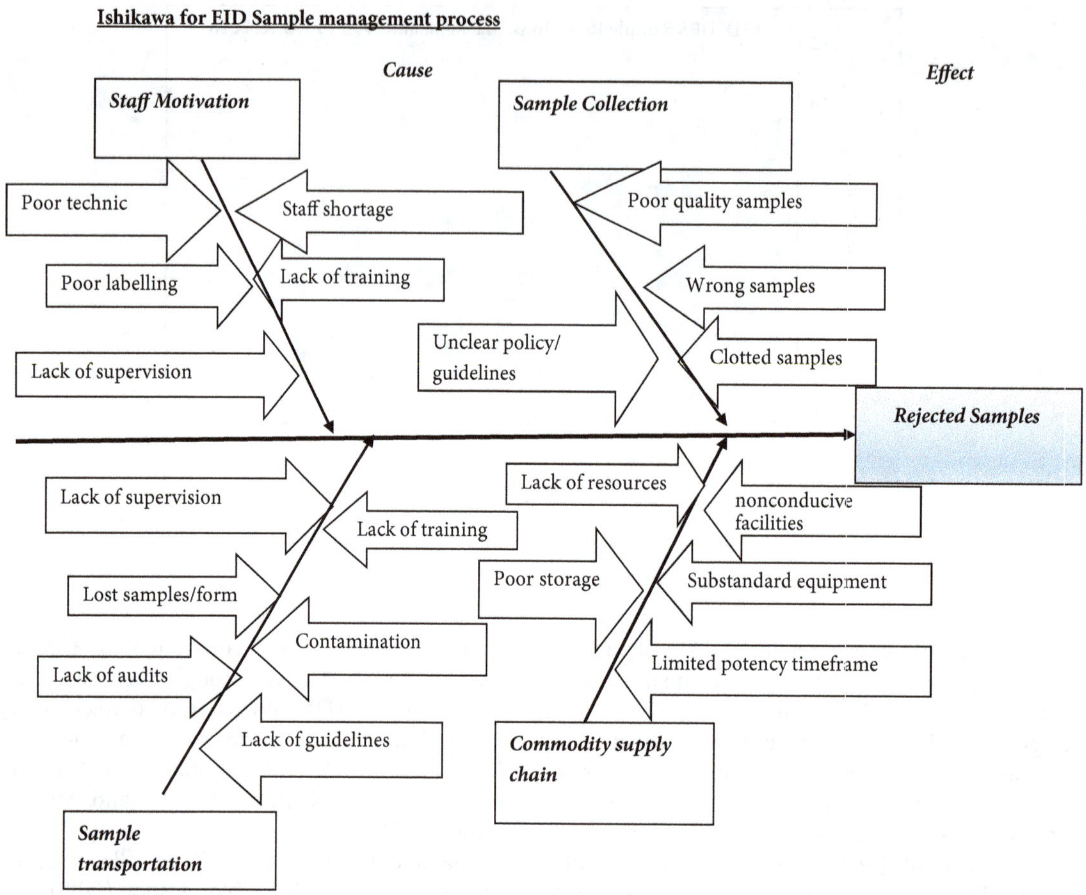


Figure 2: Ishikawa for EID sample management, Mashonaland West Province, Zimbabwe, 2017.

evaluate the existing EID sample management mechanisms and the extent of adherence to them in order to enhance paediatric ART initiations [13]. It is within this background that we sort to analyze the processes of collection and transportation of DBS specimens for EID of HIV using the SOP as a guide, in order to inform recommendations for DBS sample quality enhancement.

## 2. Material and Methods

A cause-effect analysis, using an Ishikawa diagram was conducted to evaluate factors contributing to poor quality DBS samples (Figure 2.)

This study was conducted in Mhondoro, Zvimba, and Chegutu, the leading districts on DBS rejections in Mashonaland West Province.

A total of 15 health facilities offering EID services in the three districts were randomly selected and included in the study which was conducted between October and December 2017.

The sample size was calculated using the Dobson formula: n = Za2 (p) (1-p)/delta2, where Za=1.96, p=0.5, assuming that 50% of health workers to be interviewed have adequate knowledge, at 20% precision and 80% power, a sample size of 47, adjusted for 10% nonresponse rate, and sample size of 52 was reached. A total of 53 participants were included in the study, yielding 102% response rate. Registered General Nurses (Diploma), Primary Care Nurses (PCN), and Primary Counsellors (PC) at all health facilities offering EID were recruited into the study. The District Medical officers (DMO), District Nursing Officers (DNO) from the district hospitals, and health facility Sisters in Charge (SIC) were recruited as key informants.

Timely feedback, from NMRL to sample collecting facilities, was defined as the reception of a sample acceptance or rejection decision within 10 days of submission of a sample. The definition is consistent with recommendations of the Standard Operating Procedure (SOP).

A pretested interviewer-administered questionnaire was used to collect data from healthcare workers (nurses and Primary counsellors) and key informant interviews were conducted with nurse managers. The pretest was done at three health facilities within the districts, which were then excluded from the study, and adjustments to the questionnaire were made, some questions were edited for clarity. Epi Info was used to generate frequencies, means, and proportions. DBS sample rejection results were reviewed and checklists utilized

TABLE 1: Demographic Characteristics of participants, Mhondoro, Zvimba, and Chegutu districts, Mashonaland West Province, 2017.

| Variable | Category | Mhondoro n=19 | Zvimba n=17 | Chegutu n=17 | Total (%) n=53 |
|---|---|---|---|---|---|
| Sex | Male | 6 | 7 | 5 | 18 (34) |
| | Female | 13 | 10 | 12 | 35 (66) |
| Job Position | District Medical Officer | 1 | 1 | 1 | 3 (5.7) |
| | District Nursing Officer | 1 | 1 | 1 | 3 (5.7) |
| | Sister in Charge | 2 | 1 | 3 | 17 (32.1) |
| | Registered General Nurse | 4 | 2 | 4 | 10 (18.9) |
| | Primary Care Nurse | 8 | 10 | 6 | 29 (54.7) |
| | Primary Counsellor | 3 | 2 | 2 | 7 (13.2) |
| Training | Personnel trained | 5 | 7 | 6 | 18(34) |
| Median years in service | | 6 ($Q_1$=5;$Q_3$=9) | 5 ($Q_1$=4;$Q_3$=10) | 9 ($Q_1$=6;$Q_3$=9) | 7 ($Q_1$=3;$Q_3$=11) |

TABLE 2: Compliance with Standard Operating Procedure (SOP) for DBS Sample Collection by Mhondoro, Zvimba and Chegutu Districts, 2016.

| Standard Operating Practice | Number of Compliant Facilities | Percentage Compliance n=15 |
|---|---|---|
| Only trained health care workers should collect DBS samples | 0 | 0 |
| The Charge nurse should verify the quality and completeness of collected samples before sending to the laboratory | 2 | 13.3 |
| A local register of collected samples and the received results should be kept | 4 | 26.7 |
| NMRL personnel to provide timely feedback for sub-quality samples after receiving them | 1 | 6.7 |

to evaluate SOP adherence. Permission to carry out the study was obtained from the Ministry of Health and Child Care, and Institutional review board of Mashonaland West Province. Written informed consent was obtained from key informants.

## 3. Results and Discussion

*3.1. Demographic Characteristics.* The 53 successfully recruited participants were evenly distributed across the three districts. Overall, 66% (35) were females whilst 34% (18) were males. The majority, 54.7% (29) of participants were Primary care nurses and Primary counsellors were the least at 13.2% (7). A District Nursing Officer (DNO) and District Medical Officer (DMO) from each district were recruited as key informants (Table 1).

*3.2. Compliance with Standard Operating Procedure (SOP) for DBS Sample Collection.* In all facilities visited, nurses allocated to the Family and Child Health (FCH) unit at health facilities were charged with the responsibility of collecting DBS samples regardless of prior training on the requisite technic. Only trained (formally/informally) personnel are supposed to collect DBS samples, following the Standard Operating Procedures (SOP).

Only two (13.3%) facilities observed the requirement that a second nurse or charge nurse verify the collected samples for quality and the documentation for completeness and consistency.

Facility-level documentation of collected samples was practiced at four (26.7%) of the facilities. A local register of collected samples and their results is the recommended practice. One (6.7%) facility received timely feedback from the laboratory. The rest of the facilities only obtained results when the entire batch results were received back at the facility (Table 2).

*3.3. Level of Expertise of Personnel Responsible for the Collection of DBS Samples for EID.* The level of expertise of personnel responsible for DBS collection was assessed through the checklist, interview, and observation. The majority (41; 77.4%) of the participants accurately enumerated the DBS collection process in sequence whilst 75.5% (40) were able to identify key characteristics of a potent DBS sample. Precautionary

TABLE 3: Expertise of Personnel Responsible for Collection of DBS samples for EID for Mhondoro, Zvimba, and Chegutu Districts, 2016.

| Variable | Mhondoro n=19 | Zvimba n=17 | Chegutu n=17 | Total (%) n=53 |
|---|---|---|---|---|
| **Accurately relates DBS collection sequence** | 15 | 12 | 14 | 41 (77.4) |
| **Able to identify a valid DBS sample** | 10 | 14 | 16 | 40 (75.5) |
| **Identify precautionary measures necessary for valid samples** | 10 | 9 | 11 | 30 (56.6) |
| **Accurately relates sample packaging process** | 12 | 10 | 10 | 32 (60.4) |
| **Perceive sequential DBS process essential for sample validity** | 5 | 8 | 7 | 20 (37.7) |

TABLE 4: Reasons for DBS samples rejections, reported by NMRL for Mhondoro, Zvimba, and Chegutu Districts, 2016.

| Reason for Rejection | Mhondoro N=50 | Zvimba N=48 | Chegutu N=47 | Total (%) N=145 |
|---|---|---|---|---|
| **Insufficient sample** | 38 | 35 | 40 | 113 (77.9) |
| **Clotted Blood** | 7 | 4 | 3 | 14 (9.7) |
| **Mismatching form and specimen** | 2 | 4 | 4 | 10 (6.9) |
| **Request form not submitted** | 1 | 3 | 0 | 4 (2.8) |
| **Cross-contamination** | 2 | 1 | 0 | 3 (2.1) |
| **Specimen not submitted** | 0 | 1 | 0 | 1 (0.7) |

measures necessary to obtain a valid DBS sample were identified by 56.6% (30) of the participants. Thirty-two (60.4%) of the participants accurately related the packaging process of DBS samples. Notably, only 37.7% (20) of the participants perceived the entire sequential DBS process as necessary to obtain valid specimens (Table 3).

*3.4. Reasons for DBS Sample Rejections at NMRL.* A total of 27.7% (145) Mashonaland West Province DBS rejections were shared among the 3 districts. The most prevalent reason for rejection was insufficient samples at 77.9% (113). Nearly 10% (14) of the samples were rejected because the specimen had clotted, whilst mismatching form and specimen constituted 6.9% of the rejections. Cross-contamination constituted 2.1% (3) of the rejections, and failure to submit the requisite specimen constituted less than 1% (1) of the rejections. All rejection reasons indicated divergence from the Standard Operating Procedures (SOP) for DBS sample collection (Table 4).

*3.5. Reasons for Failing to Collect Potent DBS Samples.* Ninety-four percent (50) of the participants stated that lack of training on DBS collection was the reason for the high rejection rates, whilst almost 70% (37) thought that lack of supervision resulted in errors, leading to the high rejection rates. Failing to execute the correct technic during collection process was cited by 67.9% (36) of the participants. The poor technic was implicated for failure to obtain an adequate quantity of the DBS, resulting in insufficient samples. The perceived complexity of the DBS collection process and unclear rejection criteria by the laboratory were cited by 49.1% and 50.9% of the participants, respectively.

## 4. Discussion

The study sought to determine factors associated with increased DBS sample rejections in Mashonaland West Province using an Ishikawa for cause-effect analysis.

The DBS collection process is supposed to be executed sequentially, observing the SOP prescribed precautionary measures in order to obtain valid samples. This study observed divergence from the prescribed criteria, as seen by nontrained health workers being charged with the responsibility to collect the specimen. This anomaly, coupled with the absence of effective supervision to verify what the collecting nurse would have done before sending to the laboratory, resulted in high rejections. This finding concurs with the results by Grüner et al. (2015) in a systematic review of six studies who found a correlation between sequentially following DBS collection protocol and obtaining potent samples and authentic results [13].

When received DBS specimens did not meet the testing criteria during the screening process at NMRL, feedback to collecting site was not being timely conveyed to facilitate recollection. Health facilities only learnt of the rejection of reception of the entire batch or results. This resulted in a delay in the critical diagnosis of the HIV-exposed infant, impacting negatively on the EID programme.

DBS samples were rejected for preventable reasons, which required adherence to the SOP. Insufficient sample quantity was the single most common reason for rejections despite pictorial illustrations of the required sample amount in the SOP. This could have been averted by adhering strictly to the preparatory protocol, designed to ensure that an adequate amount of blood is obtained. This finding was contrary to the results of a study by Inalegwu (2016) in Nigeria who found insufficient samples as the least rejection reason, ahead of improper sample collection (26.3%) and improper labelling (16.4%) [14].

The reasons resulting in sample rejections, as perceived by the participants indicated an underlying competence deficiency. This revealed weaknesses in the currently practicced in-service skills dissemination, from nurses trained on DBS sample collection process, to their untrained counterparts, resulting in suboptimal samples being collected. This finding was consistent with findings from a systematic review by Smit et al. (2014), who found a strong correlation between adequate process orientation and high-quality samples [15]. There is, therefore, an urgent need to train all health workers involved in the DBS collection process.

## 5. Conclusions

DBS samples were being rejected for preventable reasons that reflected nonadherence to the minimum requirements of the SOP for sample collection, drying, storage, packaging, and transportation. The absence of a designated supervisory cadre to evaluate the quality of DBS samples before transportation to NMRL resulted in suboptimal specimens being transported to the laboratory, only to be rejected. The rejection decision was not timely conveyed to the collecting facility, resulting in delayed early infant diagnosis.

As a public health action, we discussed the supervision deficiencies with District Nursing Officers for the three districts, imploring them to strengthen quality control measures in place and ensuring even distribution of trained nurses across all health facilities. Feedback was also given to the districts and to the province. Enhanced quality control measures through per-stage evaluations were recommended to ensure valid DBS samples. From the collecting sites, all DBS samples were recommended to pass through the District Laboratory Scientists for quality check before conveying them to NMRL. Suboptimal samples are timely returned to collecting facilities for recollection. Upon arrival at NMRL, DBS samples are immediately graded and substandard ones are rejected and the feedback communicated immediately to collecting facilities for recollection.

## Abbreviations

| | |
|---|---|
| ART: | Antiretroviral therapy |
| ARV: | Antiretroviral (drugs) |
| DBS: | Dried blood spot |
| DNA-PCR: | Deoxyribonucleic Acid Polymerase Chain Reaction |
| EID: | Early infant diagnosis |
| NMRL: | National Microbiology Reference Laboratory. |

## Disclosure

An earlier version of this work was presented as an oral presentation at the 9th Global TEPHINET scientific conference 7-11 August 2017, Chiang Mai, Thailand, and as a poster at ICASA 2017- The 19th International Conference on AIDS and STIs in Africa, 4-9 December 2017, Abidjan, Côte d'Ivoire.

## Conflicts of Interest

The authors declare no financial or nonfinancial conflicts of interest.

## Acknowledgments

Special gratitude goes to the Health Studies Office (HSO) with particular mention of Ms. Garande who was responsible for all administrative planning for this project. Special thanks also go to the Centers for Disease Control and Prevention (CDC) and the Provincial Health Executive (PHE), Mashonaland West Province. The authors would also want to express their gratitude to the Department of Community Medicine, University of Zimbabwe and MPH colleagues for all the help they rendered.

## References

[1] "Centers for Disease Control and Prevention (CDC) and the Association of Public Health Laboratories. Laboratory testing for the diagnosis of HIV infection: updated recommendations," http://stacks.cdc.gov/view/cdc/23447, 2016.

[2] M. Donovan and P. Palumbo, "Diagnosis of HIV: challenges and strategies for HIV prevention and detection among pregnant women and their infants," *Clinics in Perinatology*, vol. 37, no. 4, pp. 751–763, 2010.

[3] J. S. Read, "Diagnosis of HIV-1 Infection in Children Younger Than 18 Months in the United States," *Pediatrics*, vol. 120, no. 6, pp. e1547–e1562, 2007.

[4] K. Mcintosh, J. Pitt, D. Brambilla et al., "Blood culture in the first 6 months of life for the diagnosis of vertically transmitted human immunodeficiency virus infection. The women and infants transmission study group," *The Journal of Infectious Diseases*, vol. 170, no. 4, pp. 996–1000, 1994.

[5] M. Tamhane, B. Gautney, C. Shiu et al., "Analysis of the optimal cut-point for HIV-p24 antigen testing to diagnose HIV infection in HIV-exposed children from resource-constrained settings," *Journal of Clinical Virology*, vol. 50, no. 4, pp. 338–341, 2011.

[6] M. J. Wessman, Z. Theilgaard, and T. L. Katzenstein, "Determination of HIV status of infants born to HIV-infected mothers: a review of the diagnostic methods with special focus on the applicability of p24 antigen testing in developing countries," *Infectious Diseases*, vol. 44, no. 3, pp. 209–215, 2012.

[7] K. Bhowan and G. G. Sherman, "Performance of the first fourth-generation rapid human immunodeficiency virus test in children," *The Pediatric Infectious Disease Journal*, vol. 32, no. 5, pp. 486–488, 2013.

[8] P. L. Havens and L. M. Mofenson, "Evaluation and management of the infant exposed to HIV-1 in the United States," *Pediatrics*, vol. 123, no. 1, pp. 175–187, 2009.

[9] M. Burgard, S. Blanche, C. Jasseron et al., "Performance of HIV-1 DNA or HIV-1 RNA tests for early diagnosis of perinatal HIV-1 infection during anti-retroviral prophylaxis," *Journal of Pediatrics*, vol. 160, no. 1, pp. 60–e1, 2012.

[10] American Academy of Pediatrics Committee on Pediatric AIDS, "HIV testing and prophylaxis to prevent mother-to-child transmission in the United States," *Pediatrics*, vol. 122, no. 5, pp. 1127–1134, 2008.

[11] A. Saitoh, K. Hsia, T. Fenton et al., "Persistence of human immunodeficiency virus (HIV) type 1 DNA in peripheral blood despite prolonged suppression of plasma HIV-1 RNA in children," *The Journal of Infectious Diseases*, vol. 185, no. 10, pp. 1409–1416, 2002.

[12] R. J. S. Kerr, G. Player, S. A. Fiscus, and J. A. E. Nelson, "Qualitative human immunodeficiency virus RNA analysis of dried blood spots for diagnosis of infections in infants," *Journal of Clinical Microbiology*, vol. 47, no. 1, pp. 220–222, 2009.

[13] N. Grüner, O. Stambouli, and R. S. Ross, "Dried blood spots - preparing and processing for use in immunoassays and in molecular techniques," *Journal of Visualized Experiments: JoVE*, vol. 97, 2015.

[14] A. Inalegwu, S. Phillips, R. Datir et al., "Active tracking of rejected dried blood samples in a large program in Nigeria," *World Journal of Virology*, vol. 5, no. 2, pp. 73–81, 2016.

[15] P. W. Smit, K. A. Sollis, S. Fiscus et al., "Systematic review of the use of dried blood spots for monitoring HIV viral load and for early infant diagnosis," *PLoS ONE*, vol. 9, no. 3, Article ID e86461, 2014.

# 22

# Incidence and Predictors of Pregnancy among Women on ART in Debre Markos Referral Hospital, Northwest Ethiopia

**Maru Meseret,[1] Alemayehu Shimeka,[2] and Alemayehu Bekele[3]**

[1] *Amhara National Regional State Health Bureau, East Gojjam Zonal Health Department, Bahir-Dar, Ethiopia*
[2] *Department of Epidemiology and Biostatistics, College of Medicine and Health Sciences, University of Gondar, Gondar, Ethiopia*
[3] *Ethiopian Public Health Association, Addis Ababa, Ethiopia*

Correspondence should be addressed to Alemayehu Shimeka; alemayehushimeka@gmail.com

Academic Editor: Ann Duerr

Globally, death of women due to HIV/AIDS related causes during pregnancy or within 42 days after pregnancy was estimated to be 37,000. In Ethiopia, 42,900 pregnant women living with HIV gave birth in the year 2011. This study was aimed to assess incidence and predictors of pregnancy among women on ART in Debre Markos Referral Hospital, Northwest Ethiopia. A retrospective cohort study was conducted using data recorded from September 2011 to August 2015. Data was extracted from February to March, 2016, from 1,239 records and analyzed using SPSS version 16. A Kaplan-Meier survival analysis was used to estimate the probabilities of being pregnant. The Cox proportional hazards model was done and results were expressed using hazard ratios with 95% CI. A total of 1,239 women on ART were included in the study. The incidence of pregnancy was 49.2 per 1,000 person-years. Living in rural, being married, being widowed, being unemployed, and having <2 children at enrollment were found to be positively associated with being pregnant. The incidence of pregnancy among women on ART was found to be considerable. Provision of family planning and other reproductive health interventions have to be coupled with the ART service to address the problem.

## 1. Introduction

An estimated 35.3 million people were living with human immune virus (HIV) worldwide, from which 3.3 million are children. Approximately, 57% of all adults living with HIV/AIDS were women. The situation is very serious in Sub-Saharan African countries where 75% of all people with HIV in the globe are living [1]. According to UNAIDS 2013 global report, women of reproductive age in Sub-Saharan Africa were disproportionately affected by HIV/AIDS; 80% of the nearly 13 million women living with HIV worldwide live in this region [2]. According to the 2011 Ethiopian Demographic and Health Survey (EDHS), the prevalence of HIV among women aged 15–49 years was 1.9% and the prevalence increases with increasing women's age [3]. In low and middle income countries, an estimated 1.5 million women living with HIV were pregnant. Globally, death of women due to HIV/AIDS related causes during pregnancy or within 42 days after pregnancy ends was estimated to be 37,000 [4].

Women who are living with HIV should access treatment based on WHO treatment guidelines. Nowadays, antiretroviral therapy (ART) is widely available in areas with meager resources. Providing ART for women living with HIV gives women good physical functioning and an opportunity to dream a better future. ART improves health of mothers and these mothers may be motivated to have more children [5]. In most circumstances, even though it is their right to have children, women are discouraged from getting pregnant while on ART due to the fact that giving birth from HIV positive mother could result in HIV positive babies. If proper care for the mothers is not in place, maternal death due to complications related to HIV and pregnancy can be very high [6].

A meta-analysis of 23 studies showed that HIV positive women have eight times risk of pregnancy related death compared to women without HIV. One in four pregnancy related deaths in Sub-Saharan Africa was attributable to HIV [7]. Despite the fact that providing treatment to women living with HIV/AIDS has a tremendous effect on the health of a mother and her newborn, a birth from HIV positive mother who is on ART may end up with not only HIV positive baby but also with maternal death. Studies have shown that, even in the presence of ART, maternal mortality rates have been reported to be five times higher in HIV infected women than in uninfected women and HIV/AIDS was responsible for at least 20% of all deaths, a figure that is higher than any direct obstetric cause [8].

A study in Uganda estimates that, even with a projected scale-up of antiretroviral therapy (ART) based prevention of mother to child transmission (PMTCT), unwanted pregnancies among women with HIV account for almost a quarter of all HIV positive infants and about a fifth of pediatric AIDS deaths [9]. HIV positive women who seek induced abortion may be at greater risk of morbidity than HIV uninfected women [10]. ART by itself may have a negative effect on birth outcomes such as prematurity or low birth weight [11].

Women living with HIV desire additional pregnancies and thus should be assisted to conceive, carry a pregnancy to term, deliver, and care for the resulting child. However, in other cases, women living with HIV become pregnant despite not desiring. Globally, many women lack access to family planning information and modern contraceptive methods; as a result, many pregnancies are unintended. In countries with the highest HIV burden, unintended pregnancies account for 14–58% of all births, and rates of unintended pregnancy among women living with HIV are high [12].

Evidences from Canada and Malawi indicated that the desire to have more children among mothers living with HIV was 69% and 17%, respectively [13, 14]. The magnitude of the desire to have more children in Ethiopia varies from place to place. The desire to have more children among mothers living with HIV in North Wollo, Addis Ababa, Harari region, and Oromia region was 15.7%, 44%, 53%, and 92%, respectively [15–18]. The tendency of getting pregnant and having HIV negative baby is highly improved due to the introduction of ART service which reduces mother to child transmission of HIV resulting in increased incidence of pregnancy among HIV positive women [6, 19–23].

However, because of the desire to have more children or unmet needs of family planning services, the incidence of pregnancy among women living with HIV in Ethiopia was likely to be high. Therefore, the main aim of this study was to assess the magnitude of incidence of pregnancy and predictors of it among women on HIV treatment in Debre Markos Referral Hospital.

## 2. Rational of the Study

Introduction of antiretroviral therapy to women living with HIV highly improves lifestyle and the desire to have children. However, evidences have shown that even in the presence of ART maternal mortality rates have been reported to be five times higher in HIV infected women compared to uninfected women. In Ethiopia being one of the developing countries, pregnancy related complications among women on ART are among the many health challenges. Even though the country is aggressively constructing and equipping health facilities with staff and equipment, still morbidity and mortality due to complications related to pregnancy among pregnant women on ART are very high. As far as the investigators search, there is scarcity of evidences on incidence of pregnancy among reproductive age group mothers taking ART in hospitals of Ethiopia. Considering resource limitations, this study was conducted in one of the hospitals which is Debre Markos Referral Hospital.

## 3. Methods and Materials

*3.1. Study Design.* Institutional based retrospective cohort study design using five-year data from September 2011 to August 2015 was employed.

*3.2. Study Area and Period.* This study was conducted in Debre Markos Referral Hospital. Debre Markos is a city located 300 kilometers far from Addis Ababa, the capital of Ethiopia, and 256 km from Bahir-Dar, a capital of Amhara National Regional State. The hospital provides health service to more than 3.5 million populations. Currently, about 100 health centers and two district hospitals are available in the catchment area of the referral hospital. There are 109 nurses, 3 health officers, 16 general practitioners, and one emergency surgeon and five specialists. Gynecologic and obstetric ward has 19 midwives, one gynecologist, and one emergency surgeon. About 8,136 patients are admitted per year, 34% of them in obstetric ward [24]. A database from I-TECH prepared excel sheet has been seen and about 1,239 women were registered on ART from September 2011 to August 2015.

*3.2.1. Population.* All women on ART in Debre Markos Referral Hospital catchment area were the source population for this study. All women who were on antiretroviral treatment and registered for follow-up care from September 2011 to August 2015 in the hospital were taken as the study population for this study.

*3.2.2. Inclusion and Exclusion Criteria.* Mothers who were getting antiretroviral treatment in the hospital from September 2011 to August 2015 were included in the study. However, mothers who were getting pre-ART care and started ART based on option B+ and mothers with more than one pregnancy during the follow-up time in the hospital in the specified period were excluded from the study.

*3.2.3. Variables.* The dependent variable of the study was incidence of pregnancy which was labeled as yes and/or no. Independent variables included sociodemographic characteristics such as age, residence, marital status, occupation, educational status, number of children, and clinical characteristics like CD4 count, WHO staging, weight, BMI, and functional status of women on ART.

*3.3. Operational Definitions*

*3.3.1. Incidence of Pregnancy.* In this research, incidence of pregnancy was considered as the first pregnancy after ART enrollment within the follow-up time.

*3.3.2. Time to Event.* In this research, time to event was defined as the time from enrollment on ART to the conception of the first pregnancy.

*3.3.3. Exposed.* According to this research, married women were considered as exposed to pregnancy while on ART.

*3.3.4. Unexposed.* Unmarried women were considered as unexposed to pregnancy while on ART.

*3.3.5. Sampling Technique.* The total records in the hospital among women of reproductive age group were 1,239. All the records of mothers on ART follow-up during the five consecutive years with complete information were used to determine incidence and predictors of pregnancy among women on ART.

*3.3.6. Data Collection Tools.* A structured data collection checklist was prepared in English to extract data from the records.

*3.3.7. Data Collection Procedures.* Data was extracted from main excel record of the hospital. Data elements which were not included in the excel sheet were collected from ART intake forms and cards. The data was collected by two health informatics professionals of the hospital working on ART database and supervised by one B.S. nurse.

*3.3.8. Data Quality Control.* Training was given for the data collectors and the supervisor before the actual data collection. Completeness of data was checked in each day of activity and the necessary feedback was offered to data collectors the next morning. Besides this, the principal investigators and an experienced data clerk carefully entered and thoroughly cleaned the data before the commencement of the analysis.

*3.4. Data Management and Analysis.* Date extracted from the data set was entered into excel sheet. Completeness of the excel sheet data set was checked thoroughly and exported to SPSS version 16 for analysis. Descriptive statistics and incidence rate of pregnancy in person-years of follow-up were reported. A Kaplan-Meier curve with hazard and survival functions was used to estimate the probabilities of becoming pregnant. The Cox proportional hazards model was used and results were expressed as hazard ratios with 95% CIs. Variables with $p$ value $\leq 0.2$ at Kaplan-Meier survival analysis were entered into multivariable Cox proportional hazards model to identify the independent predictors of pregnancy. Adjusted hazard ratio with 95% CI was used to report the findings.

*3.5. Ethical Considerations.* A letter of ethical clearance was obtained from Ethiopian Public Health Association and Research Ethics Committee. Informed consent was obtained from East Gojjam Zonal Health Department and Debre Markos Referral Hospital. All data sets were extracted from ART database and stored with password. Full information was kept confidential.

## 4. Results

*4.1. Sociodemographic Characteristics of Women on ART.* A total of 1,951 records were reviewed. Out of these, 681 and 31 records had missing data on date of enrollment to ART and the last date of menstrual period, respectively, and thus were excluded from the analysis. Therefore, a total of 1,239 records had complete data and were considered for the final analysis. The average period for follow-up was 2.23 years with SD of 1.54. The mean age with SD of study participants was $30 \pm 10.85$ years. Among women included in the study, 550 (44.4%) were aged between 25 and 34 years, 957 (77.2%) were urban dwellers, 489 (38.7%) were married, 590 (47.6%) were unable to read and write, 692 (55.9%) have less than two children, and 975 (78.7%) were unemployed (Table 1).

*4.2. Clinical Characteristics of Women on ART.* Among the study participants, 562 (45.4%) had CD4 count less than 200 cells/mm$^2$ at enrollment, 643 (51.9%) had weight less than 50 kilograms, 440 (35.5%) were at 3rd clinical stage, 908 (73.3%) had a BMI of 18.5 to 25, and 1,030 (84.2%) of them had a functional status of working at ART enrollment (Table 2).

*4.3. Incidence of Pregnancy.* Initially, a total of 1,239 women on ART were included in the study from September 2011 to August 2015 at different entry to the cohorts. The highest number of enrollment to ART was registered during 2011 which was 355 (28.7%). The overall incidence of pregnancy was found to be 49.2 per 1000 person-years (136 pregnancies in a total of 2762.55 years of observation). The incidence of pregnancy among exposed women was 74.6 per 1000 person-years (79 pregnancies in a total of 1058.88 years of observation) while it was 33.46 per 1000 person-years (57 pregnancies in a total of 1703.67 years of observation) in unexposed. The highest rate of pregnancy was registered among the cohorts of 2015 with 109.5 per 1000 person-years.

*4.4. Kaplan-Meier Survival Analysis.* The cumulative probability of surviving from pregnancy was higher among women aged 35 and above with mean survival time 4.60 years, 95% CI (4.47–4.74). This means the cumulative hazard of pregnancy was higher among women aged 25 to 34 years (Figure 1). At Kaplan-Meier analysis, statistically significant association was observed with incidence of pregnancy at $p$ value $< 0.05$. At the beginning of the study, the probability of getting pregnant for all women was almost the same. However, the risk of getting pregnant among women having less than two children was increasing with follow-up time. The cumulative probability of surviving from pregnancy for all women was almost the same, but after follow-up it was higher among women having two and above children than those having less than two children with mean survival time of 4.56 years, 95% CI (4.44–4.68) and 4.33, 95% CI (4.20–4.46), respectively.

TABLE 1: Sociodemographic characteristics of women receiving ART treatment from Sep. 2011 to Aug. 2015 in Debre Markos Referral Hospital, Northwest Ethiopia, 2016 ($N$ = 1239).

| Variables | Pregnancy status | | Total frequency |
|---|---|---|---|
| | No | Yes | |
| Age | | | |
| 15–24 years | 267 (89.3%) | 32 (10.7%) | 299 (24.1%) |
| 25–34 years | 476 (86.5%) | 74 (13.5%) | 550 (44.4%) |
| ≥35 years | 360 (92.3%) | 30 (7.7%) | 390 (31.5%) |
| Place of residence | | | |
| Urban | 861 (90%) | 96 (10%) | 957 (77.2%) |
| Rural | 242 (85.8%) | 40 (14.2%) | 282 (22.8%) |
| Marital status | | | |
| Never married | 239 (95.2%) | 12 (4.8%) | 251 (20.3%) |
| Married | 400 (83.5%) | 79 (16.5%) | 479 (38.7%) |
| Widowed | 258 (91.5%) | 24 (8.5%) | 282 (22.8%) |
| Divorced | 206 (90.7%) | 21 (9.3%) | 227 (18.3%) |
| Educational status | | | |
| Unable to read and write | 493 (83.6%) | 97 (16.4%) | 590 (47.6%) |
| Primary (1–8) | 224 (94.5%) | 13 (5.5%) | 237 (19.1%) |
| Secondary (9–12) | 197 (92.1%) | 17 (7.9%) | 214 (17.3%) |
| Certificate and above | 189 (95.5%) | 9 (4.5%) | 198 (16%) |
| Occupational status | | | |
| Unemployed | 858 (88%) | 117 (12%) | 975 (78.7%) |
| Employed | 245 (92.8%) | 19 (7.2%) | 264 (21.3%) |
| Number of children at enrollment | | | |
| 0-1 child | 604 (87.3%) | 88 (12.7%) | 692 (55.9%) |
| ≥2 children | 499 (91.2%) | 48 (8.8%) | 547 (44.1%) |

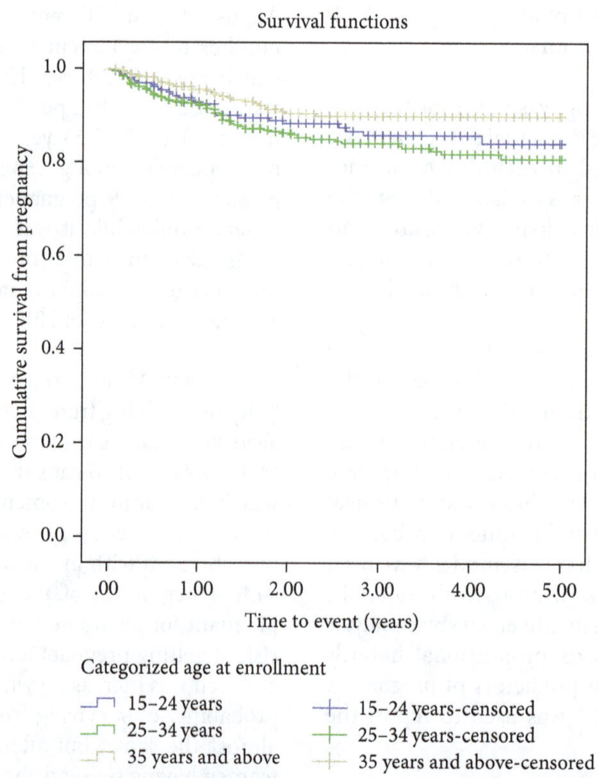


FIGURE 1: Kaplan-Meier curves of pregnancy comparing age among women receiving ART treatment from Sep. 2011 to Aug. 2015 in Debre Markos Referral Hospital, Northwest Ethiopia, 2016 ($N$ = 1,239).

Table 2: Clinical characteristics of women receiving ART treatment in Debre Markos Referral Hospital, Northwest Ethiopia, Sep. 2011 to Aug. 2015 ($N = 1239$).

| Variables | Pregnancy status | |
|---|---|---|
| | No | Yes |
| CD4 count at enrollment | | |
| <200 cell/mm$^2$ | 488 (86.8%) | 74 (13.2%) |
| 200–350 cell/mm$^2$ | 446 (91%) | 44 (9%) |
| >350 cell/mm$^2$ | 169 (90.4%) | 18 (9.6%) |
| Functional status at enrollment | | |
| Working | 913 (88.6%) | 117 (11.4%) |
| Ambulatory | 163 (91.6%) | 15 (8.4%) |
| Bedridden | 15 (100%) | 0 (0%) |
| Weight at enrollment | | |
| ≤50 kg | 580 (90.2%) | 63 (9.8%) |
| 51–60 kg | 307 (89%) | 38 (11%) |
| 61–70 kg | 100 (84%) | 19 (16%) |
| ≥71 kg | 116 (87.9%) | 16 (12.1%) |
| WHO clinical stage at enrollment | | |
| Clinical stage 1 | 367 (89.5%) | 43 (10.5%) |
| Clinical stage 2 | 258 (85.7%) | 43 (14.3%) |
| Clinical stage 3 | 395 (89.8%) | 45 (10.2%) |
| Clinical stage 4 | 83 (94.3%) | 5 (5.7%) |
| BMI at enrollment | | |
| <18.5 | 127 (91.4%) | 12 (8.6%) |
| 18.5–25 | 802 (88.3%) | 106 (11.7%) |
| >25 | 174 (90.6%) | 18 (9.4%) |

At Kaplan-Meier analysis, statistically significant association was observed with incidence of pregnancy at $p$ value < 0.05 (Figure 2).

With respect to residence, the cumulative hazard of pregnancy at year one for urban and rural residents was 5% and 9%, respectively, whereas the cumulative probability of surviving at year one for urban and rural residents was 89% and 85% with mean survival time 4.48 years, 95% CI [4.38–4.57], and 4.28 years, 95% CI [4.08–4.49], respectively. The cumulative hazard of pregnancy at year one for women with marital status never married, married, widowed, and divorced was 4%, 9%, 6%, and 3%, respectively, whereas the cumulative probability of surviving at year one for women with marital status never married, married, widowed, and divorced was 94%, 82%, 91%, and 90%, respectively. At Kaplan-Meier analysis, statistically significant association was observed with incidence of pregnancy at $p$ value < 0.05. The lowest cumulative probability of surviving from pregnancy had been observed among women with marital status married in the remaining years. Throughout follow-up period, the risk of getting pregnant was increasing among women who were unable to read and write compared to those with primary and above education. At Kaplan-Meier analysis, statistically significant association was observed with incidence of pregnancy at $p$ value < 0.05. Cumulative probability of getting pregnant among unemployed mothers was higher during early phase of the study and continued to increase throughout follow-up years compared to employed mothers whereas the cumulative probability of surviving from pregnancy among employed mothers is higher than unemployed with mean survival time of 4.63 years, 95% CI (4.46–4.78), and 4.38 years, 95% CI (4.28–4.48), respectively. At Kaplan-Meier estimate, statistically significant association was observed with incidence of pregnancy at $p$ value < 0.05.

*4.5. Predictors of Pregnancy among Mothers on ART.* Variables with a $p$ value of <0.2 at Kaplan-Meier estimate were used to assess the actual effect on incidence of pregnancy. Backward stepwise method was used. The risk of getting pregnant among rural residents women was 17.87 times higher compared to urban counterparts [AHR = 17.87, 95% CI (10.72–29.79)]. Married, widowed, and divorced women had 5.35, 3.65, and 4.34 times higher risk of pregnancy compared to women who had never married [AHR = 5.35, 95% CI (2.14–13.36), AHR = 3.65, 95% CI (1.06–12.49), and AHR = 4.34, 95% CI (1.42–13.22), resp.]. Women who had less than two children had 2.05 times higher risk of pregnancy compared to those who had two or more children [AHR = 2.05, 95% CI (1.31–3.20)]. Unemployed women had 4.37 times higher incidence of pregnancy compared to employed counterparts [AHR = 4.37, 95% CI (1.91–9.98)] (Table 3).

## 5. Discussion

This study has aimed at assessing the incidence of pregnancy and its predictors. Accordingly, the overall incidence of

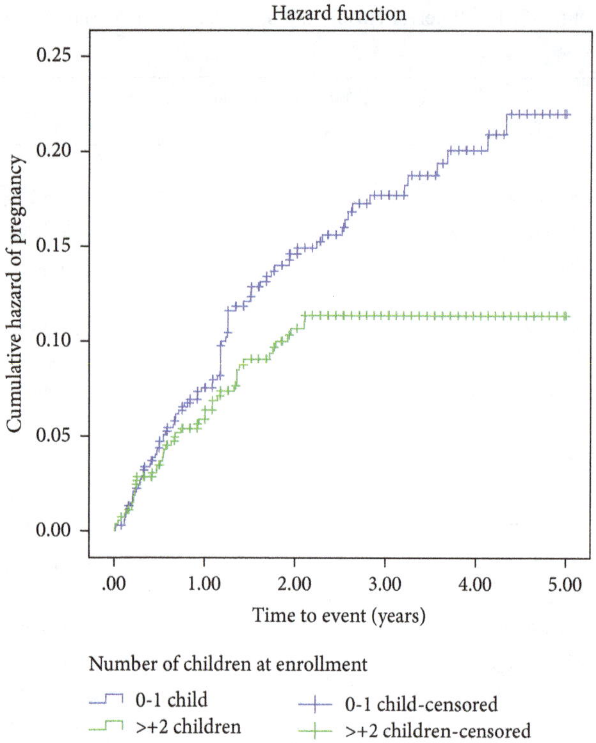


FIGURE 2: Kaplan-Meier curves of pregnancy showing hazard of pregnancy among women receiving ART treatment from Sep. 2011 to Aug. 2015 in Debre Markos Referral Hospital, Northwest Ethiopia, 2016 ($N$ = 1,239).

pregnancy was found to be 49.2 per 1000 person-years. This finding was lower than the findings of other studies such as United States of America [6], Sub-Saharan Africa [25], Uganda, and Ethiopia [26–30] with 74, 78, 90.7, and 65 per 1000 person-years, respectively.

The possible reasons for the explanation might be due to differences in the access and quality of the services, the size of records reviewed, the study period, and differences in inclusion and exclusion criteria. The risk of getting pregnant was 17.87 times higher among the rural women compared to their urban counterparts. This could be due to the fact that, in rural areas, the accessibility of family planning services was lower in the community and for mothers on ART in particular.

Married, widowed, and divorced women were 5.35, 3.65, and 4.34 times higher compared to women who never married, respectively. This finding was in line with the findings from United States of America and Sub-Saharan Arica [6, 25]; however, it was not consistent with the findings of a study of Western Uganda [26]. The possible explanation for the discrepancies might be due to differences in the size of records reviewed, the study period, and differences in inclusion and exclusion criteria.

The risk of pregnancy was 2.05 times higher among mothers who had zero or one child compared to those who had two and above children. This finding was in line with the findings of a study done in Western Uganda and Ethiopia [26, 30]. Women who had less than two children might have high fertility desire compared to those having two or more children. This might be due to the fact that mothers who had two or more children had better utilization of family planning services. The risk of pregnancy among unemployed women was also 4.37 times higher compared to the employed. It was in line with the findings of a study done in Western Uganda [26]. The possible justification of this finding might be due to the fact that in most circumstances in Ethiopia employed women are those with better educational status; in turn those women having better education may have a chance to access information from different types of media.

## 6. Limitations of the Study

Since this research was done using secondary data, all variables such as disclosure to sexual partner, adherence to ART, family planning methods uptake, open discussion with sexual partner, and other reproductive health issues which can possibly affect pregnancy among women on ART were not included. In addition to this, excluding charts with incomplete records could have an effect on the validity of the findings.

## 7. Conclusion

In light of the findings of this study, the authors forwarded the following remarks. The incidence of pregnancy among women on ART in Debre Markos Referral Hospital was found to be considerable. Living in rural areas, being married, widowed, and divorced, being unemployed, and having less than two children at enrollment on ART were found to be predictors of incidence of pregnancy among women on ART.

## 8. Recommendation

Considering the findings of this study, the Regional Health Bureau, Zonal Health Department, and health institutions should ensure that reproductive health services have to be well integrated into the HIV care system. Effective counseling strategies have to be designed focusing on rural, married, widowed, and divorced, unemployed mothers and mothers with less than two children at enrollment to reduce the risks of getting pregnant.

## Conflicts of Interest

The authors have declared that they have no conflicts of interest.

## Authors' Contributions

Maru Meseret conceptualized and designed the study, developed tools, supervised data collection, performed analysis and interpretation of data, and drafted the paper. Alemayehu Shimeka assisted in the conception and design of the study and helped in writing the proposal, developing tools, performing the analysis, and writing the paper. He has also developed the manuscript. Alemayehu Bekele assisted in the

TABLE 3: Cox's proportional hazards models examining predictors of incidence of pregnancy with 95% CIs, among women on ART in Debre Markos Referral Hospital, Northwest Ethiopia, Sept. 2011 to Aug. 2015 ($N = 1{,}239$).

| Variable | Status of pregnancy | | CHR (95% CI) | AHR (95% CI) |
|---|---|---|---|---|
| | No | Yes | | |
| Place of residence | | | | |
| Urban | 861 (90%) | 96 (10%) | 1 | 1 |
| Rural | 242 (85.8%) | 40 (14.2%) | 1.40 (0.97–2.02) | 17.87 (10.72–29.79) |
| Age | | | | |
| 15–24 | 267 (89.3%) | 32 (10.7%) | 1 | |
| 25–34 | 476 (86.5%) | 74 (13.5%) | 1.22 (0.81–1.85) | |
| ≥35 years | 360 (92.3%) | 30 (7.7%) | 0.68 (0.41–1.12) | |
| Marital status | | | | |
| Never married | 239 (95.2%) | 12 (4.8%) | 1 | 1 |
| Married | 400 (83.5%) | 79 (16.5%) | 3.61 (1.97–6.64) | 5.35 (2.14–13.36) |
| Widowed | 258 (91.5%) | 24 (8.5%) | 1.81 (0.90–3.62) | 3.65 (1.06–12.49) |
| Divorced | 206 (90.7%) | 21 (9.3%) | 2.13 (1.05–4.34) | 4.34 (1.42–13.22) |
| Educational status | | | | |
| Unable to read & write | 493 (83.6%) | 97 (16.4%) | 3.83 (1.93–7.59) | 2.28 (0.89–5.84) |
| Primary (1–8) | 224 (94.5%) | 13 (5.5%) | 1.24 (0.53–2.90) | 0.77 (0.24–2.48) |
| Secondary (9–12) | 197 (92.1%) | 17 (7.9%) | 1.81 (0.80–4.06) | 1.31 (0.37–4.61) |
| Certificate and above | 189 (95.5%) | 9 (4.5%) | 1 | 1 |
| Occupational status | | | | |
| Unemployed | 858 (88%) | 117 (12%) | 1.72 (1.06–2.80) | 4.37 (1.91–9.98) |
| Employed | 245 (92.8%) | 19 (7.2%) | 1 | 1 |
| Number of children at enrollment | | | | |
| 0-1 child | 604 (87.3%) | 88 (12.7%) | 1.55 (1.09–2.21) | 2.05 (1.31–3.20) |
| ≥2 children | 499 (91.2%) | 48 (8.8%) | 1 | 1 |

Note: level of significance was considered at a cutoff point of the $p$ value of 0.05.

conception, design, and interpretation of results and drafting the manuscript. All the authors read and approved the final manuscript.

## Acknowledgments

The authors would like to acknowledge Ethiopian Public Health Association (EPHA) for the financial support to conduct this study. They are indebted to the administration of Debre Markos Referral Hospital for allowing them to access the data. They would like to thank also the study participants.

## References

[1] HIV/AIDS, "Global fact sheet: stepping up the pace," in *Proceedings of the 20th International AIDS Conference*, Melbourne, Australia, July 2014.

[2] Joint United Nations Programs on HIV/AIDS, "Global Report: UNAIDS Report on the Global AIDS Epidemic," Tech. Rep., UNAIDS, Geneva, Switzerland, 2013.

[3] Central Statistical Agency and ICF International, "Ethiopia Demographic and Health Survey 2011," Tech. Rep., Central Statistical Agency and ICF International, Addis Ababa, Ethiopia, 2012.

[4] UNAIDS, "A progress report on the Global Plan towards the elimination of new HIV infections among children by 2015 and keeping their mothers alive, 2012".

[5] R. P. Walensky and D. R. Kuritzkes, "The impact of the President's Emergency Plan for AIDS Relief (PEPfAR) beyond HIV and why it remains essential," *Clinical Infectious Diseases*, vol. 50, no. 2, pp. 272–275, 2010.

[6] L. S. Massad, G. Springer, L. Jacobson et al., "Pregnancy rates and predictors of conception, miscarriage and abortion in US women with HIV," *AIDS*, vol. 18, no. 2, pp. 281–286, 2004.

[7] C. Calvert and C. Ronsmans, "The contribution of HIV to pregnancy-related mortality: a systematic review and meta-analysis," *AIDS*, vol. 27, no. 10, pp. 1631–1639, 2013.

[8] G. E. Gray and J. A. McIntyre, "HIV and pregnancy," *British Medical Journal*, vol. 334, no. 7600, pp. 950–953, 2007.

[9] W. Hladik, J. Stover, G. Esiru, M. Harper, and J. Tappero, "The contribution of family planning towards the prevention of vertical HIV transmission in Uganda," *PLoS ONE*, vol. 4, no. 11, article e7691, 2009.

[10] M. De Bruyn, "Safe abortion for HIV-positive women with unwanted pregnancy: a reproductive right," *Reproductive Health Matters*, vol. 11, no. 22, pp. 152–161, 2003.

[11] D. K. Ekouevi, P. A. Coffie, R. Becquet et al., "Antiretroviral therapy in pregnant women with advanced HIV disease and pregnancy outcomes in Abidjan, Côte d'Ivoire," *AIDS*, vol. 22, no. 14, pp. 1815–1820, 2008.

[12] H. W. Reynolds, B. Janowitz, R. Wilcher, and W. Cates, "Contraception to prevent HIV-positive births: current contribution and potential cost savings in PEPFAR countries," *Sexually Transmitted Infections*, vol. 84, (Suppl 2): ii49–53, no. 2, 2008.

[13] M. R. Loutfy, T. A. Hart, S. S. Mohammed et al., "Fertility desires and intentions of HIV-positive women of reproductive age in Ontario, Canada: a cross-sectional study," *PLoS ONE*, vol. 4, no. 12, article e7925, 2009.

[14] A. L. N. Dube, A. Baschieri, J. Cleland et al., "Fertility intentions and use of contraception among monogamous couples in northern malawi in the context of hiv testing: a cross-sectional analysis," *PLoS ONE*, vol. 7, no. 12, article e51861, 2012.

[15] M. Getachew, F. Alemseged, M. Abera, and A. Deribew, "Factors affecting fertility decisions of married men and women living with HIV in South Wollo Zone, Northeast Ethiopia," *Ethiopian Journal of Health Development*, vol. 24, no. 3, pp. 204–220, 2010.

[16] H. M. Asfaw and F. E. Gashe, "Fertility intentions among HIV positive women aged 18–49 years in Addis Ababa Ethiopia: a cross sectional study," *Reproductive Health*, vol. 11, no. 1, article 36, 2014.

[17] F. Haile, N. Isahak, and A. Dessie, "Fertility desire and associated factors among people living with HIV on ART, in Harari Regional State, Eastern Ethiopia," *Journal of Tropical Diseases*, vol. 2, article 2, 2014.

[18] Y.-T. Bonnenfant, M. J. Hindin, and D. Gillespie, "HIV diagnosis and fertility intentions among couple VCT clients in Ethiopia," *AIDS Care*, vol. 24, no. 11, pp. 1407–1415, 2012.

[19] C. Kilewo, K. Karlsson, M. Ngarina et al., "Prevention of mother–to–child transmission of HIV-1 through breastfeeding by treating mothers with triple antiretroviral therapy in dar es salaam, tanzania: the mitra plus study," *Journal of Acquired Immune Deficiency Syndromes*, vol. 52, no. 3, pp. 406–416, 2009.

[20] T. K. Thomas, R. Masaba, C. B. Borkowf et al., "Triple-antiretroviral prophylaxis to prevent mother–to–child HIV transmission through breastfeeding–the Kisumu Breastfeeding Study, Kenya: a clinical trial," *PLoS Medicine*, vol. 8, no. 3, Article ID e1001015, 2011.

[21] N. Siegfried, L. van der Merwe, P. Brocklehurst, and T. T. Sint, "Antiretrovirals for reducing the risk of mother–to–child transmission of HIV infection," *Cochrane Database of Systematic Reviews*, no. 7, 2011.

[22] J. J. C. Lewis, C. Ronsmans, A. Ezeh, and S. Gregson, "The population impact of HIV on fertility in Sub–Saharan Africa," *AIDS*, vol. 18, no. 2, pp. S35–S43, 2004.

[23] B. Zaba and S. Gregson, "Measuring the impact of HIV on fertility in Africa," *AIDS*, vol. 12, no. 1, pp. S41–S50, 1998.

[24] M. Gedefaw, H. Gebrehana, A. Gizachew, and F. Taddess, "Assessment of maternal near miss at debre markos referral hospital, northwest ethiopia: five years experience," *Open Journal of Epidemiology*, vol. 4, pp. 199–207, 2014.

[25] L. Myer, R. J. Carter, M. Katyal, P. Toro, W. M. El-Sadr, and E. J. Abrams, "Impact of antiretroviral therapy on incidence of pregnancy among HIV–infected women in Sub–Saharan Africa: a cohort study," *PLoS Medicine*, vol. 7, no. 2, Article ID e1000229, 2010.

[26] J. Kabami, E. Turyakira, S. Biraro, and F. Bajunirwe, "Increasing incidence of pregnancy among women receiving HIV care and treatment at a large urban facility in western Uganda," *Reproductive Health*, vol. 11, article 81, 2014.

[27] J. Homsy, R. Bunnell, D. Moore et al., "Reproductive intentions and outcomes among women on antiretroviral therapy in rural Uganda: a prospective cohort study," *PLoS ONE*, vol. 4, no. 1, Article ID e4149, 2009.

[28] A. Kaida, L. T. Matthews, S. Kanters et al., "Incidence and predictors of pregnancy among a cohort of HIV–positive women initiating antiretroviral therapy in mbarara, Uganda," *PLoS ONE*, vol. 8, no. 5, Article ID e63411, 2013.

[29] F. E. Makumbi, G. Nakigozi, S. J. Reynolds et al., "Associations between HIV antiretroviral therapy and the prevalence and incidence of pregnancy in Rakai, Uganda," *AIDS Research and Treatment*, vol. 2011, Article ID 519492, p. 10, 2011.

[30] M. Degife, G. Degu, and M. Molla, "Assessment of incidence and predictors of pregnancy among patients on antiretroviral therapy (ART) and pre-ART: a retrospective cohort study," *The Lancet*, vol. 381, article S34, 2013.

# 23

# Lipodystrophy among HIV-Infected Patients Attending Care and Treatment Clinics in Dar es Salaam

**Marina Njelekela,[1] Rose Mpembeni,[2] Alfa Muhihi,[3] Nzovu Ulenga,[3] Eric Aris,[3] and Deodatus Kakoko[4]**

[1] *Department of Physiology, Muhimbili University of Health and Allied Sciences, P.O. Box 65001, Dar es Salaam, Tanzania*
[2] *Department of Epidemiology and Biostatistics, Muhimbili University of Health and Allied Sciences, P.O. Box 65001, Dar es Salaam, Tanzania*
[3] *Management and Development for Health, Mwai Kibaki Road, Mikocheni, P.O. Box 79810, Dar es Salaam, Tanzania*
[4] *Department of Behavioral Sciences, Muhimbili University of Health and Allied Sciences, P.O. Box 65001, Dar es Salaam, Tanzania*

Correspondence should be addressed to Marina Njelekela; madaula@yahoo.com

Academic Editor: David Katzenstein

*Background.* HIV infection and long-term HAART use are associated with metabolic and morphological changes. We assessed prevalence, types, and risk factors associated with lipodystrophy among HIV-infected adults attending CTC in Dar es Salaam, Tanzania. *Methods.* Analysis included 466 HIV-infected patients. Study protocol involved administration of structured questionnaire to collect sociodemographic and clinical information. Diagnosis of lipodystrophy was based on physician clinical assessment. *Results.* Lipodystrophy was present in 95 (20.4%) of the study participants, with lipoatrophy being the most common (49.5%) followed by mixed lipodystrophy (37.9%), and lipohypertrophy was the least prevalent (12.6%). Male gender, older age, long duration on HAART, and use of Stavudine containing regimen were associated with lipodystrophy (all $p < 0.05$). The risk for lipodystrophy was 1.6 times (AOR = 1.66, 95% CI = 1.01–2.72) for male participants and 13.3 times (AOR = 13.3, 95% CI = 6.4–27.7) for those on HAART. Long duration on HAART and use of Stavudine containing regimen were also associated with increased risk for lipodystrophy. Lipodystrophy was associated with poor perception about own body image and decreased social interactions. *Conclusions.* Lipodystrophy is common among HIV-infected patients in Tanzania, especially among male patients and those on HAART. Regular screening, monitoring, and patient awareness are needed for early identification and appropriate management.

## 1. Introduction

The recent estimates by UNAIDS indicate that 36.7 million [34.0 million–39.8 million] people were living with HIV in 2015 with Sub-Saharan Africa (SSA) bearing an inordinate share (70%) of the global HIV burden [1]. The number of HIV-infected people accessing Highly Active Antiretroviral Therapy (HAART) increased from 5.2 million in 2009 to 17.0 million in 2015 [1]. Of the estimated 1.1 million AIDS-related deaths in 2015, nearly three-quarter (73%) occurred in SSA [1]. In Tanzania, HIV incidence slowed to about 3.4 per 1000 person-years between 2004 and 2008 [2]. Data from the 2012 Tanzania HIV/AIDS and Malaria Indicator Survey (THMIS) indicated the national prevalence of HIV was 5.1% among the sexually active populations (15–49 years) and was higher among women (6.2%) compared to 3.8% in men [3].

The introduction of HAART provided HIV/AIDS patients with opportunity for quality of life improvement by inhibiting disease progression and development of opportunistic infections [4, 5]. Studies have indicated decreased HIV transmission and AIDS-related morbidity and mortality in both developed and developing countries [6, 7] resulting from high coverage of HAART. The provision of HIV services including HAART in Tanzania began in October 2004 with triple therapy consisting of 2 Nucleoside Reverse Transcriptase Inhibitors (NRTIs) + 1 Non-Nucleoside Reverse Transcriptase Inhibitor (NNRTI), 2 NRTIs + 1 Protease Inhibitor (PI), or 3 NRTIs being recommended [8]. The current National

Guidelines for Management of HIV and AIDS provides drug combinations options for first-line treatment according to indications and contraindications. However, the current default first-line regimen in Tanzania is Tenofovir (TDF) 300 mg/Lamivudine (3TC) 300 mg/Efavirenz (EFV) 600 mg once daily at night [9]. Introduction of fixed dose combination therapy has significantly reduced pill burden to HIV patients and improved adherence to treatment [10, 11].

HIV infection and HAART have been associated with development of cardiovascular and metabolic complications including lipodystrophy [12, 13]. These effects are mediated through mitochondrial toxicity [13], atherosclerosis, and increased levels of inflammatory markers such as C-reactive protein, interleukin 6, cystatin C, and D-dimer all of which are associated with CVD risk [14, 15]. Lipodystrophy syndrome encompasses three clinical conditions characterized by abnormal body fat distribution; (i) lipoatrophy (peripheral fat wasting), (ii) lipohypertrophy (central fat accumulation), and (iii) mixed lipodystrophy (combination of both lipoatrophy and lipohypertrophy). Lipodystrophy patients have characteristic peripheral fat loss in the face, limbs, and buttocks, accompanied by central fat accumulation in the abdomen and breasts and over the dorsocervical spine ("buffalo hump") and lipomas [16]. Protease Inhibitors (PI) containing regimen have been most strongly linked to body fat maldistribution syndrome [17, 18]. Non-Nucleoside Reverse Transcriptase Inhibitors (NRTIs) especially Stavudine have also been associated with body fat maldistribution [19]. The overall prevalence of at least one physical abnormality related to body fat maldistribution has been estimated at about 50% after one year of using HAART [20]. Other factors, such as duration of HIV infection, age, and gender, may also contribute to the risk of development of lipodystrophy [21]. Studies have shown that body fat changes are associated with psychological trauma which may be severe enough to affect a patient's desire to continue with HAART, limit therapy options, and profoundly affect the quality of life [22].

As Tanzania scales up HAART to all HIV-infected individuals country-wide through the "test and treat" strategy, it is critical to understand the proportion of HIV-related body fat maldistribution among HIV-infected people on treatment, so as to design and institute interventions that will minimize the risk for lipodystrophy. This study was therefore conducted to determine the prevalence, types, and risk factors associated with lipodystrophy among HIV-infected adults attending Care and Treatment Clinic (CTC) at three municipal referral hospitals in Dar es Salaam, Tanzania.

## 2. Materials and Methods

*2.1. Study Design, Site, and Participants.* This cross-sectional analytical study was conducted at Amana, Temeke, and Mwananyamala Municipal Hospitals in Dar es Salaam. At the time of data collection, Amana Hospital CTC had 14,133 active clients (with 7,932 on treatment and 6,201 under care and monitoring); Temeke Hospital CTC clinic had 16,530 active clients (with 8,871 on treatment and 7,659 under care and monitoring), and Mwananyamala Hospital CTC had 17,746 active clients (with 9,193 on treatment and 8,553 under care and monitoring).

Dar es Salaam region has a population of more than 4.3 million people, with an HIV prevalence of 5.1% among sexually active age group [3]. Study participants were HIV-positive patients aged ≥ 18 years who had been attending CTC at the three aforementioned municipal referral hospitals for at least 24 months.

*2.2. Eligibility and Sampling Procedure.* Stratified sampling was used to enroll participants into the study. The daily appointment list of patients was obtained from the hospital CTC records one day in advance. From this list the two groups (HAART and HAART naïve) and duration for which the patient has been attending CTC were determined. The list of patients who had attended CTC clinic for ≥24 months formed the sampling frame. Selection of patients from each stratum was done using simple random sampling techniques. Inclusion criteria were men and women aged ≥ 18 years, had attended CTC for ≥24 months, on HAART or HAART naïve, were clinically stable with good general condition, and provided a signed informed consent to participate. Pregnant women and very sick patients (Karnofsky score ≥ 40%) [23] were excluded from the study.

*2.3. Recruitment of Research Assistants and Training.* Six research assistants (3 physicians and 3 nurses) working at the CTC in the three municipal hospitals were recruited to assist during data collection. Selected study physicians and nurses had experience working at the CTC and had good interview and communication skills. Study physicians and nurses received training on the objectives of the study, recruitment, and assessments procedures, as well as importance of ensuring data quality.

*2.4. Study Protocol.* The study protocol involved administration of a questionnaire and physical examination. Sociodemographic information including age, sex, marital status, level of education, source of income, and lifestyle related information (smoking, alcohol drinking, type of diet in the last 24 hours, and physical activity) was assessed. Dietary assessment was conducted using a 24 h recall system. Based on a list of common foods, which was provided to them at the time of interview, subjects were also asked about food and/or beverages in the past 24 hours. A quick assessment of level of physical activity was conducted using the same interview guide. Participants were then asked to rank themselves in terms of level of physical activity. Duration and type of HAART medications and for HAART naïve the duration since HIV was diagnosed were ascertained from the patient medical records.

*2.5. Anthropometric Measurement.* Anthropometric measurements including height, weight, and waist and hip circumference were obtained following standardized procedures. Body Mass Index (BMI) was calculated as weight in kilograms divided by height in meters squared (kg/m$^2$), and categorized as underweight (BMI ≤ 18.5 kg/m$^2$), normal weight (BMI:

18.5–24.9 kg/m$^2$), overweight (BMI: 25.0–29.9 kg/m$^2$), and obese (BMI ≥ 30 kg/m$^2$). Central obesity was defined as waist circumference ≥ 102 centimeters in men and ≥88 centimeters in women [24].

*2.6. Assessment and Definition of Lipodystrophy Syndrome.* In order to characterize self-rated body fat maldistribution, study participants were asked if they had noticed any changes that had alerted them in the following:

(i) Increased fat under the chin
(ii) Increased fat on the back of the neck
(iii) Increased abdominal girth
(iv) Increased chest or breast fat
(v) Loss of fat in the face
(vi) Loss of fat in the arms
(vii) Loss of fat in the buttocks
(viii) Loss of fat in the legs.

Information reported by the patient was validated by the physician after conducting a thorough physical examination. Fat maldistribution was scored as none (score = 0), mild (score = 1), moderate (score = 2), and severe (score = 3) and was recorded separately for fat losses and accumulations [25]. Lipodystrophy was categorized as

(i) *lipoatrophy*: presence of at least one site with moderate or severe fat loss,
(ii) *lipohypertrophy*: presence of at least one site with moderate or severe fat accumulation, excluding isolated abdominal fat accumulation,
(iii) *mixed lipodystrophy*: presence of signs of both lipoatrophy and lipohypertrophy.

*2.7. Ethical Clearance.* Ethical approval to conduct the study was obtained from Research Ethics Committee of the Muhimbili University of Health and Allied Sciences. Permission to conduct the study at the municipal hospitals was obtained from respective municipal medical officers of health through municipal research coordinators, who notified the medical officers in charge of the municipal hospitals. Medical officers in charge are overseers of these hospitals and facilitated to ensure that data collection was conducted smoothly.

The purpose of the study, expected duration of the participant's involvement, and description of the study procedures to be followed were clearly explained to potential participants. Description of any reasonably foreseeable benefits to the participant, such as awareness of body fat maldistribution risk factors and how they are going to be protected, for example, treatment of hypercholesterolemia, proper diet, and adequate physical activity, was done before enrolment. Risks or discomforts such as longer duration of interviews were also communicated in advance. Only those who agreed by signing informed consent were interviewed and were free to withdraw from the study during interview. To ensure confidentiality, participants were assigned unique identification numbers that were used during data collection.

*2.8. Data Collection and Management.* Data collected was edited during and after collection and adjusted for some missing information. The principal investigator scheduled visits to the study sites to observe and supervise data collection as per interview guide to ensure quality data. The principal investigator was also available for clarifications as another means of quality check. Therefore, the risk of study physicians and nurses recording wrong responses on account of misunderstanding the questions was minimized. Coding for open ended questions was done by the team and thereafter data was entered by the trained data entrant. Data cleaning and analysis were done using SPSS version 20.0 for windows.

*2.9. Data Analysis.* Frequency distribution was done to all variables to assess their distribution in the study population. Two-way tables were used to assess the association between dependent and independent variables by using the $\chi^2$-test. Multiple logistic regressions were used to assess individual contribution of each independent variable in predicting body fat maldistribution while controlling for confounding variables. In all the analyses, the $p$ values were 2-sided and $p \leq 0.05$ was considered statistically significant.

## 3. Results

*3.1. Sociodemographic and General Characteristics of Study Sample.* A total of 466 HIV-infected patients attending CTC at Amana, Temeke, and Mwananyamala Municipal Hospitals were included in the analysis. Demographic and general characteristics of the study participants are summarized in Table 1. Three-quarter (74.9%) of the participants were females. The mean age of the study participants was 41.1 ± 9.8 years, with majority (41.6%) being in the age group of 31–50 years. Nearly half (47.0%) of the participants were married or cohabiting, and majority had primary level of education (76.4%). Half of the participants (51.1%) were on HAART, with 49.6% of them being on Efavirenz based regimen, 36.1% on Stavudine based regimen, 13.0% on Nevirapine based regimen, and only 1.3% on Protease Inhibitor based second-line regimen. Majority (62.6%) of HAART patients were on treatment for 24–48 months.

*3.2. Prevalence of Lipodystrophy.* Prevalence of lipodystrophy was 20.4% with primary lipoatrophy (49.5%) being the most prevalent form of lipodystrophy followed by mixed lipodystrophy (37.9%) and primary lipohypertrophy (12.6%) was the least common (Table 1). A similar trend was observed for self-rating where 114 (24.5%) reported to have noted changes in body fat maldistribution, with more participants reporting decreased size of their body parts (17.5%) compared to increased size of body parts (14.0%).

*3.3. Factors Associated with Lipodystrophy.* Table 2 presents the characteristics of HIV-infected patients with lipodystrophy. Male participants were affected more than female participants (26.5% versus 18.3%; $p = 0.058$). However, the overall prevalence of overweight and that of obesity was significantly higher among women compared to men (25.8%

TABLE 1: Sociodemographic and general characteristics of the study participants.

| Characteristic | Number (%) |
|---|---|
| Age (years) | |
| ≤30 years | 51 (10.9) |
| 31–40 years | 194 (41.6) |
| 41–50 years | 134 (28.8) |
| ≥51 years | 67 (14.4) |
| Missing | 20 (4.3) |
| Gender | |
| Male | 117 (25.1) |
| Female | 349 (74.9) |
| Marital status | |
| Married | 219 (47.0) |
| Single | 89 (19.1) |
| Divorced/separated | 81 (17.4) |
| Widowed | 77 (16.5) |
| Education level | |
| No formal education | 27 (5.8) |
| Primary education | 356 (76.4) |
| Secondary education | 68 (14.6) |
| College/university | 15 (3.2) |
| CTC of enrolment | |
| Amana Hospital | 152 (32.6) |
| Temeke Hospital | 155 (33.3) |
| Mwananyamala Hospital | 159 (34.1) |
| HAART use | |
| On HAART | 238 (51.1) |
| HAART naïve | 228 (48.9) |
| Type of HAART | |
| Nevirapine based regimen | 31 (13.0) |
| Efavirenz based regimen | 118 (49.6) |
| Stavudine based regimen | 86 (36.1) |
| Protease Inhibitor based regimen | 3 (1.3) |
| Duration of HAART use | |
| HAART naïve | 228 (48.9) |
| 24 months | 60 (12.9) |
| 25–48 months | 149 (32.0) |
| >48 months | 29 (6.2) |
| Lipodystrophy | |
| Yes | 95 (20.4) |
| No | 371 (79.6) |
| Types of lipodystrophy | |
| Primary lipoatrophy | 47 (49.5) |
| Primary lipohypertrophy | 12 (12.6) |
| Mixed lipodystrophy | 36 (37.9) |
| Body Mass Index (BMI) | |
| Underweight | 58 (12.5) |
| Normal weight | 235 (50.5) |
| Overweight | 110 (23.7) |
| Obese | 62 (13.3) |
| Central obesity | |
| No | 301 (64.7) |
| Yes | 164 (35.7) |

BMI: Body Mass Index; CTC: Care and Treatment Clinic; HAART: Highly Active Antiretroviral Therapy.

versus 17.2%) for overweight and (16.3% versus 4.3%) for obesity (results not shown). Participants in the age group 41–50 years had the highest proportion of participants with lipodystrophy (27.6%) followed by those aged > 50 years (25.4%) and low proportion for younger participants ($p = 0.003$).

As for HAART status, lipodystrophy was higher (36.1% versus 3.9%) among participants on HAART compared to HAART naïve participants ($p < 0.001$). Differences in prevalence of lipodystrophy were also observed with the type of HAART used. Prevalence of lipodystrophy was highest for participants receiving second-line PI based regimen (66.7%) followed by Stavudine based regimen (53.5%). Nevirapine and Efavirenz based regimens had relatively similar rates of lipodystrophy (25.8% and 25.4%, resp.). The differences in the prevalence of lipodystrophy by type of HAART were statistically significant ($p < 0.001$). Duration of HAART use showed a U-shaped relationship with lipodystrophy. Patients on HAART for >48 months had highest proportion of lipodystrophy followed by those on HAART for 24 months and low in patients on HAART for 25–48 months ($p < 0.001$)

Lipodystrophy was highest among underweight patients (27.6%) followed by normal weight patients (21.7%) and least among obese patients (8.1%). The difference was statistically significant ($p = 0.048$). Although it did not attain statistical significance, prevalence of lipodystrophy was slightly higher among patients with central obesity (22.0%) compared to those without central obesity (19.6%).

*3.4. Factors Associated with Different Types of Lipodystrophy.* Table 3 presents analysis of factors associated with different types of lipodystrophy. Prevalence of primary lipoatrophy was significantly higher for patients aged more than 40 years ($p = 0.004$), male gender ($p = 0.004$), HAART use, longer duration of >48 months, and Stavudine based regimen (all $p < 0.01$). As for primary lipohypertrophy, significant association was observed with only duration of HAART use ($p = 0.025$) and was highest for patients on HAART for 24 months. Mixed type lipodystrophy was found to be associated with education level ($p = 0.039$), HAART use ($p < 0.001$), Protease Inhibitor based regimen ($p = 0.013$), and using HAART for 24–48 months.

*3.5. Determinants of Lipodystrophy.* Table 4 shows the results of multiple logistic regressions to determine the most important contributors to lipodystrophy in this population. A model for this analysis contained covariates that attained a statistically significant difference of $p < 0.05$ during bivariate analysis. These included age, gender, duration, and types of HAART used. While being in the age group of 31-40 years showed a protective effect (AOR = 0.18, 95% CI = 0.05–0.65), older age > 50 years showed a nonsignificant 12% increased risk for lipodystrophy (AOR = 1.12, 95% CI 0.58–2.19). Male gender was associated with 66% (AOR = 1.66, 95% CI = 1.01–2.72) increased risk for lipodystrophy compared to female gender. Using HAART was associated with 13 times increased risk for lipodystrophy. Similarly, long duration of Stavudine based regimen was significantly associated with 3 times increased risk for lipodystrophy (AOR = 3.22, 95% CI = 1.17–8.81).

TABLE 2: Factors associated with lipodystrophy among HIV-infected patients in Dar es Salaam.

| Characteristic | Lipodystrophy | | $p$ value |
|---|---|---|---|
| | Present | Absent | |
| Age (years) | | | |
| ≤30 | 3 (5.9) | 48 (94.1) | |
| 31–40 | 32 (16.5) | 162 (83.5) | |
| 41–50 | 37 (27.6) | 97 (72.4) | **0.003** |
| >50 | 17 (25.4) | 50 (74.6) | |
| Missing | 6 (30.0) | 14 (70.0) | |
| Gender | | | |
| Male | 31 (26.5) | 86 (73.5) | 0.058 |
| Female | 64 (18.3) | 285 (81.7) | |
| Marital status | | | |
| Married | 41 (18.7) | 178 (81.3) | |
| Single | 20 (22.5) | 69 (77.5) | 0.860 |
| Divorced/separated | 17 (21.0) | 64 (79.0) | |
| Widowed | 17 (22.1) | 60 (77.9) | |
| Education level | | | |
| No formal education | 6 (22.2) | 21 (77.8) | |
| Primary education | 68 (19.1) | 288 (80.9) | 0.484 |
| Secondary education | 16 (23.5) | 52 (76.5) | |
| College/university | 5 (33.3) | 10 (66.7) | |
| HAAT use | | | |
| On HAART | 86 (36.1) | 152 (63.9) | **<0.001** |
| HAART naïve | 9 (3.9) | 219 (96.1) | |
| Type of HAART | | | |
| Nevirapine based regimen | 8 (25.8) | 23 (74.2) | |
| Efavirenz based regimen | 30 (25.4) | 88 (74.6) | **<0.001** |
| Stavudine based regimen | 46 (53.5) | 40 (46.5) | |
| Protease Inhibitor based regimen | 2 (66.7) | 1 (33.3) | |
| Duration of HAART use | | | |
| HAART naïve | 9 (3.9) | 219 (96.1) | |
| 24 months | 23 (38.3) | 37 (61.7) | **<0.001** |
| 24–48 months | 51 (34.2) | 98 (65.8) | |
| >48 months | 12 (41.4) | 17 (58.6) | |
| Body Mass Index (BMI) | | | |
| Underweight | 16 (27.6) | 42 (72.4) | |
| Normal weight | 51 (21.7) | 184 (78.3) | **0.048** |
| Overweight | 23 (20.9) | 87 (79.1) | |
| Obese | 5 (8.1) | 57 (91.9) | |
| Central obesity | | | |
| No | 59 (19.6) | 242 (80.4) | 0.630 |
| Yes | 36 (22.0) | 128 (78.0) | |

BMI: Body Mass Index; HAART: Highly Active Antiretroviral Therapy.

3.6. *Perceptions Related to Body Image and Quality of Life.* Participants' perceptions about their body image and social life are summarized in Table 5. About 15.8% of the participants felt strongly that their current body outlook/image was worse compared to the way they looked before and 10.5% reported to dislike their mirror images. On average 24.5% of the participants with lipodystrophy avoided wearing clothing that display their body and 7.4% did so much more often. As for social aspects of life, 11.6% of the participants worried much about going into gatherings. Others reported

TABLE 3: Factors associated with different types of lipodystrophy among HIV-infected patients in Dar es Salaam.

| Characteristic | Lipoatrophy | | | Lipohypertrophy | | | Mixed lipodystrophy | | |
|---|---|---|---|---|---|---|---|---|---|
| | Yes | No | *p* value | Yes | No | *p* value | Yes | No | *p* value |
| Age categories (yrs) | | | | | | | | | |
| ≤30 | 0 (0.0) | 51 (100.0) | | 1 (2.0) | 50 (98.0) | | 2 (3.9) | 49 (96.1) | |
| 31–40 | 13 (6.7) | 181 (93.3) | | 6 (3.1) | 188 (96.9) | | 13 (6.7) | 181 (93.3) | |
| 41–50 | 18 (13.4) | 116 (86.6) | **0.004** | 5 (3.9) | 129 (96.3) | 0.463 | 14 (10.4) | 120 (89.6) | 0.436 |
| ≥51 | 11 (16.4) | 56 (83.6) | | 0 (0.0) | 67 (100.0) | | 6 (9.0) | 61 (91.0) | |
| Missing | 5 (33.3) | 15 (66.7) | | 0 (0.0) | 20 (100.0) | | 2 (9.5) | 19 (90.5) | |
| Gender | | | | | | | | | |
| Male | 20 (17.1) | 97 (82.9) | **0.004** | 3 (2.6) | 114 (97.4) | 1.000 | 8 (6.8) | 109 (93.2) | 0.699 |
| Female | 27 (7.7) | 322 (92.3) | | 9 (2.6) | 340 (97.4) | | 28 (8.0) | 321 (92.0) | |
| Education level | | | | | | | | | |
| No formal education | 3 (11.1) | 24 (88.9) | | 1 (3.7) | 26 (96.3) | | 2 (7.4) | 25 (92.6) | |
| Primary education | 34 (9.6) | 322 (90.4) | 0.797 | 7 (2.0) | 349 (98.0) | 0.204 | 27 (7.6) | 329 (92.4) | **0.039** |
| Secondary education | 9 (13.2) | 59 (86.8) | | 4 (5.9) | 64 (94.1) | | 3 (4.4) | 65 (95.6) | |
| College/university | 1 (6.7) | 14 (93.3) | | 0 (0.0) | 15 (100.0) | | 4 (26.7) | 11 (73.3) | |
| HAART use | | | | | | | | | |
| On HAART | 42 (17.6) | 196 (82.4) | **<0.001** | 9 (3.8) | 229 (96.2) | 0.142 | 35 (14.7) | 203 (85.3) | **<0.001** |
| HAART naïve | 5 (2.2) | 223 (97.8) | | 3 (1.3) | 225 (98.7) | | 1 (0.4) | 227 (99.6) | |
| Type of HAART used | | | | | | | | | |
| Nevirapine based | 1 (3.2) | 30 (96.8) | | 2 (6.5) | 29 (93.5) | | 5 (16.1) | 26 (83.9) | |
| Efavirenz based | 15 (12.7) | 103 (87.3) | **0.002** | 4 (3.4) | 114 (96.6) | 0.817 | 11 (9.3) | 107 (90.7) | **0.013** |
| Stavudine based | 26 (30.2) | 60 (69.8) | | 3 (3.5) | 83 (96.5) | | 17 (19.8) | 69 (80.2) | |
| Protease Inhibitor based | 0 (0.0) | 3 (100.0) | | 0 (0.0) | 3 (100.0) | | 2 (66.7) | 1 (33.3) | |
| Duration of HAART use | | | | | | | | | |
| HAART naïve | 5 (2.2) | 223 (97.8) | | 3 (1.3) | 225 (98.7) | | 1 (0.4) | 227 (99.6) | |
| 24 months | 11 (18.3) | 49 (81.7) | **<0.001** | 5 (8.3) | 55 (91.7) | **0.025** | 7 (11.7) | 53 (88.3) | **<0.001** |
| 24–48 months | 22 (14.8) | 127 (85.2) | | 3 (2.0) | 146 (98.0) | | 26 (17.4) | 123 (82.6) | |
| >48 months | 9 (31.0) | 20 (69.0) | | 1 (3.4) | 28 (96.6) | | 2 (6.9) | 27 (93.1) | |

HAART: Highly Active Antiretroviral Therapy.

on average lack of desire for sexual intercourse (9.7%), being afraid to be introduced to new people (13.7%), and avoiding outdoor activities like swimming (16.0%).

## 4. Discussion

This study aimed at determining the prevalence and factors associated with lipodystrophy, and assessing the perceptions towards body fat maldistribution among HIV-infected individuals attending CTC at three municipal hospitals in Dar es Salaam. Since the advent of HAART globally in 1996, HIV-related morbidity and mortality have decreased significantly. Now patients are living longer but chronic health complications such as cardiovascular diseases and lipodystrophy represent important health issues in this patient population.

In this analysis, the prevalence of physician diagnosed lipodystrophy was 20.4%. The combined prevalence of overweight and obesity was 37.0%, whereas that of central obesity was 35.7%. The precise definition and estimation of lipodystrophy are important for comparison across studies and populations. Prevalence observed in this study was low compared to findings from studies conducted in Western populations [26, 27]. Conversely, it was considerably higher than 6.6% reported among African patients after 18 months of HAART [28]. Two other studies conducted in Africa demonstrated higher prevalence rates of lipodystrophy compared to our study [29, 30]. The observed low prevalence of lipodystrophy in comparison to objective measures (BMI and waist circumference) and that of other studies conducted in Africa may be caused by clinical diagnosis by the attending physician which is subjective and compounded by malnutrition seen in HIV-positive.

Our study has demonstrated an association between lipodystrophy and demographic characteristics including age, gender, and level of education. In our study the prevalence of lipodystrophy was higher in men than women. Conversely, the prevalence of overweight and obesity as defined by BMI was higher in women compared to men. As for age, lipodystrophy was found to be higher for participants aged 41 years and above. Findings from Rwandan study indicated that age and gender were significantly associated with lipodystrophy [29]. Several other studies have also found a similar association [31, 32]. In African settings, more women

TABLE 4: Determinants of lipodystrophy among HIV-infected patients in Dar es Salaam.

| Variables | AOR | 95% CI | *p* value |
|---|---|---|---|
| Age (years) | | | |
| ≤30 | Ref | | |
| 31–40 | 0.18 | 0.05–0.65 | **0.009** |
| 41–50 | 0.59 | 0.30–1.15 | 0.120 |
| ≥51 | 1.12 | 0.58–2.19 | 0.735 |
| Gender | | | |
| Female | Ref | | |
| Male | 1.66 | 1.01–2.72 | **0.045** |
| HAAT use | | | |
| HAART naïve | Ref | | |
| On HAART | 13.3 | 6.4–27.7 | **<0.001** |
| Type of HAART used | | | |
| Nevirapine based | Ref | | |
| Efavirenz based | 0.98 | 0.36–2.66 | 0.962 |
| Stavudine based | 3.22 | 1.17–8.81 | **0.023** |
| Protease Inhibitor based | 1.06 | 0.08–9.02 | 1.00 |
| Duration of HAART use | | | |
| HAART naïve | Ref | | |
| 24 months | 12.8 | 6.0–27.6 | **<0.001** |
| 25–48 months | 13.6 | 5.7–32.4 | **<0.001** |
| >48 months | 15.3 | 5.3–43.8 | **<0.001** |

AOR: Adjusted Odds Ratio; CI: Confidence Interval; HAART: Highly Active Antiretroviral Therapy.

than men are generally obese [33] and obesity tends to increase with age and level of education [34].

Type, duration, and current use of HAART especially PI and NNRTI containing regimen are strongly associated with development of severe lipoatrophy [35]. In our study, lipodystrophy was highest for patients on PI based second-line HAART regimen, followed by patients on Stavudine based regimen and Nevirapine based regimen, and least among patients on Efavirenz based regimen. Prospective studies investigating body composition in patients starting HAART for the first time [35, 36] have demonstrated initial increases in limb fat during the first few months of therapy, followed by progressive decline during ensuing three years. In one study the decline was estimated to be 14% per year among white men receiving regimens containing Stavudine or Zidovudine with Lamivudine and either a Protease Inhibitor or Non-Nucleoside Reverse Transcriptase Inhibitor [36].

Our findings on association of Stavudine and Efavirenz with lipodystrophy are consistent with other studies that used Stavudine and Efavirenz based therapy [29, 37]. Non-Nucleoside Reverse Transcriptase Inhibitors (NNRTIs), such as Efavirenz, have been associated with in vitro altered deposition of triglycerides in the adipocyte; however its clear clinical implications is still being studied. Thymidine analog Nucleoside Reverse Transcriptase Inhibitors (tNRTIs) are risk factors for mitochondrial dysfunction associated with both dyslipidemia and lipoatrophy (particularly in subcutaneous adipocytes) [37]. Changing patients from thymidine analogs to NRTIs has demonstrated beneficial effects on lipoatrophy [38]. Stavudine, the nucleoside analog with the highest propensity for causing mitochondrial dysfunction, is relatively inexpensive and widely available in the developing world. Zidovudine is also relatively available and has many therapeutic advantages but also carries risk of producing mitochondrial toxicity. Hence the use of these drugs in the developing world will lead to mitochondrial toxicity and development of lipodystrophy as is shown in this study.

This study found diverse emotional feelings among participants regarding perception about their body image and quality of life, ranging from feeling worse than before and feeling bad about own mirror image to avoiding wearing some dressing because of fear of stigma. However, we did not explore the desire to stop treatment because of the change in body image. Other studies have also explored the psychosocial effects of lipodystrophy among HIV patients on HAART [39, 40]. Lipodystrophy might have substantial psychological repercussions with subsequent negative impact on the patient's quality of life, emergence of depressive symptoms, or anxiety [41, 42]. Moreover, body change status and subsequent stigmatization could produce social isolation and distress and, even, change in beliefs about drugs and consequently decreased adherence to HAART.

As with regard to social life, participants with lipodystrophy reported isolating themselves from other people, tending to avoid outside activities like swimming, avoiding events that will have many people, and a diminished desire for sexual intercourse. Other studies have also demonstrated altered quality of life among patients with lipodystrophy [43]. Body-shape changes may affect patients' psychosocial function and quality of life and may lead to patients considering cessation

TABLE 5: Changes in body parts and perceptions about current body image among HIV infected patients in Dar es Salaam.

| Change and perception | Extent of perceived change | | | |
|---|---|---|---|---|
| | None | Very little | Average | Very much |
| Increased body parts | | | | |
| Neck and chin | 88 (93.6) | 2 (2.1) | 4 (4.3) | 0 (0.0) |
| Back of shoulders | 83 (89.2) | 2 (2.2) | 8 (8.6) | 0 (0.0) |
| Breast and/or chest | 71 (76.3) | 7 (7.5) | 14 (15.1) | 1 (1.1) |
| Abdomen | 66 (69.5) | 7 (7.4) | 21 (22.1) | 1 (1.1) |
| Waist | 78 (85.7) | 2 (2.2) | 10 (11.0) | 1 (1.1) |
| Decreased body parts | | | | |
| Face | 53 (57.0) | 9 (9.7) | 25 (26.9) | 6 (6.5) |
| Upper limbs | 49 (53.8) | 15 (16.5) | 19 (20.9) | 8 (8.8) |
| Lower limbs | 49 (53.3) | 18 (19.6) | 17 (18.5) | 8 (8.7) |
| Buttocks | 54 (57.4) | 9 (9.6) | 24 (25.5) | 7 (7.4) |
| Perception about body image | | | | |
| Angry about own body | 60 (63.8) | 12 (12.8) | 18 (19.1) | 4 (4.3) |
| Avoiding some clothing | 50 (53.2) | 14 (14.9) | 23 (24.5) | 7 (7.4) |
| Ashamed of own body | 63 (66.3) | 9 (9.5) | 19 (20.0) | 4 (4.2) |
| Unhappy about mirror image | 49 (51.6) | 16 (16.8) | 20 (21.1) | 10 (10.5) |
| Conscious of other people | 69 (75.8) | 16 (17.6) | 5 (5.5) | 1 (1.1) |
| Bad body shape than before | 50 (52.6) | 10 (10.5) | 20 (21.1) | 15 (15.8) |
| Afraid to mix with other people | 76 (80.0) | 11 (11.6) | 8 (8.4) | 0 (0.0) |
| Perceptions related to social life | | | | |
| Avoiding outdoor activities | 67 (71.3) | 10 (10.6) | 15 (16.0) | 2 (2.1) |
| Avoiding social events with many people | 76 (78.4) | 7 (7.2) | 12 (12.4) | 2 (2.1) |
| Lack of desire for sexual intercourse | 73 (78.5) | 8 (8.6) | 9 (9.7) | 3 (3.2) |
| Afraid to be introduced to new people | 73 (76.8) | 9 (9.5) | 13 (13.7) | 0 (0.0) |
| Afraid to enter a room with new people | 79 (83.2) | 7 (7.4) | 9 (9.5) | 0 (0.0) |
| Habit to exclude himself from other people | 82 (88.2) | 6 (6.5) | 4 (4.3) | 1 (1.1) |
| Avoid going into social gatherings/parties | 61 (64.2) | 7 (7.4) | 16 (16.8) | 11 (11.6) |

of treatment [44]. However, few studies to date have formally addressed the impact of these changes on the patient. Hence this study demonstrates that there are significant variations in perceptions about body changes and the quality of life of these patients that need to be addressed in a larger and well-designed study for that purpose.

There are few limitations to our analysis. The cross-sectional design does not provide causal association of studies parameters with lipodystrophy. The study included patients who were attending CTC clinics and may not be representative of all HIV-infected individuals. However, the fact that the study was conducted in Dar es Salaam which is metropolitan with a diverse population from nearly all other regions makes it possible for the findings to be generalizable to the broader Tanzanian population. We did not collect detailed information on patient's treatment history. For participants who changed treatment due to side effects, the observed association of HAART regimen and lipodystrophy could have been caused by the previous regimen. Therefore we may have missed the true association of HAART with lipodystrophy. The detailed treatment history could also provide some insights on the quality of care in terms of management for lipodystrophy through change of regimen implicated in causing lipodystrophy. Assessments of body fat changes were done clinically, instead of using specialized instruments such as dual energy X-ray absorptiometry (DEXA) or linear calipers. Nevertheless, subjective assessment is strongly correlated with DEXA [45].

In conclusion, prevalence of lipodystrophy among HIV-infected patients is high and is worsened by HAART use. Our findings clearly demonstrate the long-term side effects of HAART, particularly Stavudine based regimen among HIV-infected patients in Tanzania. Treatment modalities among patients with lipodystrophy was not a scope of this study; however if these patients were adequately treated their perceptions against lipodystrophy could improve their quality of life. Deliberately sought efforts are needed to incorporate management of lipodystrophy and other long-term complications of HAART in Tanzania in the era of test and treat for improved adherence and overall improved patient care.

## Conflicts of Interest

The authors declare that there are no conflicts of interest regarding publication of this article.

## Acknowledgments

The authors acknowledge the contribution of the staff of the CTC of the municipal hospitals and patients who participated in the study.

## References

[1] UNAIDS, "Fact sheet," 2016, http://www.unaids.org/sites/default/files/media_asset/20150901_FactSheet_2015_en.pdf.

[2] T. B. Hallett, J. Stover, V. Mishra, P. D. Ghys, S. Gregson, and T. Boerma, "Estimates of HIV incidence from household-based prevalence surveys," *AIDS*, vol. 24, no. 1, pp. 147–152, 2010.

[3] TACAIDS, *Ministry of Health and Social Welfare: Tanzania HIV/AIDS and Malaria Indicator Survey, 2011/2012*, TACAIDS, Dar es Salaam, Tanzania, 2012.

[4] G. Greub, B. Ledergerber, M. Battegay et al., "Clinical progression, survival, and immune recovery during antiretroviral therapy in patients with HIV-1 and hepatitis C virus coinfection: the swiss HIV cohort study," *The Lancet*, vol. 356, no. 9244, pp. 1800–1805, 2000.

[5] H. Streeck, H. Jessen, G. Alter et al., "Immunological and virological impact of highly active antiretroviral therapy initiated during acute HIV-1 infection," *Journal of Infectious Diseases*, vol. 194, no. 6, pp. 734–739, 2006.

[6] V. D. Lima, L. Lourenço, B. Yip, R. S. Hogg, P. Phillips, and J. S. G. Montaner, "AIDS incidence and AIDS-related mortality in British Columbia, Canada, between 1981 and 2013: a retrospective study," *The Lancet HIV*, vol. 2, no. 3, pp. 92–97, 2015.

[7] M. Farahani, A. Vable, R. Lebelonyane et al., "Outcomes of the Botswana national HIV/AIDS treatment programme from 2002 to 2010: a longitudinal analysis," *The Lancet Global Health*, vol. 2, no. 1, pp. e44–e50, 2014.

[8] NACP, *National guideline for the management of HIV and AIDS*, NACP. The United Republic of Tanzania, Ministry of Health and Social Welfare, Dar es Salaam, Tanzania, 4th edition, 2012.

[9] NACP, *National guideline for the management of HIV and AIDS*, NACP. The United Republic of Tanzania, Ministry of Health and Social Welfare, Dar es Salaam, Tanzania, 5th edition, 2015.

[10] K. A. Van Galen, J. F. Nellen, and P. T. Nieuwkerk, "The effect on treatment adherence of administering drugs as fixed-dose combinations versus as separate pills: systematic review and meta-analysis," *AIDS Research and Treatment*, vol. 2014, Article ID 967073, pp. 1–6, 2014.

[11] A. Buscher, C. Hartman, M. A. Kallen, and T. P. Giordano, "Impact of antiretroviral dosing frequency and pill burden on adherence among newly diagnosed, antiretroviral-naïve HIV patients," *International Journal of STD and AIDS*, vol. 23, no. 5, pp. 351–355, 2012.

[12] S. M. Hammer, J. J. Eron Jr., P. Reiss et al., "Antiretroviral treatment of adult HIV infection: 2008 recommendations of the international AIDS society-USA panel," *Journal of the American Medical Association*, vol. 300, no. 5, pp. 555–570, 2008.

[13] A. J. White, "Mitochondrial toxicity and HIV therapy," *Sexually Transmitted Infections*, vol. 77, no. 3, pp. 158–173, 2001.

[14] M. J. Feinstein, M. Bogorodskaya, G. S. Bloomfield et al., "Cardiovascular complications of HIV in endemic countries," *Current Cardiology Reports*, vol. 18, no. 11, article 113, 2016.

[15] S. Subramanian, A. Tawakol, T. H. Burdo et al., "Arterial inflammation in patients with HIV," *Journal of the American Medical Association*, vol. 308, no. 4, pp. 379–386, 2012.

[16] A. Carr, S. Emery, M. Law et al., "An objective case definition of lipodystrophy in HIV-infected adults: a case-control study," *The Lancet*, vol. 361, no. 9359, pp. 726–735, 2003.

[17] A. Carr, J. Miller, M. Law, and D. A. Cooper, "A syndrome of lipoatrophy, lactic acidaemia and liver dysfunction associated with HIV nucleoside analogue therapy: contribution to protease inhibitor-related lipodystrophy syndrome," *AIDS*, vol. 14, no. 3, pp. F25–F32, 2000.

[18] A. Carr, "HIV protease inhibitor-related lipodystrophy syndrome," *Clinical Infectious Diseases*, vol. 30, no. 2, pp. S135–S142, 2000.

[19] G. A. McComsey, D. M. Paulsen, J. T. Lonergan et al., "Improvements in lipoatrophy, mitochondrial DNA levels and fat apoptosis after replacing stavudine with abacavir or zidovudine," *AIDS*, vol. 19, no. 1, pp. 15–23, 2005.

[20] A. Carr, K. Samaras, A. Thorisdottir, G. R. Kaufmann, D. J. Chisholm, and D. A. Cooper, "Diagnosis, prediction, and natural course of HIV-1 protease-inhibitor-associated lipodystrophy, hyperlipidaemia, and diabetes mellitus: a cohort study," *The Lancet*, vol. 353, no. 9170, pp. 2093–2099, 1999.

[21] D. Chen, A. Misra, and A. Garg, "Lipodystrophy in human immunodeficiency virus-infected patients," *Journal of Clinical Endocrinology and Metabolism*, vol. 87, no. 11, pp. 4845–4856, 2002.

[22] J. Blanch, A. Rousaud, E. Martínez et al., "Impact of lipodystrophy on the quality of life of HIV-1-infected patients," *Journal of Acquired Immune Deficiency Syndromes*, vol. 31, no. 4, pp. 404–407, 2002.

[23] C. C. Schag, R. L. Heinrich, and P. A. Ganz, "Karnofsky performance status revisited: reliability, validity, and guidelines," *Journal of Clinical Oncology*, vol. 2, no. 3, pp. 187–193, 1984.

[24] WHO, "Obesity: preventing and managing the global epidemic. Report of a WHO consultation," World Health Organization Technical Report Series 894:i–xii, World Health Organization, 2000.

[25] K. A. Lichtenstein, D. J. Ward, A. C. Moorman et al., "Clinical assessment of HIV-associated lipodystrophy in an ambulatory population," *AIDS*, vol. 15, no. 11, pp. 1389–1398, 2001.

[26] J. Miller, A. Carr, S. Emery et al., "HIV lipodystrophy: prevalence, severity and correlates of risk in Australia," *HIV Medicine*, vol. 4, no. 3, pp. 293–301, 2003.

[27] M. Ortu, P. Bonfanti, E. Gabrielli, L. Carenzi, R. Gulizia, G. Ferraioli et al., "Ultrasound and lipoatrophy diagnosis: experience on 295 HIV-positive outpatients in antiretroviral therapy," *Infection*, vol. 37, p. 26, 2009.

[28] P. Filippini, C. Scolastico, M. Battaglia et al., "Lipodystrophy and serum lipid abnormalities in HIV-positive sub-Saharan population on ART," *Journal of Infection*, vol. 53, no. 1, pp. e29–e33, 2006.

[29] J. van Griensven, R. Zachariah, J. Mugabo, and T. Reid, "Weight loss after the first year of stavudine-containing antiretroviral therapy and its association with lipoatrophy, virological failure, adherence and CD4 counts at primary health care level in Kigali, Rwanda," *Transactions of the Royal Society of Tropical Medicine and Hygiene*, vol. 104, no. 12, pp. 751–757, 2010.

[30] S. Mercier, N. F. N. Gueye, A. Cournil et al., "Lipodystrophy and metabolic disorders in HIV-1-infected adults on 4- to 9-year antiretroviral therapy in senegal: a case-control study," *Journal of Acquired Immune Deficiency Syndromes*, vol. 51, no. 2, pp. 224–230, 2009.

[31] M. Galli, F. Veglia, G. Angarano et al., "Gender differences in antiretroviral drug-related adipose tissue alterations: women are at higher risk than men and develop particular lipodystrophy patterns," *Journal of Acquired Immune Deficiency Syndromes*, vol. 34, no. 1, pp. 58–61, 2003.

[32] N. Andany, J. M. Raboud, S. Walmsley et al., "Ethnicity and gender differences in lipodystrophy of HIV-positive individuals taking antiretroviral therapy in Ontario, Canada," *HIV Clinical Trials*, vol. 12, no. 2, pp. 89–103, 2011.

[33] E. Sobngwi, J.-C. N. Mbanya, N. C. Unwin et al., "Physical activity and its relationship with obesity, hypertension and diabetes in urban and rural Cameroon," *International Journal of Obesity*, vol. 26, no. 7, pp. 1009–1016, 2002.

[34] P. Bovet, A. G. Ross, J.-P. Gervasoni et al., "Distribution of blood pressure, body mass index and smoking habits in the urban population of Dar es Salaam, Tanzania, and associations with socioeconomic status," *International Journal of Epidemiology*, vol. 31, no. 1, pp. 240–247, 2002.

[35] P. W. G. Mallon, J. Miller, D. A. Cooper, and A. Carr, "Prospective evaluation of the effects of antiretroviral therapy on body composition in HIV-1-infected men starting therapy," *AIDS*, vol. 17, no. 7, pp. 971–979, 2003.

[36] S. Grinspoon and A. Carr, "Cardiovascular risk and body-fat abnormalities in HIV-infected adults," *The New England Journal of Medicine*, vol. 352, no. 1, pp. 48–62, 2005.

[37] V. Joly, P. Flandre, V. Meiffredy et al., "Increased risk of lipoatrophy under stavudine in HIV-1-infected patients: Results of a substudy from a comparative trial," *AIDS*, vol. 16, no. 18, pp. 2447–2454, 2002.

[38] G. J. Moyle, C. A. Sabin, J. Cartledge et al., "A randomized comparative trial of tenofovir DF or abacavir as replacement for a thymidine analogue in persons with lipoatrophy," *AIDS*, vol. 20, no. 16, pp. 2043–2050, 2006.

[39] H. M. Crane, C. Grunfeld, R. D. Harrington, K. K. Uldall, P. S. Ciechanowski, and M. M. Kitahata, "Lipoatrophy among HIV-infected patients is associated with higher levels of depression than lipohypertrophy," *HIV Medicine*, vol. 9, no. 9, pp. 780–786, 2008.

[40] E. Collins, C. Wagner, and S. Walmsley, "Psychosocial impact of the Lipodystrophy syndrome in HIV infection," *AIDS Reader*, vol. 10, no. 9, pp. 546–550, 2000.

[41] R. Power, H. L. Tate, S. M. McGill, and C. Taylor, "A qualitative study of the psychosocial implications of lipodystrophy syndrome on HIV positive individuals," *Sexually Transmitted Infections*, vol. 79, no. 2, pp. 137–141, 2003.

[42] J. Steel, D. Landsittel, B. Calhoun, S. Wieand, and L. A. Kingsley, "Effects of lipodystrophy on quality of life and depression in HIV-infected men on HAART," *AIDS Patient Care and STDs*, vol. 20, no. 8, pp. 565–575, 2006.

[43] E. Hurley, A. Coutsoudis, J. Giddy, S. E. Knight, E. Loots, and T. M. Esterhuizen, "Weight evolution and perceptions of adults living with HIV following initiation of antiretroviral therapy in a South African urban setting," *South African Medical Journal*, vol. 101, no. 9, pp. 645–650, 2011.

[44] N. I. Paton, A. Earnest, Y. M. Ng, F. Karim, and J. Aboulhab, "Lipodystrophy in a cohort of human immunodeficiency virus-infected asian patients: prevalence, associated factors, and psychological impact," *Clinical Infectious Diseases*, vol. 35, no. 10, pp. 1244–1249, 2002.

[45] M. Tungsiripat, M. A. O'Riordan, N. Storer et al., "Subjective clinical lipoatrophy assessment correlates with DEXA-measured limb fat," *HIV Clinical Trials*, vol. 10, no. 5, pp. 314–319, 2009.

# 24

# Early Diagnosis of HIV among Infants Born to HIV-Positive Mothers on Option-B Plus in Kampala, Uganda

**Jonathan Izudi,[1,2] Sylvia Auma,[1] and John Bosco Alege[1]**

[1]*Department of Community Health, Faculty of Medicine, Mbarara University of Science and Technology, Mbarara, Uganda*
[2]*Institute of Public Health and Management, International Health Sciences University, Kampala, Uganda*

Correspondence should be addressed to Jonathan Izudi; jonahzd@gmail.com

Academic Editor: Robert R. Redfield

*Introduction.* Globally, there is delay in accessing early HIV diagnosis (EID) among HIV exposed infants (HEIs). With paucity of data on EID use at Kisenyi Health Center, this study assessed factors associated with EID use among HEIs (HIV exposed infants). *Method.* This was a cross-sectional study of 246 HIV-positive mother-baby pairs. Data was collected by structured questionnaire, double-entered in EpiData, and analyzed with STATA using multinomial logistic regression at 5% significance level. *Results.* 132 (53.7%) HEIs were not tested, 60 (24.4%) tested outside EID guideline, and 54 (21.9%) tested per the guideline. Testing per guideline was associated with maternal age above 30 years (AOR = 2.75; 95% CI: 1.20–6.34; $P = 0.017$); testing outside the guideline was associated with maternal HIV serostatus disclosure (AOR = 2.70; 95% CI: 1.10–6.63; $P = 0.003$) and four or more antenatal care (ANC) visits (AOR = 3.25; 95% CI: 1.23–8.59; $P = 0.017$). However, maternal knowledge of HIV transmission was associated with testing outside the guideline (AOR = 2.90; 95% CI: 1.10–7.65; $P = 0.032$) and per the guideline (AOR = 3.70; 95% CI: 1.39–9.88; $P = 0.009$). *Conclusion.* Timely EID testing was low. Improving maternal knowledge of EID during ANC visits and positive living empowerment is critical.

## 1. Background

Without timely access to ART (antiretroviral therapy), 20% of HIV- (Human Immunodeficiency Virus-) positive infants will die before 6 months [1], 35–40% will die before 1 year [1, 2], and over 50% will die by 2 years [3]. Early diagnosis of HIV (EID) is hence fundamental in early identification of HIV-positive infants and subsequent ART initiation. However, timely receipt of EID remains a challenge in most countries despite a 10-fold increase and improved access to ART between 2005 and 2015 [4]. In addition, the proportion of HEIs with timely access to EID varies between 30% and 90% in many countries [4]. In sub-Saharan Africa, about 75% of HEIs have delayed access to EID services resulting into substantial mortality [5]. With delayed access to EID, current progress towards zero new HIV infections and starting 90% or more HIV-positive infants on ART might be reversed [6]. EID thus facilitates timely access to ART and in so doing, it optimize viral load suppression, reduce HIV related morbidity and mortality, and improve the overall quality of life of HIV-positive children. Evidence indicates that timely initiation of ART reduces the risk of infant mortality by 76% within the first 3 months of life [7, 8] and the progression to AIDS (Acquired Immunodeficiency Syndrome), an advanced stage of HIV infection, by three quarters [8].

In June 2012, Uganda's Ministry of Health adopted Option-B plus, a strategy of starting all HIV-positive pregnant and lactating mothers on ART irrespective of their clinical and immunological stage in order to eliminate mother to child transmission of HIV (EMTCT) [9].

Via a provider initiated HIV testing and counseling (PITC), all pregnant mothers receive HIV testing during antenatal care (ANC) visits, labor, and delivery.

However, postpartum mothers receive HIV testing during postnatal-care visits. When found HIV-positive, pregnant and lactating mothers are started on ART and cotrimoxazole prophylaxis, and the viral load is monitored for response to ART [9]. From birth to 18 months, HEIs undergo routine EID care. At birth, nevirapine syrup is introduced but the dose is adjusted according to weight and age bands until 6 weeks.

At 6 weeks, nevirapine syrup is stopped, the first HIV test using Deoxyribonucleic Acid-Polymerase Chain Reaction (DNA-PCR) is performed, and cotrimoxazole prophylaxis is introduced (also adjusted according to age and weight bands) until 18 months. Exactly 6 weeks after breastfeeding cessation, the second DNA-PCR test is performed and at 18 months, a final HIV antibody test is done. Should a HEI test HIV-positive at any time point, ART is initiated alongside cotrimoxazole prophylaxis. Regarding breastfeeding, HEIs exclusively breastfeed for the first 6 months before commencing complementary feeding, and breastfeeding ceases at 1 year [6, 10]. Despite these recommendations, merely two in every five HEIs access EID by DNA-PCR tests within two months of birth (first DNA-PCR) in Uganda [11].

At Kisenyi HC (Health Center) IV, routine data indicates that a substantial number of HEIs do not receive EID by DNA-PCR test at 6 weeks. First, this presents a missed opportunity for early HIV diagnosis and ART initiation. Second, the absence of information on factors associated with receipt of DNA-PCR to inform EID programming is a big hindrance to improving EID services. In this study, we investigated factors associated with use of EID among HEIs receiving care at Kisenyi HCIV in Kampala district, Uganda.

## 2. Method

This study was conducted at Kisenyi HCIV, one of the two health facilities in Kampala Central Division, Kampala district. Kisenyi is a slum setting in the middle of down town Kampala where a mix of numerous languages in Uganda, Eastern Congo, Tanzania, Rwanda, Kenya, Somalia, and Ethiopia are spoken [12]. The study setting, Kisenyi HCIV, lies in Central Kampala along Mwanga II Road. The health facility is managed by Kampala Capital City Authority (KCCA), a new administrative body assigned with the role of managing health services delivery in Kampala City. The authority controls five divisions of Kampala Central, Nakawa, Lubaga, Makindye, and Kawempe. Each division has two health centers apart from Nakawa. In total, there are nine health centers and two hospitals [13]. According to the Uganda Bureau of Statistics 2014 data, there are 1,516,210 persons in Kampala district [14].

We used an analytical cross-sectional design to describe and analyze factors associated with use of EID among HEIs. The respondents were HIV-positive postpartum mothers or caregivers of HEIs in the EID program of Kisenyi HCIV, selected purposively. Using Kish and Leslie's formula [15], 246 respondents within 95% confidence limit, 5% precision, and 20% estimated proportion of EID use at 6 weeks were sampled and interviewed. Since we aimed to collect data over a 20-day period, first, the sample size was divided by the total number of days for data collection to get the average number of respondents to interview per day. We then used systematic sampling to establish a sampling interval by dividing the total number of expected HIV-positive mothers or caregivers on a particular clinic day by the total number of respondents required for daily interviews.

From the sampling interval, a convenience sampling method was employed to select respondents at a time until the total sample size was reached.

Prior to data collection, all data collection tools were forward and backward translated and pretested outside the study area. The data was collected by trained and supervised Research Assistants using a structured questionnaire administered by face to face interviews between December 2016 and April 2017. All interviews were conducted in a quiet room within the mother-baby care point, a clinic within the EID program where HIV-positive mothers/caregivers and HEIs are paired and followed until 18 months. Interviews were conducted from Monday to Friday between 8.30 a.m. and 12.00 p.m. All completed questionnaires were reviewed in real time for completeness and accuracy by a research team leader.

Data was collected on use of EID, maternal, and health systems-related factors. Maternal age and employment status, level of education, knowledge on HIV transmission and prevention during pregnancy, labor and delivery, distance to the nearest health facility to access EID services, ever receiving health education on HIV transmission, and knowledge of DNA-PCR test frequency and timing were variables on which data was collected. Data on use of EID was verified using EID clinical charts and registers.

Collected data was double-entered in EpiData version 3.1 (EpiData Association, Odense, Denmark) [16], checked for data quality, and exported to STATA Version 12 (StataCorp, College Station, TX, USA) for univariate, bivariate, and multivariate analysis at 5% significance level. Frequencies and percentages were calculated for categorical variables and measures of central tendency for continuous variables.

The dependent variable, EID use, was defined by three outcomes: HEIs not tested by DNA-PCR, HEIs tested by DNA-PCR outside EID guideline (early and late), and HEIs tested by DNA-PCR per EID guideline (between 6 and 8 weeks). DNA-PCR test performed before 6 weeks was considered early and that performed after 8 weeks was regarded late. The denominator was the sample size.

Tests of associations were performed using the Chi-squared test for large cell counts (when the cross-tabulations had all cell counts equal or above five) or the Fisher's exact test (when the cross-tabulations had any cell count less than five) for categorical independent variables and the $F$-test for continuous variables. Test of collinearity between variables was performed, and variables with variance inflation factor (VIF) greater than ten were excluded in the final model. Since the outcome variable was nominal, a multinomial logistic regression analysis was performed to determine factors independently associated with use of EID, with HEIs not tested by DNA-PCR being the reference category. The output of multinomial logistic regression analysis was stated in odds ratios with corresponding 95% confidence intervals (CI) and probability values ($P$ values).

This study was approved by the Research Ethics Committee of International Health Sciences University and the Health Department of Kampala Capital City Authority (KCCA). All respondents gave a written or thumb printed informed consent before participation.

TABLE 1: Sociodemographic characteristics of respondents and use of EID.

| | HEIs not tested by DNA-PCR | HEIs tested by DNA-PCR outside EID guideline | HEIs tested by DNA-PCR per EID guideline | Total | *P* value |
|---|---|---|---|---|---|
| Overall | 132 (53.7%) | 60 (24.4%) | 54 (21.9%) | 246 (100.0%) | |
| Maternal age (years) | | | | | <0.0001 |
| Less than 30 years | 103 (63.2) | 34 (20.9) | 26 (16.0) | 163 | |
| More than 30 years | 29 (34.9) | 26 (31.3) | 18 (33.7) | 83 | |
| Mean ± SD | 25.5 ± 6.12 | 29.3 ± 5.35 | 29.7 ± 5.69 | 246 | 0.0003 |
| Maternal education | | | | | <0.001 |
| None | 31 (72.1) | 9 (20.9) | 3 (7.0) | 43 | |
| Primary | 44 (80.0) | 6 (10.9) | 5 (9.1) | 55 | |
| Secondary and over | 57 (38.5) | 45 (30.4) | 46 (31.1) | 148 | |
| Marital status | | | | | 0.008 |
| Single | 101 (60.5) | 35 (21.0) | 31 (18.6) | 67 | |
| Married | 31 (39.2) | 25 (31.7) | 23 (29.1) | 79 | |
| Form of employment | | | | | <0.001 |
| None | 81 (70.4) | 20 (17.4) | 14 (12.2) | 115 | |
| Formal | 2 (7.7) | 13 (50.0) | 11 (42.3) | 26 | |
| self | 49 (46.7) | 27 (25.7) | 29 (27.6) | 105 | |
| Mother knows that HIV is transmissible during pregnancy, labor and delivery, and breastfeeding | | | | | <0.001 |
| No | 118 (68.2) | 31 (17.9) | 24 (13.9) | 173 | |
| Yes | 14 (19.2) | 29 (39.7) | 30 (41.1) | 73 | |
| Mother knows the correct frequency and timing of all HIV testing in HEIs | | | | | <0.001 |
| No | 123 (61.8) | 41 (20.6) | 35 (17.6) | 199 | |
| Yes | 9 (19.2) | 19 (40.4) | 19 (40.4) | 47 | |
| Disclosed HIV status | | | | | <0.001 |
| No | 116 (64.1) | 32 (17.7) | 33 (18.2) | 181 | |
| Yes | 16 (24.6) | 28 (43.1) | 21 (32.3) | 65 | |
| Number of ANC visits | | | | | <0.001 |
| Less than four | 85 (63.0) | 25 (18.5) | 25 (18.5) | 135 | |
| Four or more | 14 (18.7) | 33 (44.0) | 28 (37.3) | 75 | |
| Place of delivery | | | | | 0.002 |
| Outside health facility | 61 (68.5) | 14 (15.7) | 14 (15.7) | 89 | |
| In a health facility | 71 (45.2) | 46 (29.3) | 40 (25.5) | 157 | |

## 3. Results

*3.1. Sociodemographic Characteristics of Respondents and Use of EID.* The mean age of mothers with HEIs not tested for HIV by DNA-PCR was 25.5±6.12 years, that for mothers with HEIs tested outside the EID guideline was 29.3 ± 5.35 years, and that for mothers with HEIs tested per the EID guideline was 29.69 ± 5.69 years ($P < 0.0001$).

Among 163 mothers below the age of 30 years, 103 (63.2%) HEIs were not tested by DNA-PCR, 34 (20.9%) were tested outside the EID guideline, and 26 (16.0%) were tested according to the guideline. In contrast, among 83 mothers above 30 years of age, 29 (34.9%) HEIs were never tested, 26 (31.3%) were tested outside the guideline, and only 18 (33.7%) were tested per the guideline ($P < 0.001$) (Table 1).

Of 43 mothers without formal education, 31 (72.1%) HEIs were not tested, nine (20.9%) were tested outside the EID guideline, and merely three (7.0%) were tested per the guideline. Compared to 55 mothers that completed primary education, the corresponding numbers were 44 (80.0%), six (10.9%), and five (9.1%). Similarly, of 146 mothers that completed secondary education and beyond, the respective figures were 57 (38.5%), 45 (30.4%), and 46 (31.1%) ($P < 0.001$).

Regarding marital status of the mothers, 167 (67.9%) were single/unmarried while 79 (32.1%) were married. Among single/unmarried mothers, 101 (60.5%) HEIs were not tested,

35 (21.0%) were tested outside the EID guideline, and 31 (18.6%) were tested per the guideline. For married mothers, the respective figures were 31 (39.2%), 25 (31.7%), and 23 (29.1%) ($P = 0.008$).

In terms of employment, 115 (46.7%) of the mothers were unemployed, 26 (10.6%) had formal employment, and 105 (42.7%) were self-employed. Among unemployed mothers, only 14 (12.2%) HEIs were tested per the EID guideline, 20 (17.4%) were tested outside the guideline, and 81 (70.4%) were not tested. For mothers with formal employment, only two (7.7%) HEIs were not tested, 13 (50.0%) were tested outside the EID guideline, and 11 (42.3%) were tested per the guideline. Among self-employed mothers, 49 (46.7%) HEIs were not tested, 27 (25.7%) were tested outside the EID guideline, and only 29 (27.6%) were tested per the guideline ($P < 0.001$).

118 (68.2%) HEIs were not tested, 31 (17.9%) were tested outside EID guideline, and 24 (13.9%) were tested per the guideline among 173 mothers that had no knowledge of HIV transmission during pregnancy, labor and delivery, and breastfeeding. The equivalent proportion among 73 mothers with this knowledge was 14 (19.2%), 29 (39.7%), and 30 (41.1%), respectively ($P < 0.001$).

Of 199 mothers without knowledge of the correct number of times and schedules for EID testing, 123 (61.8%) HEIs were not tested, 41 (20.6%) were tested outside EID guideline, and 35 (17.6%) were tested per the guideline. Likewise, of 47 mothers with the knowledge, nine (19.2%) HEIs were not tested, 19 (40.4%) were tested outside the guideline, and another 19 (40.4%) were tested per the guideline ($P < 0.001$).

Of 118 mothers with undisclosed HIV serostatus (to a spouse, relative, friend, or significant others), 116 (64.1%) HEIs were not tested, 32 (17.7%) were tested outside the EID guideline, and 35 (17.6%) were tested per the guideline. Conversely, among 65 mothers with disclosed HIV serostatus, the proportion of testing was 16 (24.6%), 28 (43.1%), and 21 (32.3%), respectively ($P < 0.001$).

Among 135 mothers that attended less than four ANC visits during the recent pregnancy, 85 (63.0%) HEIs were not tested, 25 (18.5%) were tested outside the EID guideline, and another 25 (18.5%) were tested per the guideline. On the other hand, among 65 mothers that attended equal or more than four ANC visits, 14 (18.7%) HEIs were not tested, 33 (44.0%) were tested outside the EID guideline, and 21 (32.3%) were tested according to the guideline ($P < 0.001$).

Concerning place of delivery, among 89 mothers that did not deliver in a health facility (hospital, health center, or a health post), 61 (68.5%) HEIs were not tested, 14 (15.7%) were tested outside the EID guideline, and another 14 (15.7%) were tested per the guideline.

Similarly, of 157 mothers that delivered in a health facility, 71 (45.2%) HEIs were not tested, 46 (29.3%) were tested outside the EID guideline, and 40 (25.5%) were tested per the guideline ($P = 0.002$).

Overall, 132 (53.7%; 95% CI: 47.2–60.0) HEIs were not tested for HIV using DNA-PCR (thus EID), 60 (24.4%; 95% CI: 19.1–30.2) were tested outside the EID guideline (early and late), and 54 (21.9%; 95% CI: 16.9–27.6) were tested per the guideline (Table 1).

*3.2. Factors Associated with Testing of HEIs Outside EID Guideline Compared to Not Testing.* In multinomial unadjusted logistic regression (Table 2), testing outside EID guideline relative to no testing increased with maternal age above 30 years (UOR = 2.72; 95% CI: 1.41–5.23; $P = 0.003$), completion of primary (UOR = 0.49; 95% CI: 0.15–1.45; 0.19) and secondary (UOR = 2.72; 95% CI: 1.18–6.29; $P = 0.019$) education, being married (UOR = 2.32; 95% CI: 1.21–4.47; $P = 0.011$), and formal (UOR = 26.32; 95% CI: 5.49–26.16; $P < 0.001$) and self-employment (UOR = 2.23; 95% CI: 1.13–4.40; $P = 0.02$), maternal knowledge of HIV transmission during pregnancy, labor, and delivery, and breastfeeding (UOR = 7.88; 95% CI: 3.72–16.70; $P < 0.001$), maternal knowledge of the correct number of times and schedules of EID (UOR = 6.33; 95% CI: 6.33–15.09; $P < 0.001$), HIV serostatus disclosure (UOR = 6.34; 95% CI: 3.06–13.14; $P < 0.001$), previous attendance of four or more ANC visits (UOR = 8.01; 95% CI: 3.72–17.27; $P < 0.001$), and delivery of the HEI in a health facility: hospital, health center, or health post (UOR = 2.82; 95% CI: 1.42–5.62; $P = 0.003$).

However, it reduced by 47% with more than five-kilometer radius to the health facility (UOR = 0.53; 95% CI: 0.29–0.99; $P = 0.049$) and by 48% with equal or more than 1-hour travel time to reach the health facility on foot (UOR = 0.52; 95% CI: 0.27–0.99; $P = 0.048$).

*3.3. Factors Associated with Testing of HEIs per EID Guideline Compared to No Testing.* In unadjusted multinomial logistic regression analysis (Table 2), DNA-PCR testing per EID guideline relative to no testing increased with maternal age above 30 years (UOR = 3.82; 95% CI: 1.95–7.51; $P < 0.001$), completion of primary (UOR = 1.17; 95% CI: 0.26–5.28; $P = 0.834$) and secondary (UOR = 8.34; 95% CI: 2.34–29.0; $P = 0.001$) education, being married (UOR = 2.42; 95% CI: 1.23–4.74; $P = 0.001$), formal (UOR = 31.82; 95% CI: 6.36–59.18; $P < 0.001$) and self-employment (UOR = 3.42; 95% CI: 1.65–7.10; $P = 0.001$), knowledge of HIV transmission during pregnancy, labor, and delivery (UOR = 10.53; 95% CI: 4.87–22.79; $P < 0.001$), knowledge of the correct number of times and schedules of EID (UOR = 7.42; 95% CI: 3.09–17.84; $P < 0.001$), HIV serostatus disclosure (UOR = 4.61; 95% CI: 2.16–9.83; $P < 0.001$), attendance of equal or more than four ANC visits during recent pregnancy (UOR = 6.80; 95% CI: 3.11–14.85; $P < 0.001$), and delivery of the HEI in a health facility (UOR = 2.54; 95% CI: 1.22–4.93; $P = 0.012$).

Conversely, it decreased by 57% with more than five-kilometer radius distance to the health facility (UOR = 0.43; 95% CI: 0.22–0.82; $P = 0.011$) and by 74% with more than 1-hour travel time to the health facility on foot (UOR = 0.26; 95% CI: 0.13–0.50; $P < 0.001$).

However, two variables in this study, maternal education with VIF of 11.0 and place of delivery of the HEI with VIF of 13.53, were found to be collinear with other variables (see Supplementary Material S1 in Supplementary Material available online at https://doi.org/10.1155/2017/4654763). Consequently, they were excluded from the adjusted analysis.

Table 2: Factors associated with use of EID among HEIs, Kisenyi HC IV, Kampala, Uganda.

| Characteristics | Unadjusted multinomial logistic regression analysis | | | | Adjusted multinomial logistic regression analysis | | | |
|---|---|---|---|---|---|---|---|---|
| | HEI tested by DNA-PCR outside EID guideline versus HEI not tested UOR (95% CI) | *P* value | HEI tested by DNA-PCR per EID guideline versus HEI not tested UOR (95% CI) | *P* value | HEI tested by DNA-PCR outside EID guideline versus HEI not tested AOR (95% CI) | *P* value | HEI tested by DNA-PCR per EID guideline versus HEI not tested AOR (95% CI) | *P* value |
| Maternal age | | | | | | | | |
| ≤30 years | 1 | | 1 | | 1 | | 1 | |
| >30 years | 2.72 (1.41–5.23) | 0.003 | 3.82 (1.95–7.51) | <0.001 | 1.97 (0.87–4.49) | 0.106 | 2.75 (1.20–6.34) | **0.017** |
| Marital status | | | | | | | | |
| Single | 1 | | 1 | | 1 | | 1 | |
| Married | 2.32 (1.21–4.47) | 0.011 | 2.42 (1.23–4.74) | 0.01 | 1.28 (0.55–2.98) | 0.57 | 1.35 (0.57–3.15) | 0.494 |
| Form of employment | | | | | | | | |
| None | 1 | | 1 | | 1 | | 1 | |
| Formal | 26.32 (5.49–26.16) | <0.001 | 31.82 (6.36–9.18) | <0.001 | 7.54 (0.77–5.89) | 0.082 | 7.68 (0.75–8.99) | 0.086 |
| self | 2.23 (1.13–4.40) | 0.02 | 3.42 (1.65–7.10) | 0.001 | 1.19 (0.5–2.77) | 0.691 | 1.67 (0.68–4.08) | 0.265 |
| Mother knows HIV is transmissible at pregnancy, labor and delivery, and breastfeeding | | | | | | | | |
| No | 1 | | 1 | | 1 | | 1 | |
| Yes | 7.88 (3.72–16.70) | <0.001 | 10.53 (4.87–22.79) | <0.001 | 2.90 (1.10–7.65) | **0.032** | 3.70 (1.39–9.88) | **0.009** |
| Mother knows the correct frequency and timing of EID | | | | | | | | |
| No | 1 | | 1 | | 1 | | 1 | |
| Yes | 6.33 (2.66–15.09) | <0.001 | 7.42 (3.09–17.84) | <0.001 | 1.12 (0.36–3.54) | 0.846 | 1.61 (0.50–5.15) | 0.425 |
| Disclosed HIV serostatus | | | | | | | | |
| No | 1 | | 1 | | 1 | | 1 | |
| Yes | 6.34 (3.06–13.14) | <0.001 | 4.61 (2.16–9.83) | <0.001 | 2.70 (1.10–6.63) | **0.030** | 1.60 (0.62–4.41) | 0.332 |
| ANC visits | | | | | | | | |
| <4 visits | 1 | | 1 | | 1 | | 1 | |
| ≥4 visits | 8.01 (3.72–17.27) | <0.001 | 6.80 (3.11–14.85) | <0.001 | 3.25 (1.23–8.59) | **0.017** | 2.45 (0.88–6.81) | 0.086 |
| Distance to the health facility | | | | | | | | |
| ≤5 | 1 | | 1 | | 1 | | 1 | |
| >5 | 0.53 (0.29–0.99) | 0.049 | 0.43 (0.22–0.82) | 0.011 | 0.87 (0.26–2.95) | 0.825 | 1.81 (0.45–7.28) | 0.400 |
| Time to health facility | | | | | | | | |
| <1 hour | 1 | | 1 | | 1 | | 1 | |
| ≥1 hour | 0.52 (0.27–0.99) | 0.048 | 0.26 (0.13–0.50) | <0.001 | 1.15 (0.33–3.98) | 0.829 | 0.35 (0.09–1.42) | 0.142 |

*Note.* AOR: adjusted odds ratio; $P < 5\%$ considered statistically significant; UOR: unadjusted odds ratio; variables with significant correlation with other variables (VIF > 10) were excluded.

*3.4. Adjusted Analysis of Factors Independently Associated with Testing of HEIs.* In adjusted multinomial logistic regression analysis (Table 2), testing of HEIs outside EID guideline relative to no testing increased with maternal knowledge of HIV transmission during pregnancy, labor or delivery, and breastfeeding (AOR = 2.90; 95% CI: 1.10–7.65; $P = 0.032$), HIV serostatus disclosure to a spouse, relative or friend or significant others (AOR = 2.70; 95% CI: 1.10–6.63; $P = 0.030$), and four or more ANC visits in the last pregnancy (AOR = 3.25; 95% CI: 1.23–8.59; $P = 0.017$).

In contrast, testing of HEIs per EID guideline relative to no testing increased with maternal age above 30 years (AOR = 2.75; 95% CI: 1.20–6.34; $P = 0.017$) and with maternal knowledge of HIV transmission during pregnancy, labor or delivery, and breastfeeding (AOR = 3.70; 95% CI: 1.39–9.88; $P = 0.009$).

## 4. Discussion

This study investigated the level and factors associated with use of EID among HEIs at Kisenyi HCIV in Kampala district, Uganda. We found slightly more than half of the HEIs were not tested for HIV by DNA-PCR, almost a quarter were tested outside the EID guideline (early and late), and merely 21.9% were tested per the guideline. The proportion of HEIs that received EID by 2 months of age was lower than the standard recommendation of 100% [9] and far below 50% EID use by 8 weeks in 2014 [17]. Evidence from systematic review of 44 studies from 15 countries in sub-Saharan Africa showed that between 48 and 81% of HEIs receive EID within 2 months [18], a result not comparable to level of EID use in the present study. Without timely use of EID, the opportunity for early HIV diagnosis and ART initiation are missed out. It appears timely access to EID is a problem in most sub-Saharan countries. Evidence from a multicenter cohort study in Ethiopia found only 41% of HEIs had EID at 6 weeks and the median age at the time of the testing was 60 days [19]. In Kenya, 43% of HEIs that dropped out of the EID program within 2 months of enrolment never received EID [5], an indication that use of EID reduces with increased dropout rates.

Our study found testing of HEIs by DNA-PCR per EID guideline relative to no testing increased with maternal age above 30 years compared to below 30 years. Earlier in a Kenyan study, young mothers had increased dropout rate of HEIs from the EID program [5]. Differential dropout rates may thus account for EID use. Consistent with our results, an increase in use of maternal health services was reported with increase in maternal age in Nigeria [20].

However, the present finding is contrary to an earlier study that found high use of prevention of MTCT of HIV services among mothers aged 20–30 years that attended antenatal care at Kisenyi and Naguru Health Centers [21].

A probable explanation for the differences in use of EID services between younger and older mothers can be attributed to HIV care experiences developed over time. Mostly, young HIV-positive mothers have poor understanding of HIV transmission and prevention methods compared to older HIV-positive mothers because of their shorter stay in HIV care, treatment, and support programs. Irrespective of maternal age differences in using EID services, all mothers/caregivers of HEIs must be supported by healthcare providers to complete the 18-month follow-up of HEIs [9].

We found maternal knowledge of HIV transmission (during pregnancy, labor or delivery, and breastfeeding) was associated with increased testing of HEIs (per EID guideline and outside the EID guideline). This result highlights the importance of health education in increasing maternal knowledge thus empowering mothers to have an effective control over health determinants. Secondly, it underscores the role of health education in increasing use of available health services. In South Africa, inadequacies in knowledge of MTCT of HIV associated with maternal nonreporting for EID services at 6 weeks [22]. Consequently, HEIs missed DNA-PCR tests at required time points. In Northeastern Uganda, health education talks and counseling of mothers/caregivers of HEIs on the importance of EID significantly improved the use of EID at 6 weeks [23], probably because of enhanced maternal knowledge over determinants of health.

Our result emphasize the importance of maternal knowledge of HIV transmission during pregnancy, labor or delivery, and breastfeeding as a critical catalyst for EID services utilization. In improving utilization of EID services and ensuring HIV-free infant survival, health providers facing similar challenges should focus attention on empowering mothers/caregivers of HEIs on understanding the transmission and prevention of MTCT of HIV. Previously at both Kisenyi and Naguru Heath Centers, good counseling of mothers that attended ANC visits increased use of prevention of MTCT of HIV services [21].

Our study further indicates testing of HEIs by DNA-PCR outside EID guideline increased with maternal HIV serostatus disclosure and attendance of four or more ANC visits during the recent pregnancy. This finding indicates and confirms the importance of ANC in enhancing use of maternal, newborn and child health interventions, and the role of HIV serostatus disclosure in chronic HIV care.

First, disclosure of HIV serostatus is critical in accessing existing HIV prevention, care, treatment, and support services and in galvanizing family, spousal, friend, and relative support. This finding hence confirms the importance of HIV serostatus disclosure in general. With some HIV-positive mothers still having undisclosed HIV serostatus, health workers in EID programs should strengthen efforts in helping these mothers in disclosing their HIV serostatus (to someone they can confide in). This will assure them access to emotional, psychological, social, and medical support without hindrance. At enrolment of HIV-positive mothers into HIV care, and during adherence preparation for ART, the benefits of serostatus disclosure are further explained.

In PHDP (Positive Health, Dignity, and Prevention), a set of HIV prevention interventions that aims at keeping people living with HIV physically, mentally, and psychologically healthy, disclosure is a key component.

Second, in Uganda, all pregnant women are required to attend at least four ANC visits during which they receive routine HIV testing with same day results, and those testing HIV-positive are supported to disclosure their serostatus.

During ANC visits, all pregnant women receive health education talks on mode and prevention of mother to child transmission of HIV among others. The factors explained above might have accounted for the increased EID by DNA-PCR testing among HIV-positive mothers with disclosed serostatus [24]. However, it is surprising that attendance of four or more ANC visits did not significantly increase testing of HEIs by DNA-PCR per EID guideline, suggesting the need to continuously support HIV-positive mothers in understanding the number, schedule, and importance of EID. This is because early testing results in most HIV-positive cases being missed because of low sensitivity of DNA-PCR test before 6 weeks. Studies indicate that HIV-DNA PCR assays identify between 20% and 55% of HIV-positivity among HEIs from birth through the first week of life, but this increases to more than 90% by 2–4 weeks of age and to 100% at 3–6 months [25]. So by testing early, there is a risk of missed HIV diagnosis. Contrariwise, late testing results in late HIV diagnosis, late ART initiation, and worsened HIV morbidity and mortality.

## 5. Study Limitation

Although this study underscored critical factors associated with use of EID, the findings should be interpreted while considering certain limitations. First, we did not examine the technical competence of staffs and their availability, health facility waiting times, maternal reason(s) for choice of EID services, interpersonal relations with healthcare providers, and mode of transport among others as factors that might influence EID use. However, our results provide additional evidence for healthcare providers, healthcare managers, researchers, and other public health professionals in improving delivery of EID services in Kampala, Uganda.

## 6. Conclusion

A substantial number of HEIs were not tested by DNA-PCR, many were tested either early or late, and few were tested per EID guideline. Testing of HEIs per EID guideline was associated with maternal age above 30 years; testing outside EID guideline was associated with maternal HIV serostatus disclosure and equal or more than four ANC visits. However, maternal knowledge of HIV transmission (during pregnancy, labor or delivery, and breastfeeding) was associated with testing of HEIs per EID guideline and outside EID guideline.

## 7. Recommendation

In order to increase use of EID, improvement in maternal knowledge of EID is needed particularly on the importance of EID, the frequency, and schedule during ANC visits; the benefits of HIV serostatus disclosure so as to galvanize social, psychological, and medical support from the spouse, relatives, family members, friends, or significant others are needed. This is achievable through health education or routine counseling. In addition, EID programs should recognize maternal age differences as a key factor in use of EID services.

## Abbreviations

ANC: Antenatal care
AOR: Adjusted odds ratio
ART: Antiretroviral therapy
DNA-PCR: Deoxyribonucleic Acid-Polymerase Chain Reaction
EID: Early infant diagnosis of HIV
EPNC: Early postnatal-care
HC: Health center
HEI: HIV exposed infant
HIV: Human immunodeficiency virus
MTCT: Mother to child transmission
PHDP: Positive Health, Dignity, and Prevention
PNC: Postnatal-care
UOR: Unadjusted odds ratio
WHO: World Health Organization.

## Data Access

The data shall not be shared in order to protect participant's anonymity.

## Ethical Approval

This study was approved by the International Health Sciences University Research Ethics Committee and the Kampala Capital City Authority (KCCA) Health Department.

## Consent

All respondents gave informed consent.

## Conflicts of Interest

The authors declare that they have no conflicts of interest.

## Authors' Contributions

Jonathan Izudi performed the data analysis and wrote the draft and final manuscripts. Sylvia Auma conceptualized and designed the study. John Bosco Alege provided technical research guidance. All authors designed the data collection tool and wrote and approved the final manuscript. Jonathan Izudi is the first author.

## Acknowledgments

The Institute of Public Health and Management, International Health Sciences University, to which the authors are affiliated is acknowledged.

## References

[1] A. H. Mirkuzie, S. G. Hinderaker, M. M. Sisay, K. M. Moland, and O. Mørkve, "Current status of medication adherence and infant follow up in the prevention of mother to child HIV transmission programme in Addis Ababa: a cohort study," *Journal of the International AIDS Society*, vol. 14, article 50, 2011.

[2] R. E. Cook, P. J. Ciampa, M. Sidat et al., "Predictors of successful early infant diagnosis of HIV in a rural district hospital in

Zambézia, Mozambique," *Journal of Acquired Immune Deficiency Syndromes*, vol. 56, no. 4, pp. e104–e109, 2011.

[3] M.-L. Newell, H. Coovadia, M. Cortina-Borja, N. Rollins, P. Gaillard, and F. Dabis, "Mortality of infected and uninfected infants born to HIV-infected mothers in Africa: a pooled analysis," *The Lancet*, vol. 364, no. 9441, pp. 1236–1243, 2004.

[4] S. Essajee, R. Bhairavabhotla, M. Penazzato et al., "Scale-up of Early Infant HIV Diagnosis and Improving Access to Pediatric HIV Care in Global Plan Countries," *Journal of Acquired Immune Deficiency Syndromes*, vol. 75, pp. S51–S58, 2017.

[5] A. S. Hassan, E. M. Sakwa, H. M. Nabwera et al., "Dynamics and constraints of early infant diagnosis of HIV infection in rural Kenya," *AIDS and Behavior*, vol. 16, no. 1, pp. 5–12, 2012.

[6] E. T. Katabira, *The Integrated National Guidelines for Antiretroviral Therapy, Prevention of Mother to Child Transmission of HIV and Infant & Young Child Feeding*, vol. 134, Ministry of Health-Uganda, Kampala, Uganda, 2011.

[7] C. Motswere-Chirwa, A. Voetsch, L. Lu et al., "Follow-up of infants diagnosed with HIV-early infant diagnosis program, Francistown, Botswana, 2005–2012," *Morbidity and Mortality Weekly Report (MMWR)*, vol. 63, no. 7, pp. 158–160, 2014.

[8] A. Violari, M. F. Cotton, D. M. Gibb et al., "Early antiretroviral therapy and mortality among HIV-infected infants," *The New England Journal of Medicine*, vol. 359, no. 21, pp. 2233–2244, 2008.

[9] Republic of Uganda, *Consolidated guidelines for prevention and treatment of HIV in Uganda*, vol. 49, Minsitry of Health, Kampala, Uganda, 2016.

[10] E. T. Katabira, *National antiretroviral treatment guidelines for adults, adolescents, and children*, Uganda, Kampala, 2009.

[11] Republic of Uganda, *Uganda HIV/AIDS country progress report*, Ministry of Health, Kampala, Uganda, 2014.

[12] R. Kagumire, *Rosebells Blog "You cannot uneducate the person who has learned to read. You cannot humiliate the person who feels pride. You cannot oppress the people who are not afraid anymore" -Cesar Chavez*, Kampala, Uganda, 2012.

[13] S. Dobson, M. Fricke, and S. Vengal, *This is Kisenyi*, ACTogether Uganda, Kampala, Uganda, 2011, Melissa Fricke, and Sarital Vengal, This is Kisenyi.

[14] Republic of Uganda, *Annual Health Sector Performance Report for Financial Year 2014/2015*, Ministry of Health-Uganda, Kampala, Uganda, 2015.

[15] L. Kish, *Survey sampling*, 1965.

[16] J. Lauritsen and M. Bruus, *A comprehensive tool for validated entry and documentation of data Odense: EpiData Association*, EpiData (version 3), EpiData Association, 2003.

[17] World Health Organization, "What's new in infant diagnosis," *Fact sheet*, vol. 3, p. 4, 2015.

[18] C. Wettstein, C. Mugglin, M. Egger et al., "Missed opportunities to prevent mother-to-child-transmission in sub-Saharan Africa: systematic review and meta-analysis," *AIDS*, vol. 26, no. 18, p. 2361, 2012.

[19] B. Kebede, A. Gebeyehu, S. Jain, S. Sun, and R. Haubrich, "Delay in Early Infant Diagnosis and High Loss to Follow-Up among Infant Born to HIV-Infected Women in Ethiopia," *World Journal of AIDS*, vol. 04, no. 04, pp. 402–412, 2014.

[20] S. Adeoye, L. U. Ogbonnaya, O. U. Umeorah, and O. Asiegbu, "Concurrent use of multiple antenatal care providers by women utilising free antenatal care at Ebonyi State University Teaching Hospital, Abakaliki.," *African Journal of Reproductive Health*, vol. 9, no. 2, pp. 101–106, 2005.

[21] G. Kamugisha, "Use of PMTCT services among HIV positive womenattending ANC at Kisenyi and Naguru Health Centres, Kampala-Uganda," 2014.

[22] S. A. Woldesenbet, D. Jackson, A. E. Goga et al., "Missed opportunities for early infant HIV diagnosis: results of a national study in South Africa," *Journal of Acquired Immune Deficiency Syndromes*, vol. 68, no. 3, pp. e26–e32, 2015.

[23] J. Izudi, A. Akot, G. P. Kisitu, P. Amuge, and A. Kekitiinwa, "Quality improvement interventions for early hiv infant diagnosis in Northeastern Uganda," *BioMed Research International*, vol. 2016, pp. 1–6, 2016.

[24] The Republic of Uganda, *Consolidated Guidelines for Prevention And Treatment of HIV in Uganda*, Ministry of Health, Kampala, Uganda, 2016.

[25] AIDS Info, "Guidelines for the Use of Antiretroviral Agents in Pediatric HIV Infection," 2017, https://aidsinfo.nih.gov/guidelines/html/2/pediatric-arv-guidelines/55/diagnosis-of-hiv-infection-in-infants-and-children.

# 25

# Ritonavir-Boosted Darunavir Plus Two Nucleoside Reverse Transcriptase Inhibitors versus Other Regimens for Initial Antiretroviral Therapy for People with HIV Infection

**Tatevik Balayan,[1,2] Hacsi Horvath,[1] and George W. Rutherford[1]**

[1] *Global Health Sciences, University of California, San Francisco, San Francisco, CA, USA*
[2] *School of Public Health, American University of Armenia, Yerevan, Armenia*

Correspondence should be addressed to Hacsi Horvath; hacsi.horvath@gmail.com

Academic Editor: David Katzenstein

*Background.* Darunavir is a second-generation protease-inhibitor used with ritonavir (DRV/r) and two nucleoside reverse-transcriptase inhibitors as an option in first-line antiretroviral treatment (ART). *Methods.* We systematically reviewed randomized controlled trials (RCTs) of DRV/r versus other regimens in patients initiating ART. We searched five bibliographic databases and other key resources. We had no language limitations. We assessed bias risk with the Cochrane tool and used GRADE to assess evidence quality. We report findings in terms of risk ratio (RR) with 95% confidence intervals (CI). *Findings.* Three RCTs met inclusion criteria. In plasma viral load suppression, DRV/r outperformed ritonavir-boosted lopinavir at 48 weeks (RR 1.13, 95% CI 1.03–1.25), 96 weeks (RR 1.11, 95% CI 1.02–1.21), and 192 weeks (RR 1.20, 95% CI 1.07–1.35). DRV/r was similar to dolutegravir at 48 weeks (RR 0.96, 95% CI 0.87–1.06) but less effective at 96 weeks (RR 0.84, 95% CI 0.75–0.93). At 96 weeks, DRV/r underperformed raltegravir (RR 0.94, 95% CI 0.88–0.99) but was similar to ritonavir-boosted atazanavir (RR 1.02, 95% CI 0.96–1.09). Overall bias risk was moderate. Evidence quality was also moderate. *Interpretation.* Initial ART regimens using DRV/r should be considered in future World Health Organization guidelines.

## 1. Introduction

Darunavir (DRV) is a once-daily second-generation protease-inhibitor [1, 2] that is administered with low-dose ritonavir (DRV/r) and two nucleoside reverse transcriptase inhibitors (NRTI) for treatment of HIV infection. In vitro studies have shown that resistance to DRV develops much more slowly and that it has a higher genetic barrier for the development of resistance relative to current protease inhibitors [3]. DRV has a very low resistance profile [3], requires boosting with ritonavir, and is used in combinations with two NRTIs, such as abacavir (ABC) + lamivudine (3TC) or tenofovir (TDF) + emtricitabine (FTC).

DRV/r + two NRTIs is the third option in the United States (US) Department of Health and Human Services' and the European AIDS Clinical Society's six recommended initial regimens for antiretroviral-naïve HIV-infected patients [4, 5]. The British HIV Medical Association has also recommended it as one of six third-line agents to be used with a two-drug NRTI backbone [6]. In contrast World Health Organization (WHO) guidelines only recommend DRV/r with two NRTIs as second- and third-line regimens for adults and adolescents who have failed initial therapy [7]. Different studies have shown that DRV/r combination therapy is less expensive than other combination therapies such as ritonavir-boosted lopinavir (LPV/r) [8] and ritonavir-boosted atazanavir (ATV/r) [8] but less cost effective compared to dolutegravir (DTG) [9] and raltegravir (RAL) [10].

In this paper, we systematically review the efficacy and safety of DRV/r in combination with two NRTIs compared to the current WHO standard regimens of efavirenz (EFV), DTG, LPV/r, ATV/r, and RAL with two NRTIs.

## 2. Methods

We used Cochrane Collaboration methods throughout the review process [11]. We followed the Preferred Reporting Items for Systematic Reviews and Meta-Analyses (PRISMA) guidance in reporting our results [12]. Before beginning our review, we registered its protocol in the PROSPERO online registry (registration number CRD42016040058).

*2.1. Search Methods.* We used a comprehensive search strategy to identify all relevant studies. We searched the Cochrane Central Register of Controlled Trials, Embase, Literatura Latino Americana em Ciências da Saúde (LILACS), PubMed, and Web of Science. In our search strategy, we included Medical Subject Heading (MeSH) or other database-specific indexing terms, as well as a range of relevant keywords. Searches captured all records up to the search date (June 9, 2016). We modified our core PubMed search strategy as needed for each database. See Supplement 1 for our PubMed search strategy, modified and adapted as needed for use in the other databases (https://doi.org/10.1155/2017/2345617).

We searched available conference abstracts from three major HIV/AIDS conferences (Conference on Retroviruses and Opportunistic Infections, the International AIDS Conference, and the International AIDS Society Conference on HIV Pathogenesis, Treatment and Prevention). We searched the clinical trials registry (clinicaltrials.gov) of the US National Institutes of Health to identify ongoing trials, and any others we might have missed in searches of the peer-reviewed literature. We also examined the reference lists of our included studies and other highly relevant studies. We had no restrictions by language or publication status.

*2.2. Inclusion and Exclusion Criteria.* We included RCTs that compared clinical and laboratory outcomes in HIV-1-infected, ART-naïve adults and adolescents starting regimens of DRV/r plus two NRTIs with those starting regimens of EFV, ATV/r, LPV/r, DTG, and RAL plus two NRTIs. We excluded nonrandomized studies and studies in which participants were ART-experienced. All studies found were written in English.

*2.3. Data Extraction.* We imported search results into bibliographic citation management software (EndNote X7, Thomson Reuters, New York, New York, USA). One author (Hacsi Horvath) removed duplicate records and, by reviewing article titles, excluded all clearly irrelevant records. Following this, two authors (George W. Rutherford and Tatevik Balayan) each independently reviewed the titles, abstracts, and descriptor terms of all remaining citations. For all records deemed potentially eligible for inclusion, we obtained full-text articles. Applying the inclusion criteria, George W. Rutherford and Tatevik Balayan reviewed these articles and determined those that were indeed eligible for inclusion. In the event of disagreements during the screening process, we planned to resolve them through discussion. If necessary, a neutral third person would have contributed to the decision.

Two authors (Tatevik Balayan and Hacsi Horvath) each independently extracted data from all trials meeting inclusion criteria and separately entered these data into standardized data extraction forms. Extracted data in each author's form were then compared and were found to match.

*2.4. Risk of Bias Assessment.* We assessed risk of bias in the included RCTs by using the Cochrane Collaboration's tool [11]. This instrument assesses six domains of bias risk: sequence generation, allocation concealment, blinding, incomplete outcome data, selective outcome reporting, and other potential biases.

*2.5. Data Synthesis and Analysis.* We calculated the relative risk (RR) for dichotomous outcomes and mean difference (MD) for continuous outcomes, each with 95% confidence intervals (CI). Where appropriate and possible, we had planned to pool data across studies and estimate summary effect sizes, using a Mantel-Haenszel fixed-effects meta-analytic model. Had we been able to conduct meta-analyses, we would have used Review Manager 5.3 (Nordic Cochrane Centre, Copenhagen, Denmark).

We planned to present estimates of heterogeneity in pooled data, as determined by the $I^2$ statistic. $I^2$ statistic estimates attempt to show the percentage of variability in effect estimates that arise from statistical heterogeneity and not from chance. If we had pooled data and found high statistical heterogeneity, we would have investigated it through sensitivity analyses.

We assessed the quality of evidence for each outcome across all studies by using the GRADE methodology [13]. "Quality of evidence" in GRADE is "the extent of our confidence that the estimates of effect are correct" [13]. GRADE rates evidence quality at four levels: high, moderate, low, or very low. RCT data for a given outcome are considered at the outset to provide high quality evidence. Observational study data are deemed at the outset to provide low quality evidence. Depending on specific circumstances, evidence quality can be downgraded for high risk of bias, indirectness, inconsistency of effect estimates, statistical imprecision, or high risk of publication bias. In RCT data that have been downgraded, it can also potentially be graded up if there is a large magnitude of effect, if plausible confounding would increase confidence in an estimated effect, or if a dose-response gradient is observed. If there has been no downgrading, observational study data can potentially be graded up for the same reasons.

## 3. Results

We initially identified 660 articles (605 from bibliographic databases, 14 from conference abstracts, and 41 from registered trials). After removing 230 duplicate records and 50 clearly irrelevant records, we independently reviewed 380 titles and abstracts and excluded 350 clearly irrelevant records. We selected 30 records for full-text review. We then excluded 21 studies reporting results of other background regimens, second-line therapy, pharmacokinetics, and other topics (Figure 1).

Three trials reported in eight published articles and one conference abstract met our inclusion criteria. All studies were RCTs (Table 1). The trials were conducted in Argentina,

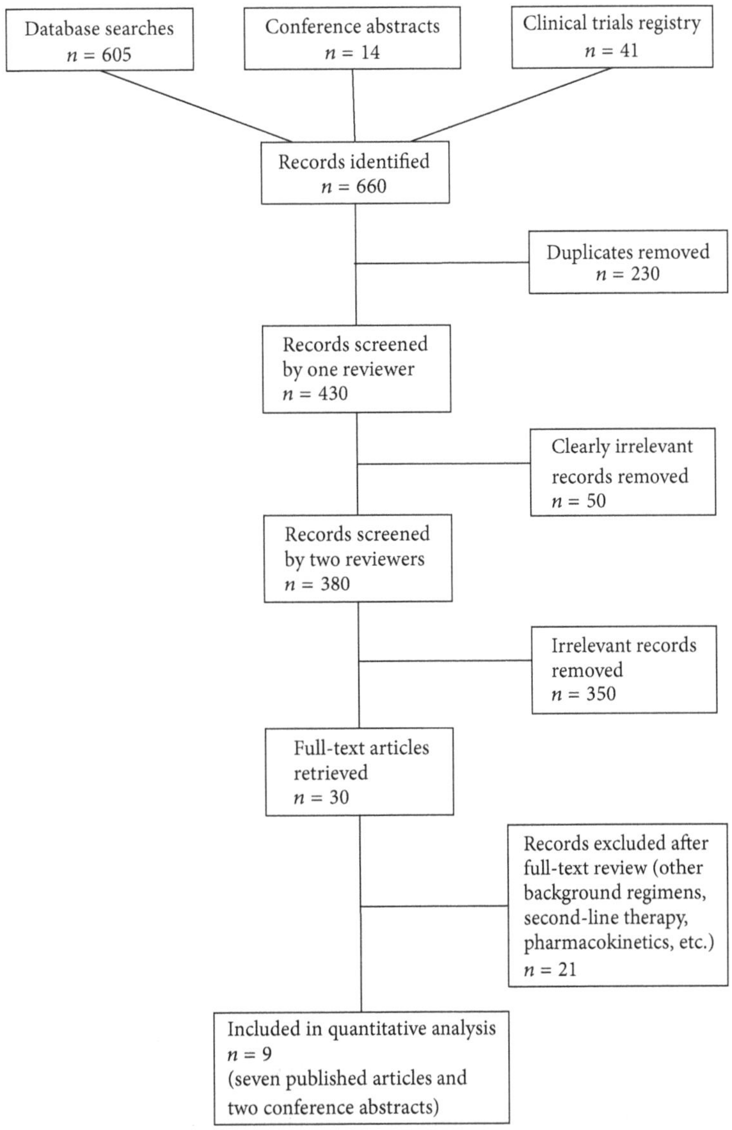


FIGURE 1: PRISMA flowchart.

Australia, Austria, Belgium, Canada, Chile, Costa Rica, Denmark, France, Germany, Greece, Guatemala, Malaysia, Mexico, Panama, Puerto Rico, Russia, Singapore, South Africa, Spain, Switzerland, Taiwan, Thailand, the United Kingdom, and the United States of America. Overall, there were 2,986 participants who were randomized. The first trial (ARTEMIS) was a two-arm Phase III trial that compared DRV/r + TDF/FTC ($N$ = 343) with LPV/RTV + TDF/FTC ($N$ = 346) [14–17]. The second trial (FLAMINGO) was a Phase IIIb two-arm trial that compared DRV/r + ABC/3TC or TDF/FTC with DTG + ABC/3TC or TDF/FTC in 488 ART-naïve patients [18, 19]. The third trial (ACTG 5257) was Phase III three-arm trial that compared DRV/RTV + FTC/TDF with ATV/RTV + FTC/TDF and RAL + FTC/TDF [20–22]. We identified no trials that compared DRV/r to EFV. ARTEMIS contributed 343 patients to the DRV/r arm and 346 to the LPV/r arm [14–17]; FLAMINGO contributed 245 patients to the DRV/r arm and 243 to the DTG arm [18, 19]; and ACTG 5272 contributed 601 patients to the DRV/r arm, 603 to the RAL arm, and 605 to the ATV arm [20–22].

Given the important differences among intervention and comparator regimens in the included trials we did not pool data in meta-analysis for any outcome.

*3.1. Viral Suppression.* The primary endpoint of all three trials was viral suppression to <50 copies/mL at 48, 96, and 192 weeks (Table 2). In the ARTEMIS trial, the DRV/r-containing regimen was superior to the LPV/r-containing regimen at 48 weeks, 96 weeks, and 192 weeks (RR 1.13, 95% CI 1.03–1.25; RR = 1.11, 95% CI 1.02–1.21; and RR 1.20, 95% CI 1.07–1.35, resp.) [14, 15]. However, among participants with baseline HIV RNA levels of >100,000 copies/mL, virologic response rates were lower in the LPV/r arm than in the DRV/r arm (ARTEMIS). In the FLAMINGO trial, the rate of virologic suppression at 48 weeks was no different in the DRV/r arm and the DTG arm (RR 0.96, 95% CI 0.87–1.06); however by 96 weeks

Table 1: Characteristics of included studies.

| Study | Clinicaltrials.gov identifier | Setting | Participants | Intervention | Comparator |
|---|---|---|---|---|---|
| ARTEMIS | NCT00258557 | Argentina, Australia, Austria, Belgium, Canada, Chile, Costa Rica, Denmark, France, Germany, Greece, Guatemala, Malaysia, Mexico, Panama, Puerto Rico, Russia, Singapore, South Africa, Spain, Switzerland, Taiwan, Thailand, United Kingdom, United States | 689 | DRV/r + TDF/FTC | LPV/r + TDF/FTC |
| FLAMINGO | NCT00951015 | France, Germany, Italy, Romania, Russia, Spain, Switzerland, United States | 286 | DRV/r + ABC/3TC or TDF/FTC | DTG + ABC/3TC or TDF/FTC |
| ACTG 5272 | NCT00811954 | Puerto Rico, United States | 1809 | DRV/RTV + FTC/TDF | ATV/r + FTC/TDF<br>RAL + FTC/TDF |

DRV/r, ritonavir-boosted darunavir; DTG, dolutegravir; ABC, abacavir; 3TC, lamivudine; FTC, emtricitabine; TDF, tenofovir; ATV/r, ritonavir-boosted atazanavir; RAL, raltegravir.

viral suppression was significantly higher in the DTG arm compared to the DRV/r arm (RR 0.84, 95% CI 0.75–0.93). The excess failure observed in the DRV/r group was primarily related to a higher rate of virologic failure among those with a viral load > 100,000 copies/mL and secondarily due to more drug discontinuations in the DRV/r group [19]. In ACTG 5257, which was a three-way comparison of DRV/r, ATV/r, and RAL, 96-week virologic suppression in the DRV/r arm was similar to that in the ATV/r arm (RR 1.02, 95% CI 0.96–1.09) but inferior to RAL (RR 0.94, 95% CI 0.88–0.99). However, more participants in the ATV/r group discontinued treatment because of adverse events [21].

Figure 2 depicts viral suppression outcomes, sorted by regimen. Figure 3 also depicts these outcomes, sorted by length of follow-up.

*3.2. Mortality.* There were no significant differences in mortality in any trial between patient arms randomized to DRV/r and those randomized to other regimens.

DRV/r versus LPV/r: at 48 weeks, one patient receiving DRV/r had died, compared to three deaths in patients receiving LPV/r (RR 0.34, 95% CI 0.04–3.22). No additional patients in either arm had died at the 96-week assessment. At 192 weeks, a total of four patients receiving DRV/r and seven receiving LPV/r had died (RR 0.58, 95% CI 0.17–1.95).

DRV/r versus RAL or ATV/r: at 96 weeks, 13 patients receiving DRV/r had died, compared to six deaths in patients receiving RAL (RR 2.17, 95% CI 0.83–5.68) and 10 deaths in patients receiving ATV/r (RR 1.31, 95% CI 0.58–2.96).

DRV/r versus DTG: at 96 weeks, no patients had died in either arm of the trial comparing DRV/r with DTG.

*3.3. Severe Adverse Events.* In the ARTEMIS trial risk of serious adverse events was lower in the DRV/r arm than in the LPV/r arm at 48 and 96 weeks (RR 0.62, 95% CI 0.38–0.99; RR 0.62, 95% CI 0.42–0.93, resp.) but similar in both arms at 192 weeks (RR 0.77, 95% CI 0.56–1.06). In the FLAMINGO trial risk of serious adverse events was lower in the DRV/r

TABLE 2: Quantitative data for trial outcomes (dichotomous).

| DRV/r versus LPV/r (ARTEMIS) | Events, DRV/r | Total, DRV/r | Events, LPV/r | Total, LPV/r | RR (95% CI) |
|---|---|---|---|---|---|
| Mortality (192 weeks) | 4 | 343 | 7 | 346 | 0.58 (0.17–1.95) |
| Mortality (96 weeks) | 1 | 343 | 3 | 346 | 0.34 (0.04–3.22) |
| Mortality (48 weeks) | 1 | 343 | 3 | 346 | 0.34 (0.04–3.22) |
| ≥1 SAE (192 weeks) | 55 | 343 | 72 | 346 | 0.77 (0.56–1.06) |
| ≥1 SAE (96 weeks) | 34 | 343 | 55 | 346 | 0.62 (0.42–0.93) |
| ≥1 SAE (48 weeks) | 25 | 343 | 41 | 346 | 0.62 (0.38–0.99) |
| PVL < 50 copies/mL (192 weeks) | 236 | 343 | 198 | 346 | 1.20 (1.07–1.35) |
| PVL < 50 copies/mL (96 weeks) | 271 | 343 | 246 | 346 | 1.11 (1.02–1.21) |
| PVL < 50 copies/mL (48 weeks) | 254 | 343 | 226 | 346 | 1.13 (1.03–1.25) |
| **DRV/r versus DTG (FLAMINGO)** | **Events, DRV/r** | **Total, DRV/r** | **Events, DTG** | **Total, DTG** | **RR (95% CI)** |
| ≥1 SAE (96 weeks) | 36 | 245 | 21 | 243 | 1.70 (1.02–2.83) |
| ≥1 SAE (48 weeks) | 13 | 245 | 26 | 243 | 0.50 (0.26–0.94) |
| PVL < 50 copies/mL (96 weeks) | 164 | 245 | 194 | 243 | 0.84 (0.75–0.93) |
| PVL < 50 copies/mL (48 weeks) | 186 | 245 | 192 | 243 | 0.96 (0.87–1.06) |
| **DRV/r versus RAL (ACTG 5257)** | **Events, DRV/r** | **Total, DRV/r** | **Events, RAL** | **Total, RAL** | **RR (95% CI)** |
| Mortality (96 weeks) | 13 | 601 | 6 | 603 | 2.17 (0.83–5.68) |
| Elevated blood bilirubin (96 weeks) | 466 | 601 | 444 | 603 | 1.05 (0.99–1.12) |
| PVL < 50 copies/mL (96 weeks) | 461 | 601 | 494 | 603 | 0.94 (0.88–0.99) |
| **DRV/r versus ATV/r (ACTG 5257)** | **Events, DRV/r** | **Total, DRV/r** | **Events, ATV/r** | **Total, ATV/r** | **RR (95% CI)** |
| Mortality (96 weeks) | 13 | 601 | 10 | 605 | 1.31 (0.58–2.96) |
| Elevated blood bilirubin (96 weeks) | 466 | 601 | 286 | 605 | 1.64 (1.49–1.80) |
| PVL < 50 copies/mL (96 weeks) | 461 | 601 | 455 | 605 | 1.02 (0.96–1.09) |

RR, risk ratio; PVL, plasma viral load; SAE, severe adverse event; CI, confidence interval; DRV/r, ritonavir boosted darunavir-based regimen; DTG, dolutegravir-based regimen; LPV/r, ritonavir boosted lopinavir-based regimen; ATV/r, ritonavir boosted atazanavir-based regimen; RAL, raltegravir-based regimen.

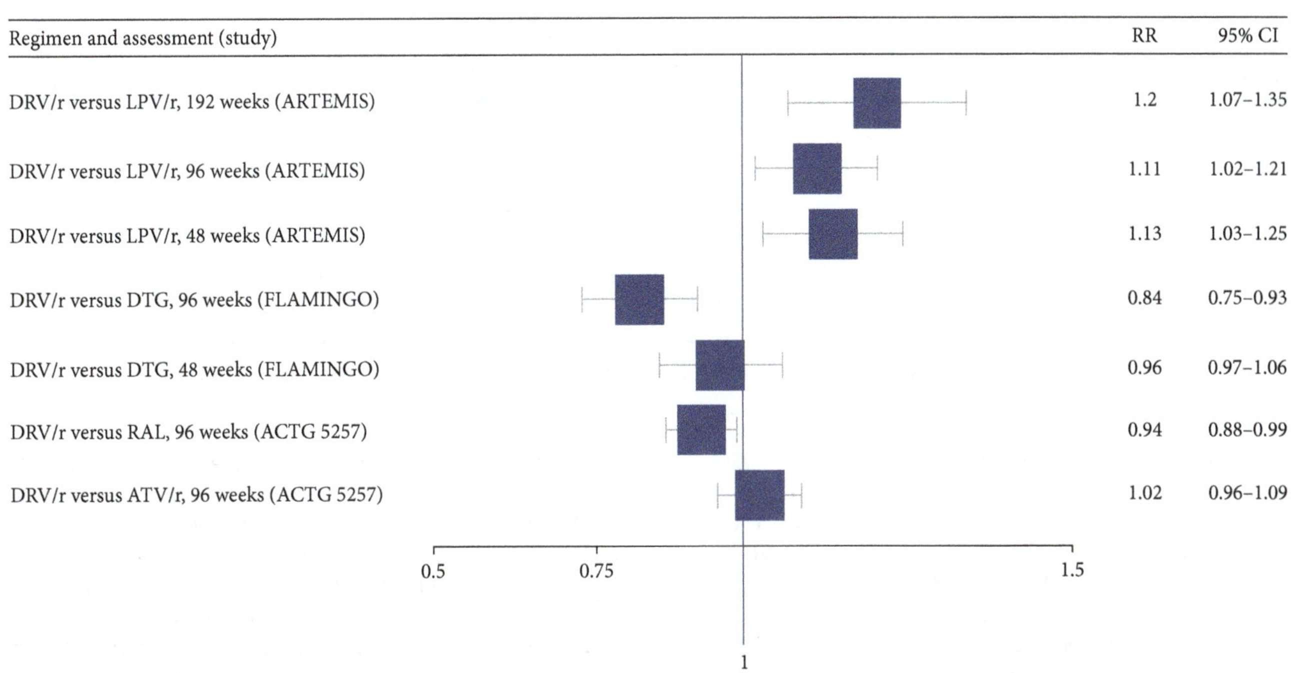


FIGURE 2: DRV/r-based regimens: efficacy in viral suppression, sorted by regimen.

TABLE 3: Quantitative data for trial outcomes (continuous).

| DRV/r versus LPV/r (ARTEMIS) | Mean change, DRV/r | Total, DRV/r | Mean change, LPV/r | Total, LPV/r |
|---|---|---|---|---|
| Immunologic recovery (192 weeks) | +258 cells/μL | 343 | +263 cells/μL | 346 |
| Immunologic recovery (96 weeks) | +171 cells/μL | 343 | +188 cells/μL | 346 |
| Immunologic recovery (48 weeks) | +137 cells/μL | 343 | +141 cells/μL | 346 |
| DRV/r versus DTG (FLAMINGO) | Mean change, DRV/r | Total, DRV/r | Mean change, DTG | Total, DTG |
| Immunologic recovery (96 weeks) | +250 cells/μL | 245 | +260 cells/μL | 243 |
| Immunologic recovery (48 weeks) | +210 cells/μL IQR 110–290 | 245 | +210 cells/μL IQR 120–350 | 243 |
| DRV/r versus RAL (ACTG 5257) | Mean change, DRV/r | Total, DRV/r | Mean change, RAL | Total, RAL |
| Immunologic recovery (96 weeks) | +256 cells/μL | 601 | +288 cells/μL | 603 |
| DRV/r versus ATV/r (ACTG 5257) | Mean change, DRV/r | Total, DRV/r | Mean change, ATV/r | Total, ATV/r |
| Immunologic recovery (96 weeks) | +256 cells/μL | 601 | +280 cells/μL | 605 |

IQR, interquartile range; DRV/r, ritonavir-boosted darunavir-based regimen; DTG, dolutegravir-based regimen; LPV/r, ritonavir-boosted lopinavir-based regimen; ATV/r, ritonavir-boosted atazanavir-based regimen; RAL, raltegravir-based regimen.

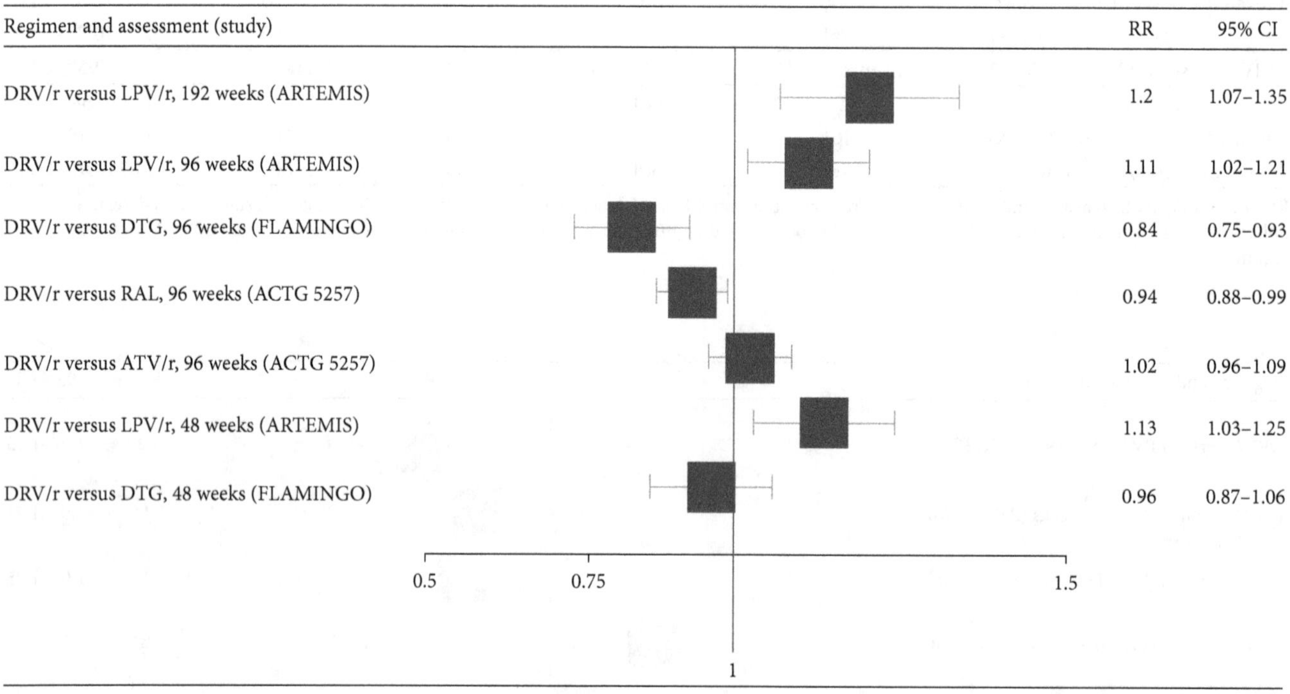


FIGURE 3: DRV/r-based regimens: efficacy in viral suppression, sorted when outcome was assessed.

arm than in the DTG arm at 48 weeks (RR 0.50, 95% CI 0.26–0.94) but higher at 96 weeks (RR 1.70, 95% CI 1.02–2.83). In the ACTG 5257 trial the risk of serious adverse events at 96 weeks was higher in DRV/r arm compared to ATV/r (hyperbilirubinaemia) (RR 1.64, 95% CI 1.49–1.80) but similar in the DRV/r and RAL arms (RR 1.05, 95% CI 0.99–1.12).

For the viral suppression, mortality, and SAE outcomes, see Table 2.

*3.4. Immunologic Recovery.* The principal secondary outcome was CD4 recovery (reaching and maintaining a higher CD4 cell count compared to baseline data). ARTEMIS contributed data to 48-, 96-, and 192-week outcomes; FLAMINGO contributed to 48- and 96-week outcomes; ACTG 5257 contributed to 96-week outcomes (Table 3). No trial reported confidence intervals for CD4 count change so it was not possible to judge the significance of the difference. Considering only reported point estimates, immune recovery was less robust among patients taking the DRV/r-based regimen in ARTEMIS study at 48, 96, and 192 weeks. The same is true for FLAMINGO at 48 and 96 weeks and ACTG 5257 at 96 weeks; see Table 3.

| | Random sequence generation (selection bias) | Allocation concealment (selection bias) | Blinding of participants and personnel (performance bias) | Blinding of outcome assessment (detection bias) | Incomplete outcome data (attrition bias) | Selective reporting (reporting bias) | Other bias |
|---|---|---|---|---|---|---|---|
| ACTG 5257 | + | − | − | − | + | + | − |
| ARTEMIS | + | − | − | − | + | + | ? |
| FLAMINGO | + | − | − | − | + | + | ? |

● = low risk of bias.
● = high risk of bias.
● = unclear risk of bias.

FIGURE 4: Risk of bias. Review authors' judgments about each risk of bias item for included studies.

*3.5. Risk of Bias in the Included Studies.* In the ARTEMIS and FLAMINGO trials, methods for sequence generation were adequate, with centralized, computer-based procedures used to randomize patients within baseline CD4 and viral load strata in ARTEMIS and within viral load strata in FLAMINGO (Figure 4). In the ACTG 5257 trial, randomization used permuted blocks stratified according to the viral load strata with balancing by institution. All trials were open label. Allocation was not concealed, and none of the studies was blinded. However, in all three trials the outcomes were biomedical and not susceptible to detection bias. There was evidence of incomplete outcome ascertainment due to differential loss to follow-up in the longer series, for instance, 24.8% of DRV/r arm participants and 32.9% of LPV/r arm participants left the trial by week 192. There was no evidence of selective reporting. All three trials were sponsored by pharmaceutical companies, although we detected no obvious problems attributable to industry involvement. Supplement 2 provides a detailed assessment of bias risk in each trial.

*3.6. Quality of the Evidence.* For the key virologic suppression outcomes, evidence quality was high for the DRV/r versus LPV/r comparison at 48 weeks but moderate at 96 and 192 weeks, graded down for risk of bias (high attrition). For the DRV/r versus DTG comparison the evidence quality for virologic suppression was high at both 48 and 96 weeks, as it was for the DRV/r versus ATV/r comparison and the DRV/r versus RAL at 96 weeks. The evidence quality was much less robust for the mortality outcomes and was rated as low or very low across all four comparisons owing to serious imprecision due to few events and in the DRV/r versus LPV/r comparison owing to risk of bias (high attrition). The evidence quality for severe adverse events was low or very low owing to few events and, again, high attrition in the trial of DRV/r versus LPV/r. See Supplement 3 for our complete GRADE evidence profile analysis of evidence quality.

## 4. Discussion

We found that DRV/r-containing regimens were associated with a greater proportion of patients being virologically suppressed up to 192 weeks after initiation of therapy compared to LPV/r-based regimens. However, we also found out that DRV/r-based regimens were inferior to DTG- and RAL-based regimens at 96 weeks. There was no difference between DRV/r and ATV/r regimens in terms of virologic suppression.

Participants in the DRV/r-containing regimens were almost three times less likely to discontinue their original regimen because of adverse events or to die than those in the LPV/r arms by 192 weeks. However, discontinuation because of adverse events or death was about 2 times higher among those in DRV/r regimen than DTG regimen, about three times higher compared with the ATV/r arm, and five times higher compared with the RAL regimen.

As with any systematic review our study is limited by the sensitivity of our search and our ability to identify studies that meet our inclusion criteria. We attempted to minimize this risk by comprehensively searching four key databases and hand searching abstracts from three major conferences as well as the bibliographies not only of included articles but also of review articles. Secondly, the three trials on which our conclusions are based were conducted across all over the world, but only South Africa was included from Africa; given that the large majority of HIV-infected patients are in Africa, this may somewhat limit the generalizability of our findings. Finally, we used the GRADE system to rate the quality of this literature. A recent evaluation of how GRADE is being used at WHO found some remaining challenges [23], but it has emerged as the gold standard for guideline development at WHO [24] and is required by the Guideline Review Committee, which approves all new guidelines.

## 5. Conclusions

We found three RCTs that directly compared DRV/r with other regimens for initial treatment of HIV infection in adults and adolescents. DRV/r appears to be superior to LPV/r in terms of durable viral suppression and immunologic recovery, inferior to DTG and RAL and similar to ATV/r. DRV/r-containing regimens should be considered in future international guidelines for initial therapy of HIV infections, but its utility has likely been eclipsed by better performing integrase inhibitor regimens.

## Conflicts of Interest

The authors have no conflicts of interest.

## Acknowledgments

The authors are grateful for the assistance of Celeste Rogers, Matthew Greenway, and all their colleagues in the Global Strategic Information group at UCSF Global Health Sciences.

## References

[1] C. L. Tremblay, "Combating HIV resistance - Focus on darunavir," *Therapeutics and Clinical Risk Management*, vol. 4, no. 4, pp. 759–765, 2008.

[2] K. McKeage, C. M. Perry, and S. J. Keam, "Darunavir: A Review of its Use in the Management of HIV Infection in Adults," *Drugs*, vol. 69, no. 4, pp. 477–503, 2009.

[3] E. Lefebvre and C. A. Schiffer, "Resilience to resistance of HIV-1 protease inhibitors: Profile of darunavir," *AIDS Reviews*, vol. 10, no. 3, pp. 131–142, 2008.

[4] *Panel on Antiretroviral Guidelines for Adults and Adolescents. Guidelines for the use of antiretroviral agents in HIV-1-infected adults and adolescents*, Department of Health and Human Services, http://aidsinfo.nih.gov/contentfiles/lvguidelines/AdultandAdolescentGL.pdf.

[5] European AIDS Clinical Society, *Guidelines 8.0*, October 2015, http://www.eacsociety.org/files/2015_eacsguidelines_8_0-english_rev-20160124.pdf.

[6] British HIV Association, *BHIVA guidelines for the treatment of HIV-1-positive adults with antiretroviral therapy 2015*, http://www.bhiva.org/documents/Guidelines/Treatment/2015/2015-treatment-guidelines.pdf.

[7] World Health Organization, "Consolidated guidelines on the use of antiretroviral drugs for treating and preventing HIV infection," http://apps.who.int/iris/bitstream/10665/85321/1/9789241505727_eng.pdf.

[8] A. Brogan, S. Soorapanth, V. Donatz, A. Hill, and E. Smets, "Comparative cost-efficacy analysis of darunavir/r and other ritonavir-boosted protease inhibitors for first-line treatment of HIV-1 infection in Germany," *Value in Health*, vol. 12, no. 7, p. A426, 2009.

[9] U. Restelli, G. Rizzardini, A. Antinori et al., "Cost-effectiveness analysis of dolutegravir plus backbone compared with raltegravir plus backbone, darunavir+ritonavir plus backbone and efavirenz/tenofovir/emtricitabine in treatment naïve and experienced HIV-positive patients," *Therapeutics and Clinical Risk Management*, vol. 13, pp. 787–797, 2017.

[10] A. Davis, A. Brogan, and B. Goodwin, "Cost analysis of raltegravir versus atazanavir/r or darunavir/r for treatment-naive adults with hIV-1 infection in the United States," *Value in Health*, vol. 19, no. 7, pp. A214–A215, 2016.

[11] "Cochrane Handbook for Systematic Reviews of Interventions Version 5.1.0 [updated March 2011]," in *The Cochrane Collaboration*, J. P. T. Higgins and S. Green, Eds., 2011, http://www.cochrane-handbook.org.

[12] D. Moher, A. Liberati, J. Tetzlaff, and D. G. Altman, "Preferred reporting items for systematic reviews and meta-analyses: the PRISMA statement," *PLoS Medicine*, vol. 6, no. 7, Article ID e1000097, 2009.

[13] G. H. Guyatt, A. D. Oxman, H. J. Schünemann, P. Tugwell, and A. Knottnerus, "GRADE guidelines: a new series of articles in the Journal of Clinical Epidemiology," *Journal of Clinical Epidemiology*, vol. 64, no. 4, pp. 380–382, 2011.

[14] C. Orkin, E. Dejesus, H. Khanlou et al., "Final 192-week efficacy and safety of once-daily darunavir/ritonavir compared with lopinavir/ritonavir in HIV-1-infected treatment-naïve patients in the ARTEMIS trial," *HIV Medicine*, vol. 14, no. 1, pp. 49–59, 2013.

[15] R. Ortiz, E. DeJesus, H. Khanlou et al., "Efficacy and safety of once-daily darunavir/ritonavir versus lopinavir/ritonavir in treatment-naïve HIV-1-infected patients at week 48," *AIDS*, vol. 22, no. 12, pp. 1389–1397, 2008.

[16] M. Nelson, P.-M. Girard, R. DeMasi et al., "Suboptimal adherence to darunavir/ritonavir has minimal effect on efficacy compared with lopinavir/ritonavir in treatment-naive, HIV-infected patients: 96 week ARTEMIS data," *Journal of Antimicrobial Chemotherapy*, vol. 65, no. 7, Article ID dkq150, pp. 1505–1509, 2010.

[17] E. Arathoon, S. Schneider, E. Baraldi et al., "Effects of once-daily darunavir/ritonavir versus lopinavir/ritonavir on metabolic parameters in treatment-naïve HIV-1-infected patients at week 96: ARTEMIS," *International Journal of STD and AIDS*, vol. 24, no. 1, pp. 12–17, 2013.

[18] B. Clotet, J. Feinberg, J. Van Lunzen et al., "Once-daily dolutegravir versus darunavir plus ritonavir in antiretroviral-naive adults with HIV-1 infection (FLAMINGO): 48 week results from the randomised open-label phase 3b study," *The Lancet*, vol. 383, no. 9936, pp. 2222–2231, 2014.

[19] J.-M. Molina, B. Clotet, J. van Lunzen et al., "Once-daily dolutegravir versus darunavir plus ritonavir for treatment-naive adults with HIV-1 infection (FLAMINGO): 96 week results from a randomised, open-label, phase 3b study," *The Lancet HIV*, vol. 2, no. 4, pp. e127–e136, 2015.

[20] R. Landovitz, H. Ribaudo, I. Ofotukin, H. Wang, B. P. Baugh, R. Y. Leavitt et al., "Efficacy and tolerability of atazanavir, raltegravir, or darunavir with FTC/tenofovir: ACTG 5257," in *in proceedings of 21st Conference on Retroviruses and Opportunistic Infection (CROI)*, Boston, Massachusetts, USA, 3-6 March 2014.

[21] J. Lennox, R. Landovitz, H. Ribaudo, I. Ofotokun, L. H. Na, C. Godfrey et al., "Efficacy and tolerability of 3 nonnucleoside reverse transcriptase inhibitor-sparing antiretroviral regimens

for treatment-naïve volunteers infected with HIV-1," *Annals of Internal Medicine*, vol. 161, pp. 161–461, 2014.

[22] I. Ofotukin, L. Na, R. Landovitz, H. J. Ribaudo, G. A. McComsey, C. Godfrey et al., "Comparison of the Metabolic Effects of Ritonavir-Boosted Darunavir or Atazanavir Versus Raltegravir, and the Impact of Tironavir Plazma Exposure: ACTG 5257," *Clinical Infectious Diseases*, vol. 60, pp. 1842–1851, 2015.

[23] D. Sinclair, R. Isba, T. Kredo, B. Zani, H. Smith, and P. Garner, "World Health Organization guideline development: an evaluation," *PLoS ONE*, vol. 8, no. 5, Article ID e63715, 2013.

[24] World Health Organization, *WHO Handbook for Guideline Development*, http://apps.who.int/iris/bitstream/10665/75146/1/9789241548441_eng.pdf?ua=1.

# Permissions

All chapters in this book were first published in AIDS R&T, by Hindawi Publishing Corporation; hereby published with permission under the Creative Commons Attribution License or equivalent. Every chapter published in this book has been scrutinized by our experts. Their significance has been extensively debated. The topics covered herein carry significant findings which will fuel the growth of the discipline. They may even be implemented as practical applications or may be referred to as a beginning point for another development.

The contributors of this book come from diverse backgrounds, making this book a truly international effort. This book will bring forth new frontiers with its revolutionizing research information and detailed analysis of the nascent developments around the world.

We would like to thank all the contributing authors for lending their expertise to make the book truly unique. They have played a crucial role in the development of this book. Without their invaluable contributions this book wouldn't have been possible. They have made vital efforts to compile up to date information on the varied aspects of this subject to make this book a valuable addition to the collection of many professionals and students.

This book was conceptualized with the vision of imparting up-to-date information and advanced data in this field. To ensure the same, a matchless editorial board was set up. Every individual on the board went through rigorous rounds of assessment to prove their worth. After which they invested a large part of their time researching and compiling the most relevant data for our readers.

The editorial board has been involved in producing this book since its inception. They have spent rigorous hours researching and exploring the diverse topics which have resulted in the successful publishing of this book. They have passed on their knowledge of decades through this book. To expedite this challenging task, the publisher supported the team at every step. A small team of assistant editors was also appointed to further simplify the editing procedure and attain best results for the readers.

Apart from the editorial board, the designing team has also invested a significant amount of their time in understanding the subject and creating the most relevant covers. They scrutinized every image to scout for the most suitable representation of the subject and create an appropriate cover for the book.

The publishing team has been an ardent support to the editorial, designing and production team. Their endless efforts to recruit the best for this project, has resulted in the accomplishment of this book. They are a veteran in the field of academics and their pool of knowledge is as vast as their experience in printing. Their expertise and guidance has proved useful at every step. Their uncompromising quality standards have made this book an exceptional effort. Their encouragement from time to time has been an inspiration for everyone.

The publisher and the editorial board hope that this book will prove to be a valuable piece of knowledge for researchers, students, practitioners and scholars across the globe.

# List of Contributors

**Nurilign Abebe Moges and Habtamu Mellie Bizuayehu**
Public Health Department, Medicine and Health Sciences College, DebreMarkos University, Debre Markos, Ethiopia

**Vaidehi Mujumdar and Doris Berman**
Wake Forest School of Medicine, 1 Medical Center Blvd,Winston-Salem, NC 27157, USA

**Katherine R. Schafer**
Section on Infectious Diseases,Wake Forest University Health Sciences,Winston-Salem, NC, USA

**Bonaventura C. T. Mpondo**
Department of Internal Medicine, School of Medicine, College of Health Sciences,The University of Dodoma, Dodoma, Tanzania

**Daniel W. Gunda and Semvua B. Kilonzo**
Department of Internal Medicine, School of Medicine, Catholic University of Health and Allied Sciences, Mwanza, Tanzania

**Ferdinand C. Mukumbang, Joyce Chali Mwale, and Brian van Wyk**
School of Public Health, University of the Western Cape, Cape Town, South Africa

**Cecilia T. Costiniuk, Vikram Mehraj, Jean-Pierre Routy, Christina de Castro, Syim Salahuddin, Bertrand Lebouché, Joseph Cox, Jason Szabo and Marina Klein**
Chronic Viral Illnesses Service and Research Institute, McGill University Health Centre (MUHC), Montreal, QC, Canada

**Natale Wasef**
Department of Medicine, National University of Ireland, Galway, Ireland

**Mohammad-Ali Jenabian**
Department of Biological Sciences and BioMed Research Centre, Universit´e du Québecà Montré al (UQAM), Montreal, QC, Canada

**Larry Lands and Adam J. Shapiro**
Division of Pediatric Respiratory Medicine, McGill University Health Center Research Institute, Montreal, QC, Canada

**Patrick Igulot**
University of Sunderland in London, UK

**Monica A. Magadi**
University of Hull, UK

**Mohammed Biset Ayalew**
Department of Clinical Pharmacy, School of Pharmacy, College of Medicine and Health Sciences, University of Gondar, Gondar, Ethiopia

**Tadele Amare, Wondale Getinet, Shegaye Shumet and Biksegn Asrat**
Department of Psychiatry, College of Medicine and Health Science, University of Gondar, Gondar, Ethiopia

**Degefa Tadele Belato**
Hadiya Zone Health Department, Hadiya Zone, Ethiopia

**Abera Beyamo Mekiso**
Public Health Department, College of Health Sciences, Wolayta Sodo University, Wolayta Sodo, Ethiopia

**Bayu Begashaw**
Public Health Department, College of Health Sciences, Mizan-Tepi University, Mizan-Aman, Ethiopia
College of Medicine and Health Sciences, Institute of Public Health, University of Gondar, Gondar, Ethiopia

**Woudneh Gereme Desta**
Health Promotion and Disease Prevention Core Process, Amhara National Regional State Health Bureau, Bahir Dar, Ethiopia

**Mulusew Alemneh Sinishaw**
Clinical Chemistry, Amhara Public Health Institute, Bahir Dar, Ethiopia

**Kelemu Dessie Bizuneh**
Public Health Emergency Management, Awi Zone Health Department, Injibara, Ethiopia

**Adama Baguiya**
Institut de Recherche en Sciences de la Santé (IRSS), Ouagadougou, West Africa, Burkina Faso

**Henri Gautier Ouedraogo**
Institut de Recherche en Sciences de la Sant´e (IRSS), Ouagadougou, West Africa, Burkina Faso
University Ouaga Joseph Ki-Zerbo, Ouagadougou,West Africa, Burkina Faso
Institut Africain de Sant´e Publique, Ouagadougou, West Africa, Burkina Faso

**Seni Kouanda**
Institut de Recherche en Sciences de la Sant´e (IRSS), Ouagadougou, West Africa, Burkina Faso
Institut Africain de Sant´e Publique, Ouagadougou, West Africa, Burkina Faso

**Yves Traore and Nicolas Barro**
University Ouaga Joseph Ki-Zerbo, Ouagadougou, West Africa, Burkina Faso

**Odette Ky-Zerbo, Benoît Cesaire Samadoulougou and Marcel Lougue**
Programme d'Appui au Monde Associatif et Communautaire, Ouagadougou, West Africa, Burkina Faso

**Ashley Grosso, Sara Goodman and Stefan Baral**
Department of Epidemiology, Johns Hopkins Bloomberg School of Public Health, Baltimore, MD, USA

**Nongoba Sawadogo**
Centre Hospitalier Regional de Kaya, West Africa, Burkina Faso

**Judith G. Rabkin and Martin C. McElhiney**
New York State Psychiatric Institute, New York, NY, USA
Department of Psychiatry, Columbia University, New York, NY, USA

**Mark Harrington and Tim Horn**
Treatment Action Group, New York, NY,USA

**Hannah N. Gilbert**
Department of Global Health and Social Medicine, Harvard Medical School, Boston, MA, USA

**Monique A. Wyatt**
Department of Global Health and Social Medicine, Harvard Medical School, Boston, MA, USA
Harvard Global, Cambridge, MA, USA

**Norma C. Ware**
Department of Global Health and Social Medicine, Harvard Medical School, Boston, MA, USA
Division of Global Health Equity, Department of Medicine, Brigham and Women's Hospital, Boston, MA, USA

**Stephen Asiimwe, Bosco Turyamureeba and Elioda Tumwesigye**
Integrated Community Based Initiatives, Kabwohe, Uganda

**Heidi Van Rooyen**
Human Sciences Research Council, Durban, South Africa
School of Clinical Medicine, Faculty of Health Sciences, University of theWitwatersrand, Johannesburg, South Africa

**Ruanne V. Barnabas and Connie L. Celum**
Department of Global Health, School of Medicine and School of Public Health, University ofWashington, Seattle, WA, USA

**Clifford O. Odimegwu**
Demography and Population Studies Programme, Schools of Public Health and Social Sciences, University of theWitwatersrand, Johannesburg, South Africa

**Joshua O. Akinyemi**
Demography and Population Studies Programme, Schools of Public Health and Social Sciences, University of theWitwatersrand, Johannesburg, South Africa
Department of Epidemiology and Medical Statistics, Faculty of PublicHealth, College of Medicine, University of Ibadan, Ibadan, Nigeria

**Olatunji O. Alabi**
Demography and Population Studies Programme, Schools of Public Health and Social Sciences, University of theWitwatersrand, Johannesburg, South Africa
Department of Demography and Social Statistics, Federal University, Birnin Kebbi, Nigeria

**David W. Pittman, Alexandra M. Brantly, Alexandra L. Drobonick, Hannah T. King, Daniel C. Mesta and Caroline G. Richards**
Department of Psychology,Wofford College, 429 North Church Street, Spartanburg, SC 29303, USA

**Manjari Lal and Manshun Lai**
PATH, 2201 Westlake Avenue, Suite 200, Seattle, WA 98121, USA

**Nooshin Zarei**
Shiraz HIV/AIDS Research Center, Institute of Health, Shiraz University of Medical Sciences, Shiraz, Iran

**Hassan Joulaei**
Health Policy Research Center, Institute of Health, Shiraz University of Medical Sciences, Shiraz, Iran

**James Osei-Yeboah, Sylvester Yao Lokpo, Emmanuel Alote Allotey, John Gameli Deku, Emmanuel Akomanin Asiamah, Nana Yaw Barimah Manaphraim, Prince Senyo Kwasi Nyamadi, Edward Yiadom Boakye Tibemponi Ntoni, Roseline Avorkliyah and Romeo Asumbasiya Aduko**
Department of Medical Laboratory Sciences, School of Allied Health Sciences, University of Health and Allied Sciences, Ho, Ghana

**Christian Obirikorang**
Department of Molecular Medicine, School of Medical Sciences, Kwame Nkrumah University of Science and Technology, Kumasi, Ghana

**William K. B. A. Owiredu**
Department of Molecular Medicine, School of Medical Sciences, Kwame Nkrumah University of Science and Technology, Kumasi, Ghana
Department of Clinical Biochemistry, Diagnostic Directorate, Komfo Anokye Teaching Hospital, Kumasi, Ghana

**Gameli Kwame Norgbe**
School of Allied Health Sciences, University of Health and Allied Sciences, Ho, Ghana

**Seyram Tetteh Quarshie**
Health Information Unit, Ho Municipal Hospital, Ghana Health Service, Ho, Volta Region, Ghana

**Maxwell Jenkins Gbemu**
Laboratory Department, Volta Regional Hospital, Ghana Health Service, Ho, Volta Region, Ghana

**Harry D. J. Knights**
Brasenose College, University of Oxford, Oxford, UK

**Stefanie Hornschuh, Janan Janine Dietrich, Celokuhle Tshabalala and Fatima Laher**
Perinatal HIV Research Unit, Chris Hani Baragwanath Academic Hospital, Faculty of Health Sciences, University of the Witwatersrand, Gauteng 1864, South Africa

**Charles Peter Osingada and Rose Chalo Nabirye**
Makerere University College of Health Sciences, School of Health Sciences, Department of Nursing, Kampala, Uganda

**Monica Okuga**
Makerere University School of Public Health, Department of Health Policy Planning and Management, Kampala, Uganda

**Nelson Kaulukusi Sewankambo and Damalie Nakanjako**
Department of Internal Medicine, School of Medicine, Makerere College of Health Sciences, Kampala, Uganda

**Hamufare Mugauri, Tsitsi Juru, Notion Tafara Gombe, Gerald Shambira and Mufuta Tshimanga**
Department of Community Medicine, University of Zimbabwe, Zimbabwe

**Owen Mugurungi**
Ministry of Health and Child Care, Zimbabwe

**Addmore Chadambuka**
Elizabeth Glaser Paediatric AIDS Foundation (EGPAF), Zimbabwe

**Maru Meseret**
Amhara National Regional State Health Bureau, East Gojjam Zonal Health Department, Bahir-Dar, Ethiopia

**Alemayehu Shimeka**
Department of Epidemiology and Biostatistics, College of Medicine and Health Sciences, University of Gondar, Gondar, Ethiopia

**Alemayehu Bekele**
Ethiopian Public Health Association, Addis Ababa, Ethiopia

**Marina Njelekela**
Department of Physiology, Muhimbili University of Health and Allied Sciences, Dar es Salaam, Tanzania

**Rose Mpembeni**
Department of Epidemiology and Biostatistics, Muhimbili University of Health and Allied Sciences, Dar es Salaam, Tanzania

**Alfa Muhihi, Nzovu Ulenga and Eric Aris**
Management and Development for Health, Mwai Kibaki Road, Mikocheni, Dar es Salaam, Tanzania

**Deodatus Kakoko**
Department of Behavioral Sciences, Muhimbili University of Health and Allied Sciences, Dar es Salaam, Tanzania

**Sylvia Auma and John Bosco Alege**
Department of Community Health, Faculty of Medicine, Mbarara University of Science and Technology, Mbarara, Uganda

**Jonathan Izudi**
Department of Community Health, Faculty of Medicine, Mbarara University of Science and Technology, Mbarara, Uganda

Institute of Public Health and Management, International Health Sciences University, Kampala, Uganda

**Hacsi Horvath and George W. Rutherford**
Global Health Sciences, University of California, San Francisco, San Francisco, CA, USA

**Tatevik Balayan**
Global Health Sciences, University of California, San Francisco, San Francisco, CA, USA
School of Public Health, American University of Armenia, Yerevan, Armenia

# Index

www.ingramcontent.com/pod-product-compliance
Lightning Source LLC
LaVergne TN
LVHW060534210926
848485LV00005B/1195